FREE Study Skills DVD Offer

Dear Customer,

Thank you for your purchase from Mometrix! We consider it an honor and a privilege that you have purchased our product and we want to ensure your satisfaction.

As a way of showing our appreciation and to help us better serve you, we have developed a Study Skills DVD that we would like to give you for <u>FREE</u>. This DVD covers our *best practices* for getting ready for your exam, from how to use our study materials to how to best prepare for the day of the test.

All that we ask is that you email us with feedback that would describe your experience so far with our product. Good, bad, or indifferent, we want to know what you think!

To get your FREE Study Skills DVD, email <u>freedvd@mometrix.com</u> with *FREE STUDY SKILLS DVD* in the subject line and the following information in the body of the email:

- The name of the product you purchased.

- Your product rating on a scale of 1-5, with 5 being the highest rating.

- Your feedback. It can be long, short, or anything in between. We just want to know your impressions and experience so far with our product. (Good feedback might include how our study material met your needs and ways we might be able to make it even better. You could highlight features that you found helpful or features that you think we should add.)

- Your full name and shipping address where you would like us to send your free DVD.

If you have any questions or concerns, please don't hesitate to contact me directly.

Thanks again!

Sincerely,

Jay Willis
Vice President
<u>jay.willis@mometrix.com</u>
1-800-673-8175

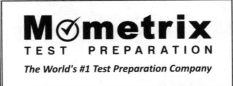

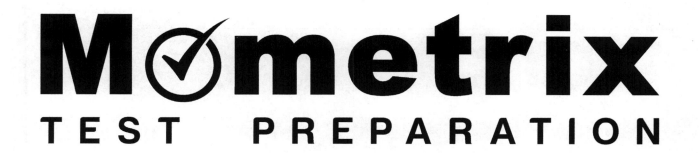

PAX

Exam Prep Study Guide 2020 and 2021

Pre-Admission Test Secrets
Study Guide for the NLN
Pre Entrance Exam

Practice Test Questions

Detailed Explanations

ISBN 13: 978-1-5167-3642-3
ISBN 10: 1-5167-3642-7

DEAR FUTURE EXAM SUCCESS STORY

First of all, **THANK YOU** for purchasing Mometrix study materials!

Second, congratulations! You are one of the few determined test-takers who are committed to doing whatever it takes to excel on your exam. **You have come to the right place.** We developed these study materials with one goal in mind: to deliver you the information you need in a format that's concise and easy to use.

In addition to optimizing your guide for the content of the test, we've outlined our recommended steps for breaking down the preparation process into small, attainable goals so you can make sure you stay on track.

We've also analyzed the entire test-taking process, identifying the most common pitfalls and showing how you can overcome them and be ready for any curveball the test throws you.

Standardized testing is one of the biggest obstacles on your road to success, which only increases the importance of doing well in the high-pressure, high-stakes environment of test day. Your results on this test could have a significant impact on your future, and this guide provides the information and practical advice to help you achieve your full potential on test day.

Your success is our success

We would love to hear from you! If you would like to share the story of your exam success or if you have any questions or comments in regard to our products, please contact us at **800-673-8175** or **support@mometrix.com**.

Thanks again for your business and we wish you continued success!

Sincerely,
The Mometrix Test Preparation Team

Need more help? Check out our flashcards at:
http://mometrixflashcards.com/nursing

TABLE OF CONTENTS

Introduction

Thank you for purchasing this resource! You have made the choice to prepare yourself for a test that could have a huge impact on your future, and this guide is designed to help you be fully ready for test day. Obviously, it's important to have a solid understanding of the test material, but you also need to be prepared for the unique environment and stressors of the test, so that you can perform to the best of your abilities.

For this purpose, the first section that appears in this guide is the **Secret Keys**. We've devoted countless hours to meticulously researching what works and what doesn't, and we've boiled down our findings to the five most impactful steps you can take to improve your performance on the test. We start at the beginning with study planning and move through the preparation process, all the way to the testing strategies that will help you get the most out of what you know when you're finally sitting in front of the test.

We recommend that you start preparing for your test as far in advance as possible. However, if you've bought this guide as a last-minute study resource and only have a few days before your test, we recommend that you skip over the first two Secret Keys since they address a long-term study plan.

If you struggle with **test anxiety**, we strongly encourage you to check out our recommendations for how you can overcome it. Test anxiety is a formidable foe, but it can be beaten, and we want to make sure you have the tools you need to defeat it.

Secret Key #1 – Plan Big, Study Small

There's a lot riding on your performance. If you want to ace this test, you're going to need to keep your skills sharp and the material fresh in your mind. You need a plan that lets you review everything you need to know while still fitting in your schedule. We'll break this strategy down into three categories.

Information Organization

Start with the information you already have: the official test outline. From this, you can make a complete list of all the concepts you need to cover before the test. Organize these concepts into groups that can be studied together, and create a list of any related vocabulary you need to learn so you can brush up on any difficult terms. You'll want to keep this vocabulary list handy once you actually start studying since you may need to add to it along the way.

Time Management

Once you have your set of study concepts, decide how to spread them out over the time you have left before the test. Break your study plan into small, clear goals so you have a manageable task for each day and know exactly what you're doing. Then just focus on one small step at a time. When you manage your time this way, you don't need to spend hours at a time studying. Studying a small block of content for a short period each day helps you retain information better and avoid stressing over how much you have left to do. You can relax knowing that you have a plan to cover everything in time. In order for this strategy to be effective though, you have to start studying early and stick to your schedule. Avoid the exhaustion and futility that comes from last-minute cramming!

Study Environment

The environment you study in has a big impact on your learning. Studying in a coffee shop, while probably more enjoyable, is not likely to be as fruitful as studying in a quiet room. It's important to keep distractions to a minimum. You're only planning to study for a short block of time, so make the most of it. Don't pause to check your phone or get up to find a snack. It's also important to **avoid multitasking**. Research has consistently shown that multitasking will make your studying dramatically less effective. Your study area should also be comfortable and well-lit so you don't have the distraction of straining your eyes or sitting on an uncomfortable chair.

The time of day you study is also important. You want to be rested and alert. Don't wait until just before bedtime. Study when you'll be most likely to comprehend and remember. Even better, if you know what time of day your test will be, set that time aside for study. That way your brain will be used to working on that subject at that specific time and you'll have a better chance of recalling information.

Finally, it can be helpful to team up with others who are studying for the same test. Your actual studying should be done in as isolated an environment as possible, but the work of organizing the information and setting up the study plan can be divided up. In between study sessions, you can discuss with your teammates the concepts that you're all studying and quiz each other on the details. Just be sure that your teammates are as serious about the test as you are. If you find that your study time is being replaced with social time, you might need to find a new team.

Secret Key #2 – Make Your Studying Count

You're devoting a lot of time and effort to preparing for this test, so you want to be absolutely certain it will pay off. This means doing more than just reading the content and hoping you can remember it on test day. It's important to make every minute of study count. There are two main areas you can focus on to make your studying count:

Retention

It doesn't matter how much time you study if you can't remember the material. You need to make sure you are retaining the concepts. To check your retention of the information you're learning, try recalling it at later times with minimal prompting. Try carrying around flashcards and glance at one or two from time to time or ask a friend who's also studying for the test to quiz you.

To enhance your retention, look for ways to put the information into practice so that you can apply it rather than simply recalling it. If you're using the information in practical ways, it will be much easier to remember. Similarly, it helps to solidify a concept in your mind if you're not only reading it to yourself but also explaining it to someone else. Ask a friend to let you teach them about a concept you're a little shaky on (or speak aloud to an imaginary audience if necessary). As you try to summarize, define, give examples, and answer your friend's questions, you'll understand the concepts better and they will stay with you longer. Finally, step back for a big picture view and ask yourself how each piece of information fits with the whole subject. When you link the different concepts together and see them working together as a whole, it's easier to remember the individual components.

Finally, practice showing your work on any multi-step problems, even if you're just studying. Writing out each step you take to solve a problem will help solidify the process in your mind, and you'll be more likely to remember it during the test.

Modality

Modality simply refers to the means or method by which you study. Choosing a study modality that fits your own individual learning style is crucial. No two people learn best in exactly the same way, so it's important to know your strengths and use them to your advantage.

For example, if you learn best by visualization, focus on visualizing a concept in your mind and draw an image or a diagram. Try color-coding your notes, illustrating them, or creating symbols that will trigger your mind to recall a learned concept. If you learn best by hearing or discussing information, find a study partner who learns the same way or read aloud to yourself. Think about how to put the information in your own words. Imagine that you are giving a lecture on the topic and record yourself so you can listen to it later.

For any learning style, flashcards can be helpful. Organize the information so you can take advantage of spare moments to review. Underline key words or phrases. Use different colors for different categories. Mnemonic devices (such as creating a short list in which every item starts with the same letter) can also help with retention. Find what works best for you and use it to store the information in your mind most effectively and easily.

Secret Key #3 – Practice the Right Way

Your success on test day depends not only on how many hours you put into preparing, but also on whether you prepared the right way. It's good to check along the way to see if your studying is paying off. One of the most effective ways to do this is by taking practice tests to evaluate your progress. Practice tests are useful because they show exactly where you need to improve. Every time you take a practice test, pay special attention to these three groups of questions:

- The questions you got wrong
- The questions you had to guess on, even if you guessed right
- The questions you found difficult or slow to work through

This will show you exactly what your weak areas are, and where you need to devote more study time. Ask yourself why each of these questions gave you trouble. Was it because you didn't understand the material? Was it because you didn't remember the vocabulary? Do you need more repetitions on this type of question to build speed and confidence? Dig into those questions and figure out how you can strengthen your weak areas as you go back to review the material.

Additionally, many practice tests have a section explaining the answer choices. It can be tempting to read the explanation and think that you now have a good understanding of the concept. However, an explanation likely only covers part of the question's broader context. Even if the explanation makes sense, **go back and investigate** every concept related to the question until you're positive you have a thorough understanding.

As you go along, keep in mind that the practice test is just that: practice. Memorizing these questions and answers will not be very helpful on the actual test because it is unlikely to have any of the same exact questions. If you only know the right answers to the sample questions, you won't be prepared for the real thing. **Study the concepts** until you understand them fully, and then you'll be able to answer any question that shows up on the test.

It's important to wait on the practice tests until you're ready. If you take a test on your first day of study, you may be overwhelmed by the amount of material covered and how much you need to learn. Work up to it gradually.

On test day, you'll need to be prepared for answering questions, managing your time, and using the test-taking strategies you've learned. It's a lot to balance, like a mental marathon that will have a big impact on your future. Like training for a marathon, you'll need to start slowly and work your way up. When test day arrives, you'll be ready.

Start with the strategies you've read in the first two Secret Keys—plan your course and study in the way that works best for you. If you have time, consider using multiple study resources to get different approaches to the same concepts. It can be helpful to see difficult concepts from more than one angle. Then find a good source for practice tests. Many times, the test website will suggest potential study resources or provide sample tests.

Practice Test Strategy

If you're able to find at least three practice tests, we recommend this strategy:

UNTIMED AND OPEN-BOOK PRACTICE

Take the first test with no time constraints and with your notes and study guide handy. Take your time and focus on applying the strategies you've learned.

TIMED AND OPEN-BOOK PRACTICE

Take the second practice test open-book as well, but set a timer and practice pacing yourself to finish in time.

TIMED AND CLOSED-BOOK PRACTICE

Take any other practice tests as if it were test day. Set a timer and put away your study materials. Sit at a table or desk in a quiet room, imagine yourself at the testing center, and answer questions as quickly and accurately as possible.

Keep repeating timed and closed-book tests on a regular basis until you run out of practice tests or it's time for the actual test. Your mind will be ready for the schedule and stress of test day, and you'll be able to focus on recalling the material you've learned.

Secret Key #4 – Pace Yourself

Once you're fully prepared for the material on the test, your biggest challenge on test day will be managing your time. Just knowing that the clock is ticking can make you panic even if you have plenty of time left. Work on pacing yourself so you can build confidence against the time constraints of the exam. Pacing is a difficult skill to master, especially in a high-pressure environment, so **practice is vital**.

Set time expectations for your pace based on how much time is available. For example, if a section has 60 questions and the time limit is 30 minutes, you know you have to average 30 seconds or less per question in order to answer them all. Although 30 seconds is the hard limit, set 25 seconds per question as your goal, so you reserve extra time to spend on harder questions. When you budget extra time for the harder questions, you no longer have any reason to stress when those questions take longer to answer.

Don't let this time expectation distract you from working through the test at a calm, steady pace, but keep it in mind so you don't spend too much time on any one question. Recognize that taking extra time on one question you don't understand may keep you from answering two that you do understand later in the test. If your time limit for a question is up and you're still not sure of the answer, mark it and move on, and come back to it later if the time and the test format allow. If the testing format doesn't allow you to return to earlier questions, just make an educated guess; then put it out of your mind and move on.

On the easier questions, be careful not to rush. It may seem wise to hurry through them so you have more time for the challenging ones, but it's not worth missing one if you know the concept and just didn't take the time to read the question fully. Work efficiently but make sure you understand the question and have looked at all of the answer choices, since more than one may seem right at first.

Even if you're paying attention to the time, you may find yourself a little behind at some point. You should speed up to get back on track, but do so wisely. Don't panic; just take a few seconds less on each question until you're caught up. Don't guess without thinking, but do look through the answer choices and eliminate any you know are wrong. If you can get down to two choices, it is often worthwhile to guess from those. Once you've chosen an answer, move on and don't dwell on any that you skipped or had to hurry through. If a question was taking too long, chances are it was one of the harder ones, so you weren't as likely to get it right anyway.

On the other hand, if you find yourself getting ahead of schedule, it may be beneficial to slow down a little. The more quickly you work, the more likely you are to make a careless mistake that will affect your score. You've budgeted time for each question, so don't be afraid to spend that time. Practice an efficient but careful pace to get the most out of the time you have.

Secret Key #5 – Have a Plan for Guessing

When you're taking the test, you may find yourself stuck on a question. Some of the answer choices seem better than others, but you don't see the one answer choice that is obviously correct. What do you do?

The scenario described above is very common, yet most test takers have not effectively prepared for it. Developing and practicing a plan for guessing may be one of the single most effective uses of your time as you get ready for the exam.

In developing your plan for guessing, there are three questions to address:

- When should you start the guessing process?
- How should you narrow down the choices?
- Which answer should you choose?

When to Start the Guessing Process

Unless your plan for guessing is to select C every time (which, despite its merits, is not what we recommend), you need to leave yourself enough time to apply your answer elimination strategies. Since you have a limited amount of time for each question, that means that if you're going to give yourself the best shot at guessing correctly, you have to decide quickly whether or not you will guess.

Of course, the best-case scenario is that you don't have to guess at all, so first, see if you can answer the question based on your knowledge of the subject and basic reasoning skills. Focus on the key words in the question and try to jog your memory of related topics. Give yourself a chance to bring the knowledge to mind, but once you realize that you don't have (or you can't access) the knowledge you need to answer the question, it's time to start the guessing process.

It's almost always better to start the guessing process too early than too late. It only takes a few seconds to remember something and answer the question from knowledge. Carefully eliminating wrong answer choices takes longer. Plus, going through the process of eliminating answer choices can actually help jog your memory.

Summary: Start the guessing process as soon as you decide that you can't answer the question based on your knowledge.

How to Narrow Down the Choices

The next chapter in this book (**Test-Taking Strategies**) includes a wide range of strategies for how to approach questions and how to look for answer choices to eliminate. You will definitely want to read those carefully, practice them, and figure out which ones work best for you. Here though, we're going to address a mindset rather than a particular strategy.

Your chances of guessing an answer correctly depend on how many options you are choosing from.

How many choices you have	How likely you are to guess correctly
5	20%
4	25%
3	33%
2	50%
1	100%

You can see from this chart just how valuable it is to be able to eliminate incorrect answers and make an educated guess, but there are two things that many test takers do that cause them to miss out on the benefits of guessing:

- Accidentally eliminating the correct answer
- Selecting an answer based on an impression

We'll look at the first one here, and the second one in the next section.

To avoid accidentally eliminating the correct answer, we recommend a thought exercise called **the $5 challenge**. In this challenge, you only eliminate an answer choice from contention if you are willing to bet $5 on it being wrong. Why $5? Five dollars is a small but not insignificant amount of money. It's an amount you could afford to lose but wouldn't want to throw away. And while losing $5 once might not hurt too much, doing it twenty times will set you back $100. In the same way, each small decision you make—eliminating a choice here, guessing on a question there—won't by itself impact your score very much, but when you put them all together, they can make a big difference. By holding each answer choice elimination decision to a higher standard, you can reduce the risk of accidentally eliminating the correct answer.

The $5 challenge can also be applied in a positive sense: If you are willing to bet $5 that an answer choice *is* correct, go ahead and mark it as correct.

Summary: Only eliminate an answer choice if you are willing to bet $5 that it is wrong.

Which Answer to Choose

You're taking the test. You've run into a hard question and decided you'll have to guess. You've eliminated all the answer choices you're willing to bet $5 on. Now you have to pick an answer. Why do we even need to talk about this? Why can't you just pick whichever one you feel like when the time comes?

The answer to these questions is that if you don't come into the test with a plan, you'll rely on your impression to select an answer choice, and if you do that, you risk falling into a trap. The test writers know that everyone who takes their test will be guessing on some of the questions, so they intentionally write wrong answer choices to seem plausible. You still have to pick an answer though, and if the wrong answer choices are designed to look right, how can you ever be sure that you're not falling for their trap? The best solution we've found to this dilemma is to take the decision out of your hands entirely. Here is the process we recommend:

Once you've eliminated any choices that you are confident (willing to bet $5) are wrong, select the first remaining choice as your answer.

Whether you choose to select the first remaining choice, the second, or the last, the important thing is that you use some preselected standard. Using this approach guarantees that you will not be enticed into selecting an answer choice that looks right, because you are not basing your decision on how the answer choices look.

This is not meant to make you question your knowledge. Instead, it is to help you recognize the difference between your knowledge and your impressions. There's a huge difference between thinking an answer is right because of what you know, and thinking an answer is right because it looks or sounds like it should be right.

Summary: To ensure that your selection is appropriately random, make a predetermined selection from among all answer choices you have not eliminated.

Test-Taking Strategies

This section contains a list of test-taking strategies that you may find helpful as you work through the test. By taking what you know and applying logical thought, you can maximize your chances of answering any question correctly!

It is very important to realize that every question is different and every person is different: no single strategy will work on every question, and no single strategy will work for every person. That's why we've included all of them here, so you can try them out and determine which ones work best for different types of questions and which ones work best for you.

Question Strategies

READ CAREFULLY

Read the question and answer choices carefully. Don't miss the question because you misread the terms. You have plenty of time to read each question thoroughly and make sure you understand what is being asked. Yet a happy medium must be attained, so don't waste too much time. You must read carefully, but efficiently.

CONTEXTUAL CLUES

Look for contextual clues. If the question includes a word you are not familiar with, look at the immediate context for some indication of what the word might mean. Contextual clues can often give you all the information you need to decipher the meaning of an unfamiliar word. Even if you can't determine the meaning, you may be able to narrow down the possibilities enough to make a solid guess at the answer to the question.

PREFIXES

If you're having trouble with a word in the question or answer choices, try dissecting it. Take advantage of every clue that the word might include. Prefixes and suffixes can be a huge help. Usually they allow you to determine a basic meaning. Pre- means before, post- means after, pro - is positive, de- is negative. From prefixes and suffixes, you can get an idea of the general meaning of the word and try to put it into context.

HEDGE WORDS

Watch out for critical hedge words, such as *likely, may, can, sometimes, often, almost, mostly, usually, generally, rarely,* and *sometimes.* Question writers insert these hedge phrases to cover every possibility. Often an answer choice will be wrong simply because it leaves no room for exception. Be on guard for answer choices that have definitive words such as *exactly* and *always.*

SWITCHBACK WORDS

Stay alert for *switchbacks.* These are the words and phrases frequently used to alert you to shifts in thought. The most common switchback words are *but, although,* and *however.* Others include *nevertheless, on the other hand, even though, while, in spite of, despite, regardless of.* Switchback words are important to catch because they can change the direction of the question or an answer choice.

FACE VALUE

When in doubt, use common sense. Accept the situation in the problem at face value. Don't read too much into it. These problems will not require you to make wild assumptions. If you have to go beyond creativity and warp time or space in order to have an answer choice fit the question, then you should move on and consider the other answer choices. These are normal problems rooted in reality. The applicable relationship or explanation may not be readily apparent, but it is there for you to figure out. Use your common sense to interpret anything that isn't clear.

Answer Choice Strategies

ANSWER SELECTION

The most thorough way to pick an answer choice is to identify and eliminate wrong answers until only one is left, then confirm it is the correct answer. Sometimes an answer choice may immediately seem right, but be careful. The test writers will usually put more than one reasonable answer choice on each question, so take a second to read all of them and make sure that the other choices are not equally obvious. As long as you have time left, it is better to read every answer choice than to pick the first one that looks right without checking the others.

ANSWER CHOICE FAMILIES

An answer choice family consists of two (in rare cases, three) answer choices that are very similar in construction and cannot all be true at the same time. If you see two answer choices that are direct opposites or parallels, one of them is usually the correct answer. For instance, if one answer choice says that quantity x increases and another either says that quantity x decreases (opposite) or says that quantity y increases (parallel), then those answer choices would fall into the same family. An answer choice that doesn't match the construction of the answer choice family is more likely to be incorrect. Most questions will not have answer choice families, but when they do appear, you should be prepared to recognize them.

ELIMINATE ANSWERS

Eliminate answer choices as soon as you realize they are wrong, but make sure you consider all possibilities. If you are eliminating answer choices and realize that the last one you are left with is also wrong, don't panic. Start over and consider each choice again. There may be something you missed the first time that you will realize on the second pass.

AVOID FACT TRAPS

Don't be distracted by an answer choice that is factually true but doesn't answer the question. You are looking for the choice that answers the question. Stay focused on what the question is asking for so you don't accidentally pick an answer that is true but incorrect. Always go back to the question and make sure the answer choice you've selected actually answers the question and is not merely a true statement.

EXTREME STATEMENTS

In general, you should avoid answers that put forth extreme actions as standard practice or proclaim controversial ideas as established fact. An answer choice that states the "process should be used in certain situations, if…" is much more likely to be correct than one that states the "process should be discontinued completely." The first is a calm rational statement and doesn't even make a definitive, uncompromising stance, using a hedge word *if* to provide wiggle room, whereas the second choice is a radical idea and far more extreme.

11

BENCHMARK

As you read through the answer choices and you come across one that seems to answer the question well, mentally select that answer choice. This is not your final answer, but it's the one that will help you evaluate the other answer choices. The one that you selected is your benchmark or standard for judging each of the other answer choices. Every other answer choice must be compared to your benchmark. That choice is correct until proven otherwise by another answer choice beating it. If you find a better answer, then that one becomes your new benchmark. Once you've decided that no other choice answers the question as well as your benchmark, you have your final answer.

PREDICT THE ANSWER

Before you even start looking at the answer choices, it is often best to try to predict the answer. When you come up with the answer on your own, it is easier to avoid distractions and traps because you will know exactly what to look for. The right answer choice is unlikely to be word-for-word what you came up with, but it should be a close match. Even if you are confident that you have the right answer, you should still take the time to read each option before moving on.

General Strategies

TOUGH QUESTIONS

If you are stumped on a problem or it appears too hard or too difficult, don't waste time. Move on! Remember though, if you can quickly check for obviously incorrect answer choices, your chances of guessing correctly are greatly improved. Before you completely give up, at least try to knock out a couple of possible answers. Eliminate what you can and then guess at the remaining answer choices before moving on.

CHECK YOUR WORK

Since you will probably not know every term listed and the answer to every question, it is important that you get credit for the ones that you do know. Don't miss any questions through careless mistakes. If at all possible, try to take a second to look back over your answer selection and make sure you've selected the correct answer choice and haven't made a costly careless mistake (such as marking an answer choice that you didn't mean to mark). This quick double check should more than pay for itself in caught mistakes for the time it costs.

PACE YOURSELF

It's easy to be overwhelmed when you're looking at a page full of questions; your mind is confused and full of random thoughts, and the clock is ticking down faster than you would like. Calm down and maintain the pace that you have set for yourself. Especially as you get down to the last few minutes of the test, don't let the small numbers on the clock make you panic. As long as you are on track by monitoring your pace, you are guaranteed to have time for each question.

DON'T RUSH

It is very easy to make errors when you are in a hurry. Maintaining a fast pace in answering questions is pointless if it makes you miss questions that you would have gotten right otherwise. Test writers like to include distracting information and wrong answers that seem right. Taking a little extra time to avoid careless mistakes can make all the difference in your test score. Find a pace that allows you to be confident in the answers that you select.

KEEP MOVING

Panicking will not help you pass the test, so do your best to stay calm and keep moving. Taking deep breaths and going through the answer elimination steps you practiced can help to break through a stress barrier and keep your pace.

Final Notes

The combination of a solid foundation of content knowledge and the confidence that comes from practicing your plan for applying that knowledge is the key to maximizing your performance on test day. As your foundation of content knowledge is built up and strengthened, you'll find that the strategies included in this chapter become more and more effective in helping you quickly sift through the distractions and traps of the test to isolate the correct answer.

Now it's time to move on to the test content chapters of this book, but be sure to keep your goal in mind. As you read, think about how you will be able to apply this information on the test. If you've already seen sample questions for the test and you have an idea of the question format and style, try to come up with questions of your own that you can answer based on what you're reading. This will give you valuable practice applying your knowledge in the same ways you can expect to on test day.

Good luck and good studying!

Reading Comprehension

Reading in Context

UNDERSTANDING LITERATURE

One of the most important skills in reading comprehension is the identification of **topics** and **main ideas.** There is a subtle difference between these two features. The topic is the **subject** of a text, or what the text is about. The main idea, on the other hand, is the **most important point** being made by the author. The topic is usually expressed in a few words at the most, while the main idea often needs a full sentence to be completely defined. As an example, a short passage might have the topic of penguins and the main idea *Penguins are different from other birds in many ways*. In most nonfiction writing, the topic and the main idea will be stated directly, often in a sentence at the very **beginning** or **end** of the text. When being tested on an understanding of the author's topic, the reader can quickly *skim* the passage for the general idea, stopping to read only the first sentence of each paragraph. A paragraph's first sentence is often (but not always) the main topic sentence, and it gives you a summary of the content of the paragraph. However, there are cases in which the reader must figure out an **unstated** topic or main idea. In these instances, the student must read every sentence of the text, and try to come up with an overarching idea that is supported by each of those sentences.

> **Review Video: Topics and Main Ideas**
> Visit mometrix.com/academy and enter code: 407801

While the main idea is the overall premise of a story, **supporting details** provide evidence and backing for the main point. In order to show that a main idea is correct, or valid, the author needs to add details that prove their point. All texts contain details, but they are only classified as supporting details when they serve to reinforce some larger point. Supporting details are most commonly found in **informative** and **persuasive** texts. In some cases, they will be clearly indicated with words like *for example* or *for instance*, or they will be enumerated with words like *first*, *second*, and *last*. However, they may not be indicated with special words. As a reader, it is important to consider whether the author's supporting details really back up his or her **main point**. Supporting details can be factual and correct but still not relevant to the author's point. Conversely, supporting details can seem pertinent but be ineffective because they are based on opinion or assertions that cannot be proven.

pertinent — relevant or applicable to a particular matter

syn: relevant, to the point, appropriate

> **Review Video: Supporting Details**
> Visit mometrix.com/academy and enter code: 396297

An example of a main idea is: "Giraffes live in the Serengeti of Africa." A supporting detail about giraffes could be: "A giraffe uses its long neck to reach twigs and leaves on trees." The main idea gives the general idea that the text is about giraffes. The supporting detail gives a specific fact about how the giraffes eat.

Topic and summary sentences are a convenient way to encapsulate the **main idea** of a text. In some textbooks and academic articles, the author will place a **topic** or **summary sentence** at the beginning of each section as a means of preparing the reader for what is to come. Research suggests that the brain is more receptive to new information when it has been prepared by the presentation of the main idea or some key words. The phenomenon is somewhat akin to the primer coat of paint that allows subsequent coats of paint to absorb more easily. A good topic sentence will be **clear** and not contain any **jargon**. When topic or summary sentences are not provided, good readers can jot down their own so that they can find their place in a text and refresh their memory.

As opposed to a main idea, themes are seldom expressed directly in a text, so they can be difficult to identify. A **theme** is an issue, an idea, or a question raised by the text. For instance, a theme of William Shakespeare's *Hamlet* is indecision, as the title character explores his own psyche and the results of his failure to make bold choices. A great work of literature may have many themes, and the reader is justified in identifying any for which he or she can find support. One common characteristic of themes is that they raise more questions than they answer. In a good piece of fiction, the author is not always trying to convince the reader, but is instead trying to elevate the reader's perspective and encourage him to consider the themes more deeply. When reading, one can identify themes by constantly asking what general issues the text is addressing. A good way to evaluate an author's approach to a theme is to begin reading with a question in mind (for example, how does this text approach the theme of love?) and then look for evidence in the text that addresses that question.

> **Review Video: Theme**
> Visit mometrix.com/academy and enter code: 732074

PURPOSES FOR WRITING

In order to be an effective reader, one must pay attention to the author's position and purpose. Even those texts that seem objective and impartial, like textbooks, have some sort of **position** and **bias**. Readers need to take these positions into account when considering the author's message. When an author uses emotional language or clearly favors one side of an argument, his position is clear. However, the author's position may be evident not only in what he writes, but in what he doesn't write. For this reason, it is sometimes necessary to review some other texts on the same topic in order to develop a view of the author's position. If this is not possible, then it may be useful to acquire a little background personal information about the author. When the only source of information is the text, however, the reader should look for language and argumentation that seems to indicate a particular stance on the subject.

> **Review Video: Author's Position**
> Visit mometrix.com/academy and enter code: 827954

Identifying the **purpose** of an author is usually easier than identifying her position. In most cases, the author has no interest in hiding his or her purpose. A text that is meant to entertain, for instance, should be obviously written to please the reader. Most narratives, or stories, are written to entertain, though they may also inform or persuade. Informative texts are easy to identify as well. The most difficult purpose of a text to identify is persuasion, because the author has an interest in making this purpose *hard to detect*. When a person knows that the author is trying to convince him, he is automatically more wary and skeptical of the argument. For this reason, persuasive texts often try to establish an entertaining tone, hoping to amuse the reader into agreement, or an informative tone, hoping to create an appearance of authority and objectivity.

An author's purpose is often evident in the **organization** of the text. For instance, if the text has headings and subheadings, if key terms are in bold, and if the author makes his main idea clear from the beginning, then the likely purpose of the text is to **inform**. If the author begins by making a claim and then makes various arguments to support that claim, the purpose is probably to **persuade**. If the author is telling a story, or is more interested in holding the attention of the reader than in making a particular point or delivering information, then his purpose is most likely to **entertain**. As a reader, it is best to judge an author on how well he accomplishes his purpose. In other words, it is not entirely fair to complain that a textbook is boring: if the text is clear and easy to understand, then the author has done his job. Similarly, a storyteller should not be judged too harshly for getting some facts wrong, so long as he is able to give pleasure to the reader.

Review Video: Purpose of an Author
Visit mometrix.com/academy and enter code: 497555

The author's purpose for writing will affect his writing style and the response of the reader. In a **persuasive essay**, the author is attempting to change the reader's mind or convince him of something he did not believe previously. There are several identifying characteristics of persuasive writing. One is **opinion presented as fact**. When an author attempts to persuade the reader, he often presents his or her opinions as if they were fact. A reader must be on guard for statements that sound factual but which cannot be subjected to research, observation, or experiment. Another characteristic of persuasive writing is **emotional language**. An author will often try to play on the reader's emotion by appealing to his sympathy or sense of morality. When an author uses colorful or evocative language with the intent of arousing the reader's passions, it is likely that he is attempting to persuade. Finally, in many cases a persuasive text will give an **unfair explanation of opposing positions,** if these positions are mentioned at all.

An **informative text** is written to **educate** and **enlighten** the reader. Informative texts are almost always nonfiction, and are rarely structured as a story. The intention of an informative text is to deliver information in the most *comprehensible* way possible, so the structure of the text is likely to be very clear. In an informative text, the **thesis statement** is often in the first sentence. The author may use some colorful language, but is likely to put more emphasis on **clarity** and **precision**. Informative essays do not typically appeal to the emotions. They often contain *facts* and *figures*, and rarely include the opinion of the author. Sometimes a persuasive essay can resemble an informative essay, especially if the author maintains an even tone and presents his or her views as if they were established fact.

The success or failure of an author's intent to **entertain** is determined by those who read the author's work. Entertaining texts may be either fiction or nonfiction, and they may describe real or imagined people, places, and events. Entertaining texts are often narratives, or stories. A text that is written to entertain is likely to contain **colorful language** that engages the imagination and the emotions. Such writing often features a great deal of figurative language, which typically enlivens its subject matter with images and analogies. Though an entertaining text is not usually written to persuade or inform, it may accomplish both of these tasks. An entertaining text may **appeal to the reader's emotions a**nd cause him or her to think differently about a particular subject. In any case, entertaining texts tend to showcase the personality of the author more so than do other types of writing.

When an author intends to **express feelings,** she may use colorful and evocative language. An author may write emotionally for any number of reasons. Sometimes, the author will do so because she is describing a personal situation of great pain or happiness. Sometimes an author is attempting to persuade the reader, and so will use emotion to stir up the passions. It can be easy to identify this kind of expression when the writer uses phrases like *I felt* and *I sense*. However, sometimes the author will simply describe feelings without introducing them. As a reader, it is important to recognize when an author is expressing emotion, and not to become overwhelmed by sympathy or passion. A reader should maintain some **detachment** so that he or she can still evaluate the strength of the author's argument or the quality of the writing.

In a sense, almost all writing is descriptive, insofar as it seeks to describe events, ideas, or people to the reader. Some texts, however, are primarily concerned with **description**. A descriptive text focuses on a particular subject, and attempts to depict it in a way that will be clear to the reader. Descriptive texts contain many **adjectives** and **adverbs**, words that give shades of meaning and create a more detailed mental picture for the reader. A descriptive text fails when it is unclear or vague to the reader. On the other hand, however, a descriptive text that compiles too much detail can be boring and overwhelming to the reader. A descriptive text will certainly be informative, and it may be persuasive and entertaining as well. Descriptive writing is a challenge for the author, but when it is done well, it can be fun to read.

WRITING DEVICES

Authors will use different stylistic and writing devices to make their meaning more clearly understood. One of those devices is comparison and contrast. When an author describes the ways in which two things are alike, he or she is **comparing** them. When the author describes the ways in which two things are different, he or she is **contrasting** them. The "compare and contrast" essay is one of the most common forms in nonfiction. It is often signaled with certain words: a comparison may be indicated with such words as *both*, *same*, *like*, *too*, and *as well*; while a contrast may be indicated by words like *but*, *however*, *on the other hand*, *instead*, and *yet*. Of course, comparisons and contrasts may be implicit without using any such signaling language. A single sentence may both compare and contrast. Consider the sentence *Brian and Sheila love ice cream, but Brian prefers vanilla and Sheila prefers strawberry*. In one sentence, the author has described both a similarity (love of ice cream) and a difference (favorite flavor).

> **Review Video: <u>Compare and Contrast</u>**
> Visit mometrix.com/academy and enter code: 798319

One of the most common text structures is **cause and effect**. A cause is an **act** or **event** that makes something happen, and an effect is the thing that happens as a **result** of that cause. A cause-and-effect relationship is not always explicit, but there are some words in English that signal causality, such as *since*, *because*, and *as a result*. As an example, consider the sentence *Because the sky was clear, Ron did not bring an umbrella*. The cause is the clear sky, and the effect is that Ron did not bring an umbrella. However, sometimes the cause-and-effect relationship will not be clearly noted. For instance, the sentence *He was late and missed the meeting* does not contain any signaling words, but it still contains a cause (he was late) and an effect (he missed the meeting). It is possible for a single cause to have multiple effects, or for a single effect to have multiple causes. Also, an effect can in turn be the cause of another effect, in what is known as a cause-and-effect chain.

Authors often use analogies to add meaning to the text. An **analogy** is a comparison of two things. The words in the analogy are connected by a certain, often undetermined relationship. Look at this analogy: moo is to cow as quack is to duck. This analogy compares the sound that a cow makes with the sound that a duck makes. Even if the word 'quack' was not given, one could figure out it is the correct word to complete the analogy based on the relationship between the words 'moo' and 'cow'. Some common relationships for analogies include synonyms, antonyms, part to whole, definition, and actor to action.

Another element that impacts a text is the author's point of view. The **point of view** of a text is the perspective from which it is told. The author will always have a point of view about a story before he draws up a plot line. The author will know what events they want to take place, how they want the characters to interact, and how the story will resolve. An author will also have an opinion on the topic, or series of events, which is presented in the story, based on their own prior experience and beliefs.

The two main points of view that authors use are first person and third person. If the narrator of the story is also the main character, or *protagonist*, the text is written in **first-person point of view**. In first person, the author writes with the word *I*. **Third-person point of view** is probably the most common point of view that authors use. Using third person, authors refer to each character using the words *he* or *she*. In third-person omniscient, the narrator is not a character in the story and tells the story of all of the characters at the same time.

> **Review Video: Point of View**
> Visit mometrix.com/academy and enter code: 383336

A good writer will use **transitional words** and phrases to guide the reader through the text. You are no doubt familiar with the common transitions, though you may never have considered how they operate. Some transitional phrases (*after, before, during, in the middle of*) give information about time. Some indicate that an example is about to be given (*for example, in fact, for instance*). Writers use them to compare (*also, likewise*) and contrast (*however, but, yet*). Transitional words and phrases can suggest addition (*and, also, furthermore, moreover*) and logical relationships (*if, then, therefore, as a result, since*). Finally, transitional words and phrases can demarcate the steps in a process (*first, second, last*). You should incorporate transitional words and phrases where they will orient your reader and illuminate the structure of your composition.

> **Review Video: Transitional Words and Phrases**
> Visit mometrix.com/academy and enter code: 197796

TYPES OF PASSAGES

A **narrative passage** is a story. Narratives can be fiction or nonfiction. However, there are a few elements that a text must have in order to be classified as a narrative. To begin with, the text must have a **plot**. That is, it must describe a series of events. If it is a good narrative, these events will be interesting and emotionally engaging to the reader. A narrative also has **characters**. These could be people, animals, or even inanimate objects, so long as they participate in the plot. A narrative passage often contains **figurative language**, which is meant to stimulate the imagination of the reader by making comparisons and observations. A metaphor, which is a description of one thing in terms of another, is a common piece of figurative language. *The moon was a frosty snowball* is an example of a metaphor: it is obviously untrue in the literal sense, but it suggests a certain mood for the reader. Narratives often proceed in a clear sequence, but they do not need to do so.

An **expository passage** aims to **inform and enlighten** the reader. It is nonfiction and usually centers around a simple, easily defined topic. Since the goal of exposition is to teach, such a passage should be as clear as possible. It is common for an expository passage to contain helpful organizing words, like *first, next, for example*, and *therefore*. These words keep the reader **oriented** in the text. Although expository passages do not need to feature colorful language and artful writing, they are often more effective when they do. For a reader, the challenge of expository passages is to maintain steady attention. Expository passages are not always about subjects in which a reader will naturally be interested, and the writer is often more concerned with **clarity and comprehensibility** than with engaging the reader. For this reason, many expository passages are dull. Making notes is a good way to maintain focus when reading an expository passage.

A **technical passage** is written to describe a complex object or process. Technical writing is common in medical and technological fields, in which complicated mathematical, scientific, and engineering ideas need to be explained simply and clearly. To ease comprehension, a technical passage usually proceeds in a very logical order. Technical passages often have clear headings and subheadings, which are used to keep the reader oriented in the text. It is also common for these passages to break sections up with numbers or letters. Many technical passages look more like an outline than a piece of prose. The amount of **jargon** or difficult vocabulary will vary in a technical passage depending on the intended audience. As much as possible, technical passages try to avoid language that the reader will have to research in order to understand the message. Of course, it is not always possible to avoid jargon.

A **persuasive passage** is meant to change the reader's mind or lead her into agreement with the author. The persuasive intent may be obvious, or it may be quite difficult to discern. In some cases, a persuasive passage will be indistinguishable from an informative passage: it will make an assertion and offer supporting details. However, a persuasive passage is more likely to make claims based on **opinion** and to appeal to the reader's **emotions**. Persuasive passages may not describe alternate positions and, when they do, they often display significant **bias**. It may be clear that a persuasive passage is giving the author's viewpoint, or the passage may adopt a seemingly objective tone. A persuasive passage is successful if it can make a convincing argument and win the trust of the reader.

A persuasive essay will likely focus on one **central argument**, but it may make many smaller claims along the way. These are **subordinate arguments** with which the reader must agree if he or she is going to agree with the central argument. The central argument will only be as strong as the subordinate claims. These claims should be rooted in fact and observation, rather than subjective judgment. The best persuasive essays provide enough supporting detail to justify claims without overwhelming the reader. Remember that a fact must be susceptible to **independent verification**: that is, it must be something the reader could confirm. Also, **statistics** are only effective when they take into account possible objections. For instance, a statistic on the number of foreclosed houses would only be useful if it was taken over a defined interval and in a defined area. Most readers are wary of statistics, because they are so often misleading. If possible, a persuasive essay should always include **references** so that the reader can obtain more information. Of course, this means that the writer's accuracy and fairness may be judged by the inquiring reader.

Opinions are formed by **emotion** as well as reason, and persuasive writers often appeal to the feelings of the reader. Although readers should always be skeptical of this technique, it is often used in a proper and ethical manner. For instance, there are many subjects that have an obvious emotional component, and therefore cannot be completely treated without an appeal to the emotions. Consider an article on drunk driving: it makes sense to include some specific examples that will alarm or sadden the reader. After all, drunk driving often has serious and tragic consequences. Emotional appeals are not appropriate, however, when they attempt to **mislead** the reader. For instance, in political advertisements it is common to emphasize the patriotism of the preferred candidate, because this will encourage the audience to link their own positive feelings about the country with their opinion of the candidate. However, these ads often imply that the other candidate is unpatriotic, which in most cases is far from the truth. Another common and improper emotional appeal is the use of loaded language, as for instance referring to an avidly religious person as a "fanatic" or a passionate environmentalist as a "tree hugger." These terms introduce an emotional component that detracts from the argument.

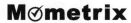

Finding the Meaning and Assessing the Text

RESPONDING TO LITERATURE

When reading good literature, the reader is moved to engage actively in the text. One part of being an active reader involves making predictions. A **prediction** is a guess about what will happen next. Readers are constantly making predictions based on what they have read and what they already know. Consider the following sentence: *Staring at the computer screen in shock, Kim blindly reached over for the brimming glass of water on the shelf to her side.* The sentence suggests that Kim is agitated and that she is not looking at the glass she is going to pick up, so a reader might predict that she is going to knock the glass over. Of course, not every prediction will be accurate: perhaps Kim will pick the glass up cleanly. Nevertheless, the author has certainly created the expectation that the water might be spilled. Predictions are always subject to revision as the reader acquires more information.

> **Review Video: <u>Predictions</u>**
> Visit mometrix.com/academy and enter code: 437248

Test-taking tip: To respond to questions requiring future predictions, the answers should be based on evidence of past or present behavior.

Readers are often required to understand text that claims and suggests ideas without stating them directly. An **inference** is a piece of information that is implied but not written outright by the author. For instance, consider the following sentence: *Mark made more money that week than he had in the previous year.* From this sentence, the reader can infer that Mark either has not made much money in the previous year or made a great deal of money that week. Often, a reader can use information he or she already knows to make inferences. Take as an example the sentence *When his coffee arrived, he looked around the table for the silver cup.* Many people know that cream is typically served in a silver cup, so using their own base of knowledge they can infer that the subject of this sentence takes his coffee with cream. Making inferences requires concentration, attention, and practice.

> **Review Video: <u>Inference</u>**
> Visit mometrix.com/academy and enter code: 379203

Test-taking tip: While being tested on his ability to make correct inferences, the student must look for **contextual clues**. An answer can be *true* but not *correct*. The contextual clues will help you find the answer that is the **best answer** out of the given choices. Understand the context in which a phrase is stated. When asked for the implied meaning of a statement made in the passage, the student should immediately locate the statement and read the **context** in which it was made. Also, look for an answer choice that has a similar phrase to the statement in question.

In addition to inferring and predicting things about the text, the reader must often **draw conclusions** about the information he has read. When asked for a *conclusion* that may be drawn, look for critical "hedge" phrases, such as *likely, may, can, will often*, among many others. When you are being tested on this knowledge, remember that question writers insert these hedge phrases to cover every possibility. Often an answer will be wrong simply because it leaves no room for exception. Extreme positive or negative answers (such as always, never, etc.) are usually not correct. The reader should not use any outside knowledge that is not gathered from the reading passage to answer the related questions. Correct answers can be derived straight from the reading passage.

A reader must be able to identify a text's **sequence**, or the order in which things happen. Often, and especially when the sequence is very important to the author, it is indicated with signal words like *first*, *then*, *next*, and *last*. However, sometimes a sequence is merely implied and must be noted by the reader. Consider the sentence *He walked in the front door and switched on the hall lamp*. Clearly, the man did not turn the lamp on before he walked in the door, so the implied sequence is that he first walked in the door and then turned on the lamp. Texts do not always proceed in an **orderly** sequence from first to last: sometimes, they begin at the end and then start over at the beginning. As a reader, it can be useful to make brief **notes** to clarify the sequence.

OPINIONS, FACTS, AND FALLACIES

Critical thinking skills are mastered through understanding various types of writing and the different purposes that authors have for writing the way they do. Every author writes for a purpose. Understanding that purpose, and how they accomplish their goal, will allow you to critique the writing and determine whether or not you agree with their conclusions.

Readers must always be conscious of the distinction between fact and opinion. A **fact** can be subjected to analysis and can be either proved or disproved. An **opinion**, on the other hand, is the author's personal feeling, which may not be alterable by research, evidence, or argument. If the author writes that the distance from New York to Boston is about two hundred miles, he is stating a fact. But if he writes that New York is too crowded, then he is giving an opinion, because there is no objective standard for overpopulation. An opinion may be indicated by words like *believe*, *think*, or *feel*. Also, an opinion may be **supported** by facts: for instance, the author might give the population density of New York as a reason for why it is overcrowded. An opinion supported by fact tends to be more convincing. When authors support their opinions with other opinions, the reader is unlikely to be moved.

Facts should be presented to the reader from **reliable sources**. An opinion is what the author thinks about a given topic. An opinion is not common knowledge or proven by expert sources, but it is information that the author believes and wants the reader to consider. To distinguish between fact and opinion, a reader needs to look at the type of source that is presenting information, what information backs-up a claim, and whether or not the author may be motivated to have a certain point of view on a given topic. For example, if a panel of scientists has conducted multiple studies on the effectiveness of taking a certain vitamin, the results are more likely to be factual than if a company selling a vitamin claims that taking the vitamin can produce positive effects. The company is motivated to sell its product, while the scientists are using the scientific method to prove a theory. If the author uses words such as "I think...", the statement is an opinion.

Review Video: Fact or Opinion
Visit mometrix.com/academy and enter code: 870899

In their attempt to persuade, writers often make mistakes in their thinking patterns and writing choices. It's important to understand these so you can make an informed decision. Every author has a point of view, but when an author ignores reasonable counterarguments or distorts opposing viewpoints, she is demonstrating a **bias**. A bias is evident whenever the author is **unfair** or **inaccurate** in his or her presentation. Bias may be intentional or unintentional, but it should always alert the reader to be skeptical of the argument being made. It should be noted that a biased author may still be correct. However, the author will be correct in spite of her bias, not because of it. A **stereotype** is like a bias, except that it is specifically applied to a **group** or place. Stereotyping is considered to be particularly abhorrent because it promotes negative generalizations about people. Many people are familiar with some of the hateful stereotypes of certain ethnic, religious, and cultural groups. Readers should be very wary of authors who stereotype. These faulty assumptions typically reveal the author's ignorance and lack of curiosity.

Review Video: Bias and Stereotype
Visit mometrix.com/academy and enter code: 644829

Sometimes, authors will **appeal to the reader's emotion** in an attempt to persuade or to distract the reader from the **weakness** of the argument. For instance, the author may try to inspire the **pity** of the reader by delivering a heart-rending story. An author also might use the **bandwagon** approach, in which he suggests that his opinion is correct because it is held by the majority. Some authors resort to **name-calling**, in which insults and harsh words are delivered to the opponent in an attempt to distract. In advertising, a common appeal is the **testimonial**, in which a famous person endorses a product. Of course, the fact that a celebrity likes something should not really mean anything to the reader. These and other emotional appeals are usually evidence of poor reasoning and a weak argument.

Review Video: Appeal to Emotion
Visit mometrix.com/academy and enter code: 163442

Certain **logical fallacies** are frequent in writing. A logical fallacy is a failure of reasoning. As a reader, it is important to recognize logical fallacies, because they diminish the value of the author's message. The four most common logical fallacies in writing are the false analogy, circular reasoning, false dichotomy, and overgeneralization. In a **false analogy**, the author suggests that two things are similar, when in fact they are different. This fallacy is often committed when the author is attempting to convince the reader that something unknown is like something relatively familiar. The author takes advantage of the reader's ignorance to make this false comparison. One example might be the following statement: *Failing to tip a waitress is like stealing money out of somebody's wallet.* Of course, failing to tip is very rude, especially when the service has been good, but people are not arrested for failing to tip as they would for stealing money from a wallet. To compare stingy diners with thieves is a false analogy.

Review Video: False Analogy
Visit mometrix.com/academy and enter code: 865045

Circular reasoning is one of the more difficult logical fallacies to identify, because it is typically hidden behind dense language and complicated sentences. Reasoning is described as circular when it offers no support for assertions other than **restating them in different words**. Put another way, a circular argument refers to itself as evidence of truth. A simple example of circular argument is when a person uses a word to define itself, such as saying *Niceness is the state of being nice.* If the reader does not know what *nice* means, then this definition will not be very useful. In a text, circular reasoning is usually more complex. For instance, an author might say *Poverty is a problem for society because it creates trouble for people throughout the community.* It is redundant to say that poverty is a problem because it creates trouble. When an author engages in circular reasoning, it is often because he or she has not fully thought out the argument, or cannot come up with any legitimate justifications.

Review Video: Circular Reasoning
Visit mometrix.com/academy and enter code: 398925

One of the most common logical fallacies is the **false dichotomy**, in which the author creates an artificial sense that there are only **two possible alternatives** in a situation. This fallacy is common when the author has an agenda and wants to give the impression that his view is the only sensible one. A false dichotomy has the effect of limiting the reader's options and imagination. An example of a false dichotomy is the statement _You need to go to the party with me, otherwise you'll just be bored at home_. The speaker suggests that the only other possibility besides being at the party is being bored at home. But this is not true, as it is perfectly possible to be entertained at home, or even to go somewhere other than the party. Readers should always be wary of the false dichotomy: when an author limits alternatives, it is always wise to ask whether he is being valid.

> **Review Video: <u>False Dichotomy</u>**
> Visit mometrix.com/academy and enter code: 484397

Overgeneralization is a logical fallacy in which the author makes a claim that is so broad it **cannot be proved or disproved**. In most cases, overgeneralization occurs when the author wants to create an illusion of authority, or when he is using sensational language to sway the opinion of the reader. For instance, in the sentence _Everybody knows that she is a terrible teacher_, the author makes an assumption that cannot really be believed. This kind of statement is made when the author wants to create the illusion of consensus when none actually exists: it may be that most people have a negative view of the teacher, but to say that _everybody_ feels that way is an exaggeration. When a reader spots overgeneralization, she should become skeptical about the argument that is being made, because an author will often try to hide a weak or unsupported assertion behind authoritative language.

> **Review Video: <u>Overgeneralization</u>**
> Visit mometrix.com/academy and enter code: 367357

Two other types of logical fallacies are slippery slope arguments and hasty generalizations. In a **slippery slope argument**, the author says that if something happens, it automatically means that something else will happen as a result, even though this may not be true. (i.e., just because you study hard does not mean you are going to ace the test). **Hasty generalization** is drawing a conclusion too early, without finishing analyzing the details of the argument. Writers of persuasive texts often use these techniques because they are very effective. In order to **identify logical fallacies**, readers need to read carefully and ask questions as they read. Thinking critically means not taking everything at face value. Readers need to critically evaluate an author's argument to make sure that the logic used is sound.

The **"straw man" fallacy** is an **oversimplification or distortion of opposing views**. This fallacy is one of the most obvious and easily uncovered. The reason is that it relies on gross distortions. The name refers to a side that is set up so weak--like a straw man--that it is easily refuted.

ORGANIZATION OF THE TEXT

The way a text is organized can help the reader to understand more clearly the author's intent and his conclusions. There are various ways to organize a text, and each one has its own purposes and uses.

Some nonfiction texts are organized to present a **problem** followed by a **solution**. In this type of text, it is common for the problem to be explained before the solution is offered. In some cases, as when the problem is well known, the solution may be briefly introduced at the beginning. The entire passage may focus on the solution, and the problem will be referenced only occasionally. Some texts will outline multiple solutions to a problem, leaving the reader to choose among them. If the author has an interest or an allegiance to one solution, he may fail to mention or may describe inaccurately some of the other solutions. Readers should be careful of the author's **agenda** when reading a problem-solution text. Only by understanding the author's point of view and interests can one develop a proper judgment of the proposed solution.

Authors need to organize information logically so the reader can follow it and locate information within the text. Two common organizational structures are cause and effect and chronological order. When using **chronological order**, the author presents information in the order that it happened. For example, biographies are written in chronological order; the subject's birth and childhood are presented first, followed by their adult life, and lastly by the events leading up to the person's death.

In **cause and effect**, an author presents one thing that makes something else happen. For example, if one were to go to bed very late, they would be tired. The cause is going to bed late, with the effect of being tired the next day.

It can be tricky to identify the cause-and-effect relationships in a text, but there are a few ways to approach this task. To begin with, these relationships are often **signaled** with certain terms. When an author uses words like *because*, *since*, *in order*, and *so*, she is likely describing a cause-and-effect relationship. Consider the sentence, "He called her because he needed the homework." This is a simple causal relationship, in which the cause was his need for the homework and the effect was his phone call. Not all cause-and-effect relationships are marked in this way, however. Consider the sentences, "He called her. He needed the homework." When the cause-and-effect relationship is not indicated with a keyword, it can be discovered by asking why something happened. He called her: why? The answer is in the next sentence: He needed the homework.

Persuasive essays, in which an author tries to make a convincing argument and change the reader's mind, usually include cause-and-effect relationships. However, these relationships should not always be taken at face value. An author frequently will assume a cause or take an effect for granted. To read a persuasive essay effectively, one needs to judge the **cause-and-effect relationships** the author is presenting. For instance, imagine an author wrote the following: "The parking deck has been unprofitable because people would prefer to ride their bikes." The relationship is clear: the cause is that people prefer to ride their bikes, and the effect is that the parking deck has been unprofitable. However, a reader should consider whether this argument is conclusive. Perhaps there are other reasons for the failure of the parking deck: a down economy, excessive fees, etc. Too often, authors present causal relationships as if they are fact rather than opinion. Readers should be on the alert for these dubious claims.

Thinking critically about ideas and conclusions can seem like a daunting task. One way to make it easier is to understand the basic elements of ideas and writing techniques. Looking at the way different ideas relate to each other can be a good way for the reader to begin his analysis. For instance, sometimes writers will write about two different ideas that are in opposition to each other. The analysis of these opposing ideas is known as **contrast**. Contrast is often marred by the author's obvious partiality to one of the ideas. A discerning reader will be put off by an author who does not engage in a fair fight. In an analysis of opposing ideas, both ideas should be presented in their clearest and most reasonable terms. If the author does prefer a side, he should avoid indicating this preference with pejorative language. An analysis of opposing ideas should proceed through the major differences point by point, with a full explanation of each side's view. For instance, in an analysis of capitalism and communism, it would be important to outline each side's view on labor, markets, prices, personal responsibility, etc. It would be less effective to describe the theory of communism and then explain how capitalism has thrived in the West. An analysis of opposing views should present each side in the same manner.

Many texts follow the **compare-and-contrast model**, in which the similarities and differences between two ideas or things are explored. Analysis of the similarities between ideas is called comparison. In order for a comparison to work, the author must place the ideas or things in an equivalent structure. That is, the author must present the ideas in the same way. Imagine an author wanted to show the similarities between cricket and baseball. The correct way to do so would be to summarize the equipment and rules for each game. It would be incorrect to summarize the equipment of cricket and then lay out the history of baseball, since this would make it impossible for the reader to see the similarities. It is perhaps too obvious to say that an analysis of similar ideas should emphasize the similarities. Of course, the author should take care to include any differences that must be mentioned. Often, these small differences will only reinforce the more general similarity.

DRAWING CONCLUSIONS

Authors should have a clear purpose in mind while writing. Especially when reading informational texts, it is important to understand the logical conclusion of the author's ideas. Identifying this **logical conclusion** can help the reader understand whether he agrees with the writer or not. Identifying a logical conclusion is much like making an inference: it requires the reader to combine the information given by the text with what he already knows to make a supportable assertion. If a passage is written well, then the conclusion should be obvious even when it is unstated. If the author intends the reader to draw a certain conclusion, then all of his argumentation and detail should be leading toward it. One way to approach the task of drawing conclusions is to make brief notes of all the points made by the author. When these are arranged on paper, they may clarify the logical conclusion. Another way to approach conclusions is to consider whether the reasoning of the author raises any pertinent questions. Sometimes it will be possible to draw several conclusions from a passage, and on occasion these will be conclusions that were never imagined by the author. It is essential, however, that these conclusions be **supported** directly by the text.

> **Review Video: Identifying Logical Conclusions**
> Visit mometrix.com/academy and enter code: 281653

The term **text evidence** refers to information that supports a **main point or minor points** in a story, and can help lead the reader to a conclusion. Information used as text evidence is precise, descriptive, and factual. A main point is often followed by **supporting details** that provide evidence to back-up a claim. For example, a story may include the claim that winter occurs during opposite months in the Northern and Southern hemispheres. Text evidence based on this claim may include countries where winter occurs in opposite months, along with reasons that winter occurs at different times of the year in separate hemispheres (due to the tilt of the Earth as it rotates around the sun).

Readers **interpret** text and **respond** to it in a number of ways. Using textual support helps defend your response or interpretation because it roots your thinking in the text. You are interpreting based on information in the text and not simply your own ideas. When crafting a response, look for important quotes and details from the text to help bolster your argument. If you are writing about a character's personality trait, for example, use details from the text to show that the character acted in such a way. You can also include statistics and facts from a nonfiction text to strengthen your response. For example, instead of writing, "A lot of people use cell phones," use statistics to provide the exact number. This strengthens your argument because it is more precise.

A reader should always be drawing conclusions from the text. Sometimes conclusions are implied from written information, and other times the information is **stated directly** within the passage. It is always more comfortable to draw **conclusions** from information stated within a passage, rather than to draw them from mere implications. At times an author may provide some information and then describe a **counterargument**. The reader should be alert for direct statements that are subsequently rejected or weakened by the author. The reader should always read the **entire passage** before drawing conclusions. Many readers are trained to expect the author's conclusions at either the beginning or the end of the passage, but many texts do not adhere to this format.

Drawing conclusions from information implied within a passage requires confidence on the part of the reader. **Implications** are things the author does not state directly, but which can be assumed based on what the author does say. For instance, consider the following simple passage: "I stepped outside and opened my umbrella. By the time I got to work, the cuffs of my pants were soaked." The author never states that it is raining, but this fact is clearly implied. Conclusions based on implication must be well supported by the text. In order to draw a solid conclusion, a reader should have multiple pieces of **evidence**, or, if he only has one, must be assured that there is no other possible explanation than his conclusion. A good reader will be able to draw many conclusions from information implied by the text, which enriches the reading experience considerably.

As an aid to drawing conclusions, the reader should be adept at **outlining** the information contained in the passage; an effective outline will reveal the structure of the passage, and will lead to solid conclusions. An effective outline will have a title that refers to the basic subject of the text, though it need not recapitulate the main idea. In most outlines, the **main idea** will be the first major section. It will have each major idea of the passage established as the head of a category. For instance, the most common outline format calls for the main ideas of the passage to be indicated with Roman numerals. In an effective outline of this kind, each of the main ideas will be represented by a Roman numeral and none of the Roman numerals will designate minor details or secondary ideas. Moreover, all **supporting ideas and details** should be placed in the appropriate place on the outline. An outline does not need to include every detail listed in the text, but it should feature all of those that are central to the argument or message. Each of these details should be listed under the appropriate main idea.

It is also helpful to **summarize** the information you have read in a paragraph or passage format. This process is similar to creating an effective outline. To begin with, a summary should accurately define the **main idea** of the passage, though it does not need to explain this main idea in exhaustive detail. It should continue by laying out the most important **supporting details** or arguments from the passage. All of the significant supporting details should be included, and none of the details included should be irrelevant or insignificant. Also, the summary should accurately report all of these details. Too often, the desire for brevity in a summary leads to the sacrifice of clarity or veracity. Summaries are often difficult to read, because they omit all of graceful language, digressions, and asides that distinguish great writing. However, if the summary is effective, it should contain much the same message as the original text.

Paraphrasing is another method the reader can use to aid in comprehension. When paraphrasing, one puts what they have read into their own words, rephrasing what the author has written to

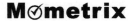

make it their own, to "translate" all of what the author says to their own words, including as many details as they can.

CREDIBILITY

The text used to support an argument can be the argument's downfall if it is not credible. A text is **credible**, or believable, when the author is knowledgeable and objective, or unbiased. The author's **motivations** for writing the text play a critical role in determining the credibility of the text and must be evaluated when assessing that credibility. The author's motives should be for the dissemination of information. The purpose of the text should be to inform or describe, not to persuade. When an author writes a persuasive text, he has the motivation that the reader will do what they want. The extent of the author's knowledge of the topic and their motivation must be evaluated when assessing the credibility of a text. Reports written about the Ozone layer by an environmental scientist and a hairdresser will have a different level of credibility.

After determining your own opinion and evaluating the credibility of your supporting text, it is sometimes necessary to communicate your ideas and findings to others. When writing a **response** to a text, it is important to use elements of the text to support your assertion or defend your position. Using supporting evidence from the text strengthens the argument because the reader can see how in depth the writer read the original piece and based their response on the details and facts within that text. Elements of text that can be used in a response include: facts, details, statistics, and direct quotations from the text. When writing a response, one must make sure they indicate which information comes from the original text and then base their discussion, argument, or defense around this information.

Additional Parts of Literature

INFORMATIONAL SOURCES

Informational sources often come in short forms like a memo or recipe, or longer forms like books, magazines, or journals. These longer sources of information each have their own way of organizing information, but there are some similarities that the reader should be aware of.

Most books, magazines, and journals have a **table of contents** at the beginning. This helps the reader find the different parts of the book. The table of contents is usually found a page or two after the title page in a book, and on the first few pages of a magazine. However, many magazines now place the table of contents in the midst of an overabundance of advertisements, because they know readers will have to look at the ads as they search for the table. The standard orientation for a table of contents is the sections of the book listed along the left side, with the initial page number for each along the right. It is common in a book for the **prefatory material** (preface, introduction, etc.) to be numbered with Roman numerals. The contents are always listed in order from the beginning of the book to the end.

A nonfiction book will also typically have an **index** at the end so that the reader can easily find information about particular topics. An index lists the topics in alphabetical order. The names of people are listed with the last name first. For example, *Adams, John* would come before *Washington, George*. To the right of the entry, the relevant page numbers are listed. When a topic is mentioned over several pages, the index will often connect these pages with a dash. For instance, if the subject is mentioned from pages 35 to 42 and again on 53, then the index entry will be labeled as *35-42, 53*. Some entries will have subsets, which are listed below the main entry, indented slightly, and placed in alphabetical order. This is common for subjects that are discussed frequently in the book. For instance, in a book about Elizabethan drama, William Shakespeare will likely be an important topic.

Beneath Shakespeare's name in the index, there might be listings for *death of, dramatic works of, life of*, etc. These more specific entries help the reader refine his search.

Many informative texts, especially textbooks, use **headings** and **subheadings** for organization. Headings and subheadings are typically printed in larger and bolder fonts, and are often in a different color than the main body of the text. Headings may be larger than subheadings. Also, headings and subheadings are not always complete sentences. A heading announces the **topic** that will be addressed in the text below. Headings are meant to alert the reader to what is about to come. Subheadings announce the **topics of smaller sections** within the entire section indicated by the heading. For instance, the heading of a section in a science textbook might be *AMPHIBIANS*, and within that section might be subheadings for *Frogs*, *Salamanders*, and *Newts*. Readers should always pay close attention to headings and subheadings, because they prime the brain for the information that is about to be delivered, and because they make it easy to go back and find particular details in a long text.

REFERENCE MATERIALS

Knowledge of reference materials such as dictionaries, encyclopedias, and manuals are vital for any reader. **Dictionaries** contain information about words. A standard dictionary entry begins with a pronunciation guide for the word. The entry will also give the word's **part of speech**: that is, whether it is a noun, verb, adjective, etc. A good dictionary will also include the word's origins, including the language from which it is derived and its meaning in that language. This information is known as the word's **etymology**.

Dictionary entries are in alphabetical order. Many words have more than one definition, in which case the definitions will be numbered. Also, if a word can be used as different parts of speech, its various definitions in those different capacities may be separated. A sample entry might look like this:

WELL: (adverb) 1. in a good way (noun) 1. a hole drilled into the earth

The correct definition of a word will vary depending on how it is **used in a sentence**. When looking up a word found while reading, the best way to determine the relevant definition is to substitute the dictionary's definitions for the word in the text, and select the definition that seems most appropriate.

Encyclopedias used to be the best source for general information on a range of common subjects. Many people took pride in owning a set of encyclopedias, which were often written by top researchers. Now, encyclopedias largely exist online. Although they no longer have a preeminent place in general scholarship, these digital encyclopedias now often feature audio and video clips. A good encyclopedia remains the best place to obtain basic information about a well-known topic. There are also specialty encyclopedias that cover more obscure or expert information. For instance, there are many medical encyclopedias that contain the detail and sophistication required by doctors. For a regular person researching a subject like ostriches, Pennsylvania, or the Crimean War, an encyclopedia is a good source.

A **thesaurus** is a reference book that gives synonyms of words. It is different from a dictionary because a thesaurus does not give definitions, only lists of synonyms. A thesaurus can be helpful in finding the meaning of an unfamiliar word when reading. If the meaning of a synonym is known, then the meaning of the unfamiliar word will be known. The other time a thesaurus is helpful is when writing. Using a thesaurus helps authors to vary their word choice.

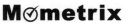

ORGANIZING AND UNDERSTANDING GRAPHIC INFORMATION

Two of the most common ways to organize ideas from a text, paraphrasing and summarizing, are **verbal** ways to organize data. Ideas from a text can also be organized using **graphic organizers**. A graphic organizer is a way to simplify information and just take key points from the text. A graphic organizer such as a timeline may have an event listed for a corresponding date on the timeline, whereas an outline may have an event listed under a key point that occurs in the text. Each reader needs to create the type of graphic organizer that works the best for him or her in terms of being able to recall information from a story. Examples include a *spider-map,* which takes a main idea from the story and places it in a bubble, with supporting points branching off the main idea, an *outline,* useful for diagramming the main and supporting points of the entire story, and a *Venn diagram,* which classifies information as separate or overlapping.

These graphic organizers can also be used by authors to enliven their presentation or text, but this may be counterproductive if the graphics are confusing or misleading. A graph should strip the author's message down to the **essentials**. It should have a clear **title**, and should be in the appropriate **format**. Authors may elect to use tables, line or bar graphs, or pie charts to illustrate their message. Each of these formats is correct for different types of data. The graphic should be large enough to read, and should be divided into appropriate categories. For instance, if the text is about the differences between federal spending on the military and on the space program, a pie chart or a bar graph would be the most effective choices. The pie chart could show each type of spending as a portion of total federal spending, while the bar graph would be better for directly comparing the amounts of money spent on these two programs.

In most cases, the work of **interpreting information** presented in graphs, tables, charts, and diagrams is done for the reader. The author will usually make explicit his or her reasons for presenting a certain set of data in such a way. However, an effective reader will avoid taking the author's claims for granted. Before considering the information presented in the graphic, the reader should consider whether the author has chosen the correct format for presentation, or whether the author has omitted variables or other information that might undermine his case. Interpreting the graphic itself is essentially an exercise in spotting **trends**. On a graph, for instance, the reader should be alert for how one variable responds to a change in the other. If education level increases, for example, does income increase as well? The same can be done for a table. Readers should be alert for values that break or exaggerate a trend; these may be meaningless outliers or indicators of a change in conditions.

When a reader is required to draw conclusions from the information presented in graphs, tables, charts, or diagrams, it is important to limit these conclusions to the terms of the graphic itself. In other words, the reader should avoid extrapolating from the data to make claims that are not supportable. As an example, consider a graph that compares the price of eggs to the demand. If the price and demand rise and fall together, a reader would be justified in saying that the demand for eggs and the price are tied together. However, this simple graph does not indicate which of these variables causes the other, so the reader would not be justified in concluding that the price of eggs raises or lowers the demand. In fact, demand could be tied to all sorts of other factors not included in this chart.

Review Video: <u>Graphic Organizers</u>
Visit mometrix.com/academy and enter code: 665513

TYPES OF TABLES AND CHARTS

Tables are presented in a standard format so that they will be easy to read and understand. At the top of the table, there will be a **title**. This will be a short phrase indicating the information the table or graph intends to convey. The title of a table could be something like "Average Income for Various Education Levels" or "Price of Milk Compared to Demand." A table is composed of information laid out in vertical **columns** and horizontal **rows**. Typically, each column will have a label. If "Average Income for Various Education Levels" was placed in a table format, the two columns could be labeled "Education Level" and "Average Income." Each location on the table is called a **cell**. Cells are defined by their column and row (e.g., second column, fifth row). The table's information is placed in these cells.

Like a table, a **graph** will typically have a title on top. This title may simply state the identities of the two axes: e.g., "Income vs. Education." However, the title may also be something more descriptive, like "A comparison of average income with level of education." In any case, bar and line graphs are laid out along two perpendicular lines, or axes. The vertical axis is called the *y-axis*, and the horizontal axis is called the *x-axis*. It is typical for the *x*-axis to be the independent variable and the *y*-axis to be the dependent variable. The **independent variable** is the one manipulated by the researcher or whoever put together the graph. In the above example, the independent variable would be "level of education," since the maker of the graph will define these values (high school, college, master's degree, etc.). The **dependent variable** is not controlled by the researcher.

A **line graph** is a type of graph that is typically used for measuring trends over time. It is set up along a vertical and a horizontal axis. The variables being measured are listed along the left side and the bottom side of the axes. Points are then plotted along the graph, such that they correspond with their values for each variable. For instance, imagine a line graph measuring a person's income for each month of the year. If the person earned $1500 in January, there would be a point directly above January, perpendicular to the horizontal axis, and directly to the right of $1500, perpendicular to the vertical axis. Once all of the lines are plotted, they are connected with a line from left to right. This line provides a nice visual illustration of the general trends. For instance, using the earlier example, if the line sloped up, it would be clear that the person's income had increased over the course of the year.

The **bar graph** is one of the most common visual representations of information. Bar graphs are used to illustrate sets of numerical data. The graph has a vertical axis, along which numbers are listed, and a horizontal axis, along which categories, words, or some other indicators are placed. One example of a bar graph is a depiction of the respective heights of famous basketball players: the vertical axis would contain numbers ranging from five to eight feet, and the horizontal axis would contain the names of the players. The length of the bar above the player's name would illustrate his height, as the top of the bar would stop perpendicular to the height listed along the left side. In this representation, then, it would be easy to see that Yao Ming is taller than Michael Jordan, because Yao's bar would be higher.

A **pie chart**, also known as a **circle graph**, is useful for depicting how a single unit or category is divided. The standard pie chart is a circle within which wedges have been cut and labeled. Each of these wedges is proportional in size to its part of the whole. For instance, consider a pie chart representing a student's budget. If the student spends half her money on rent, then the pie chart will represent that amount with a line through the center of the pie. If she spends a quarter of her money on food, there will be a line extending from the edge of the circle to the center at a right angle to the line depicting rent. This illustration would make it clear that the student spends twice

31

as much money on rent as she does on food. The pie chart is only appropriate for showing how a whole is divided.

A pie chart is effective at showing how a single entity is divided into **parts**. They are not effective at demonstrating the relationships between parts of different wholes. For example, it would not be as helpful to use a pie chart to compare the respective amounts of state and federal spending devoted to infrastructure, since these values are only meaningful in the context of the entire budget.

Plot lines are another way to visual represent information. Every plot line follows the same **stages**. One can identify each of these stages in every story they read. These stages are: the introduction, rising action, conflict, climax, falling action, and resolution. The introduction tells the reader what the story will be about and sets up the plot. The rising action is what happens that leads up to the conflict, which is some sort of problem that arises, with the climax at its peak. The falling action is what happens after the climax of the conflict. The resolution is the conclusion and often has the final solution to the problem in the conflict. A plot line looks like this:

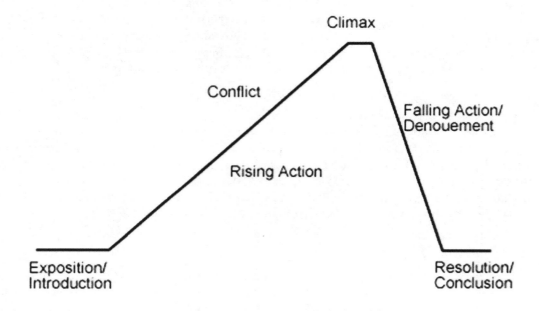

Review Video: Plot Line
Visit mometrix.com/academy and enter code: 944011

Word Knowledge

Determining Word Meaning

An understanding of the basics of language is helpful, and often vital, to understanding what you read. The term **structural analysis** refers to looking at the parts of a word and breaking it down into its different **components** to determine the word's meaning. Parts of a word include prefixes, suffixes, and the root word. By learning the meanings of prefixes, suffixes, and other word fundamentals, you can decipher the meaning of words which may not yet be in your vocabulary. **Prefixes** are common letter combinations at the beginning of words, while **suffixes** are common letter combinations at the end. The main part of the word is known as the **root**. Visually, it would look like this: prefix + root word + suffix. Look first at the individual meanings of the root word, prefix and/or suffix. Using knowledge of the meaning(s) of the prefix and/or suffix to see what information it adds to the root. Even if the meaning of the root is unknown, one can use knowledge of the prefix's and/or suffix's meaning(s) to determine an **approximate meaning** of the word. For example, if one sees the word *uninspired* and does not know what it means, they can use the knowledge that *un-* means 'not' to know that the full word means "not inspired." Understanding the common prefixes and suffixes can illuminate at least part of the meaning of an unfamiliar word.

Below is a list of common prefixes and their meanings:

Prefix	Definition	Examples
a	in, on, of, up, to	abed, afoot
a-	without, lacking	atheist, agnostic
ab-	from, away, off	abdicate, abjure
ad-	to, toward	advance
am-	friend, love	amicable, amatory
ante-	before, previous	antecedent, antedate
anti-	against, opposing	antipathy, antidote
auto-	self	autonomy, autobiography
belli-	war, warlike	bellicose
bene-	well, good	benefit, benefactor
bi-	two	bisect, biennial
bio-	life	biology, biosphere
cata-	down, away, thoroughly	catastrophe, cataclysm
chron-	time	chronometer, synchronize
circum-	around	circumspect, circumference
com-	with, together, very	commotion, complicate
contra-	against, opposing	contradict, contravene
cred-	belief, trust	credible, credit
de-	from	depart
dem-	people	demographics, democracy
dia-	through, across, apart	diameter, diagnose
dis-	away, off, down, not	dissent, disappear
epi-	upon	epilogue
equi-	equal, equally	equivalent

33

Prefix	Definition	Examples
ex-	out	extract
for-	away, off, from	forget, forswear
fore-	before, previous	foretell, forefathers
homo-	same, equal	homogenized
hyper-	excessive, over	hypercritical, hypertension
hypo-	under, beneath	hypodermic, hypothesis
in-	in, into	intrude, invade
in-	not, opposing	incapable, ineligible
inter-	among, between	intercede, interrupt
intra-	within	intramural, intrastate
magn-	large	magnitude, magnify
mal-	bad, poorly, not	malfunction
micr-	small	microbe, microscope
mis-	bad, poorly, not	misspell, misfire
mono-	one, single	monogamy, monologue
mor-	die, death	mortality, mortuary
neo-	new	neolithic, neoconservative
non-	not	nonentity, nonsense
ob-	against, opposing	objection
omni-	all, everywhere	omniscient
ortho-	right, straight	orthogonal, orthodox
over-	above	overbearing
pan-	all, entire	panorama, pandemonium
para-	beside, beyond	parallel, paradox
per-	through	perceive, permit
peri-	around	periscope, perimeter
phil-	love, like	philosophy, philanthropic
poly-	many	polymorphous, polygamous
post-	after, following	postpone, postscript
pre-	before, previous	prevent, preclude
prim-	first, early	primitive, primary
pro-	forward, in place of	propel, pronoun
re-	back, backward, again	revoke, recur
retro-	back, backward	retrospect, retrograde
semi-	half, partly	semicircle, semicolon
sub-	under, beneath	subjugate, substitute
super-	above, extra	supersede, supernumerary
sym-	with, together	sympathy, symphony
trans-	across, beyond, over	transact, transport
ultra-	beyond, excessively	ultramodern, ultrasonic, ultraviolet
un-	not, reverse of	unhappy, unlock
uni-	one	uniform, unity
vis-	to see	visage, visible

Below is a list of common suffixes and their meanings:

Suffix	Definition	Examples
-able	able to, likely	capable, tolerable
-age	process, state, rank	passage, bondage
-ance	act, condition, fact	acceptance, vigilance
-arch	to rule	monarch
-ard	one that does excessively	drunkard, wizard
-ate	having, showing	separate, desolate
-ation	action, state, result	occupation, starvation
-cy	state, condition	accuracy, captaincy
-dom	state, rank, condition	serfdom, wisdom
-en	cause to be, become	deepen, strengthen
-er	one who does	teacher
-esce	become, grow, continue	convalesce, acquiesce
-esque	in the style of, like	picturesque, grotesque
-ess	feminine	waitress, lioness
-fic	making, causing	terrific, beatific
-ful	full of, marked by	thankful, zestful
-fy	make, cause, cause to have	glorify, fortify
-hood	state, condition	manhood, statehood
-ible	able, likely, fit	edible, possible, divisible
-ion	action, result, state	union, fusion
-ish	suggesting, like	churlish, childish
-ism	act, manner, doctrine	barbarism, socialism
-ist	doer, believer	monopolist, socialist
-ition	action, state, result	sedition, expedition
-ity	state, quality, condition	acidity, civility
-ize	make, cause to be, treat with	sterilize, mechanize, criticize
-less	lacking, without	hopeless, countless
-like	like, similar	childlike, dreamlike
-logue	type of written/spoken language	prologue
-ly	like, of the nature of	friendly, positively
-ment	means, result, action	refreshment, disappointment
-ness	quality, state	greatness, tallness
-or	doer, office, action	juror, elevator, honor
-ous	marked by, given to	religious, riotous
-ship	the art or skill of	statesmanship
-some	apt to, showing	tiresome, lonesome
-th	act, state, quality	warmth, width
-tude	quality, state, result	magnitude, fortitude
-ty	quality, state	enmity, activity
-ward	in the direction of	backward, homeward

When defining words in a text, words often have a meaning that is more than the dictionary definition. The **denotative** meaning of a word is the **literal** meaning. The **connotative** meaning goes beyond the denotative meaning to include the **emotional reaction** a word may invoke. The connotative meaning often takes the denotative meaning a step further due to associations which the reader makes with the denotative meaning. The reader can differentiate between the denotative and connotative meanings by first recognizing when authors use each meaning. Most non-fiction, for example, is fact-based, the authors not using flowery, figurative language. The reader can assume that the writer is using the denotative, or literal, meaning of words. In fiction, on the other hand, the author may be using the connotative meaning. Connotation is one form of figurative language. The reader should use **context clues** to determine if the author is using the denotative or connotative meaning of a word.

Readers of all levels will encounter words with which they are somewhat unfamiliar. The best way to define a word in **context** is to look for nearby words that can help. For instance, unfamiliar nouns are often accompanied by examples that furnish a definition. Consider the following sentence: "Dave arrived at the party in hilarious garb: a leopard-print shirt, buckskin trousers, and high heels." If a reader was unfamiliar with the meaning of garb, he could read the examples and quickly determine that the word means "clothing." Examples will not always be this obvious. For instance, consider this sentence: "Parsley, lemon, and flowers were just a few of items he used as garnishes." Here, the possibly unfamiliar word *garnishes* is exemplified by parsley, lemon, and flowers. Readers who have eaten in a few restaurants will probably be able to identify a garnish as something used to decorate a plate.

In addition to looking at the context of a passage, readers can often use **contrasts** to define an unfamiliar word in context. In many sentences, the author will not describe the unfamiliar word directly, but will instead describe the opposite of the unfamiliar word. Of course, this provides information about the word the reader needs to define. Consider the following example: "Despite his intelligence, Hector's low brow and bad posture made him look obtuse." The author suggests that Hector's appearance was opposite to his actual intelligence. Therefore, *obtuse* must mean unintelligent or stupid. Here is another example: "Despite the horrible weather, we were beatific about our trip to Alaska." The word *despite* indicates that the speaker's feelings were at odds with the weather. Since the weather is described as "horrible," *beatific* must mean something good.

In some cases, there will be very few contextual clues to help a reader define the meaning of an unfamiliar word. When this happens, one strategy the reader may employ is **substitution**. A good reader will brainstorm some possible synonyms for the given word, and then substitute these words into the sentence. If the sentence and the surrounding passage continue to make sense, the substitution has revealed at least some information about the unfamiliar word. Consider the sentence, "Frank's admonition rang in her ears as she climbed the mountain." A reader unfamiliar with *admonition* might come up with some substitutions like "vow," "promise," "advice," "complaint," or "compliment." All of these words make general sense of the sentence, though their meanings are diverse. The process has suggested, however, that an admonition is some sort of message. The substitution strategy is rarely able to pinpoint a precise definition, but can be effective as a last resort.

It is sometimes possible to define an unfamiliar word by looking at the **descriptive words** in the context. Consider the following sentence: "Fred dragged the recalcitrant boy kicking and screaming up the stairs." *Dragged*, *kicking*, and *screaming* all suggest that the boy does not want to go up the stairs. The reader may assume that *recalcitrant* means something like unwilling or protesting. In that example, an unfamiliar adjective was identified. It is perhaps more typical to use description to define an unfamiliar noun, as in this sentence: "Don's wrinkled frown and constantly shaking fist identified him as a curmudgeon of the first order." Don is described as having a "wrinkled frown and constantly shaking fist," suggesting that a *curmudgeon* must be a grumpy old man. Contrasts do not always provide detailed information about the unfamiliar word, but they at least give the reader some clues.

When a word has **more than one meaning**, it can be tricky to determine how it is being used in a given sentence. Consider the verb *cleave*, which bizarrely can mean either "join" or "separate." When a reader comes upon this word, she will have to select the definition that makes the most sense. So, take as an example the following sentence: "The birds cleaved together as they flew from the oak tree." Immediately, the presence of the word *together* should suggest that in this sentence *cleave* is being used to mean "*join*." A slightly more difficult example would be the sentence, "Hermione's knife cleaved the bread cleanly." It doesn't make sense for a knife to join bread together, so the word must be meant to indicate separation. Discovering the meaning of a word with multiple meanings requires the same tricks as defining an unknown word: looking for contextual clues and evaluating substituted words.

Literary Devices

Understanding how words relate to each other can often add meaning to a passage. This is explained by understanding **synonyms** (words that mean the same thing) and **antonyms** (words that mean the opposite of one another). As an example, *dry* and *arid* are synonyms, and *dry* and *wet* are antonyms. There are many pairs of words in English that can be considered synonyms, despite having slightly different definitions. For instance, the words *friendly* and *collegial* can both be used to describe a warm interpersonal relationship, so it would be correct to call them synonyms. However, *collegial* (kin to *colleague*) is more often used in reference to professional or academic relationships, while *friendly* has no such connotation. Nevertheless, it would be appropriate to call these words synonyms. If the difference between the two words is too great, however, they may not be called synonyms. *Hot* and *warm* are not synonyms, for instance, because their meanings are too distinct. A good way to determine whether two words are synonyms is to substitute one for the other and see if the sentence means the same thing. Substituting *warm* for *hot* in a sentence would convey a different meaning.

Antonyms are opposites. *Light* and *dark*, *up* and *down*, *right* and *left*, *good* and *bad*: these are all sets of antonyms. It is important to distinguish between antonyms and pairs of words that are simply different. *Black* and *gray*, for instance, are not antonyms because gray is not the opposite of black. *Black* and *white*, on the other hand, are antonyms. Not every word has an antonym. For instance, many nouns do not. What would be the antonym of *chair*, after all? On a standardized test, the questions related to antonyms are more likely to concern adjectives. Remember that adjectives

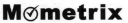

are words that describe a noun. Some common adjectives include *red*, *fast*, *skinny*, and *sweet*. Of these four examples, only *red* lacks a group of obvious antonyms.

There are many types of language devices that authors use to convey their meaning in a more descriptive or interesting way. Understanding these concepts will help you understand what you read. These types of devices are called **figurative language** – language that goes beyond the literal meaning of the words. **Descriptive language** that evokes imagery in the reader's mind is one type of figurative language. **Exaggeration** is also one type of figurative language. Also, when you compare two things, you are using figurative language. **Similes** and **metaphors** are ways of comparing things, and both are types of figurative language commonly found in poetry. An example of figurative language (a simile in this case) is: "The child howled like a coyote when her mother told her to pick up the toys." In this example, the child's howling is compared to that of a coyote. Figurative language is descriptive in nature and helps the reader understand the sound being made in this sentence.

A **figure of speech**, sometimes termed a rhetorical figure or device, or elocution, is a word or phrase that departs from straightforward, literal language. Figures of speech are often used and crafted for emphasis, freshness of expression, or clarity. However, clarity may also suffer from their use.

Note that not all theories of meaning necessarily have a concept of "literal language" (see literal and figurative language). Under theories that do not, figure of speech is not an entirely coherent concept.

As an example of the figurative use of a word, consider the sentence, "I am going to crown you." It may mean:

- I am going to place a literal crown on your head.
- I am going to symbolically exalt you to the place of kingship.
- I am going to punch you in the head with my clenched fist.
- I am going to put a second checker on top of your checker to signify that it has become a king.

A **metaphor** is a type of figurative language in which the writer equates one thing with a different thing. For instance, in the sentence "The bird was an arrow arcing through the sky," the arrow is serving as a metaphor for the bird. The point of a metaphor is to encourage the reader to think about the thing being described in a different way. Using this example, we are being asked to envision the bird's flight as being similar to the arc of an arrow, so we will imagine it to be swift, bending, etc. Metaphors are a way for the author to describe without being direct and obvious. Metaphors are a more lyrical and suggestive way of providing information. Note that the thing to which a metaphor refers will not always be mentioned explicitly by the author. For instance, consider the following description of a forest in winter: "Swaying skeletons reached for the sky and groaned as the wind blew through them." The author is clearly using *skeletons* as a metaphor for leafless trees. This metaphor creates a spooky tone while inspiring the reader's imagination.

Review Video: Metaphor
Visit mometrix.com/academy and enter code: 133295

Metonymy is referring to one thing in terms of another, closely related thing. This is similar to metaphor, but there is less distance between the description and the thing being described. An example of metonymy is referring to the news media as the "press," when of course the press is only the device by which newspapers are printed. Metonymy is a way of referring to something without having to repeat its name constantly. **Synecdoche**, on the other hand, is referring to a whole by one of its parts. An example of synecdoche would be calling a police officer a "badge." Synecdoche, like metonymy, is a handy way of referring without having to overuse certain words. It also allows the writer to emphasize aspects of the thing being described. For instance, referring to businessmen as "suits" suggests professionalism, conformity, and drabness.

Hyperbole is overstatement for effect. The following sentence is an example of hyperbole: *He jumped ten feet in the air when he heard the good news.* Obviously, no person has the ability to jump ten feet in the air. The author hyperbolizes not because he believes the statement will be taken literally, but because the exaggeration conveys the extremity of emotion. Consider how much less colorful the sentence would be if the author simply said, "He jumped when he heard the good news." Hyperbole can be dangerous if the author does not exaggerate enough. For instance, if the author wrote, "He jumped two feet in the air when he heard the good news," the reader might not be sure whether this is actually true or just hyperbole. Of course, in many situations this distinction will not really matter. However, an author should avoid confusing or vague hyperbole when he needs to maintain credibility or authority with readers.

Understatement is the opposite of hyperbole: that is, it is describing something as less than it is, for effect. As an example, consider a person who climbs Mount Everest and then describes the journey as "a little stroll." This is an almost extreme example of understatement. Like other types of figurative language, understatement has a range of uses. It may convey self-deprecation or modesty, as in the above example. Of course, some people might interpret understatement as false modesty, a deliberate attempt to call attention to the magnitude of what is being discussed. For example, a woman is complimented on her enormous diamond engagement ring and says, "Oh, this little thing?" Her understatement might be viewed as snobby or insensitive. Understatement can have various effects, but it always calls attention to itself.

Review Video: Hyperbole and Understatement
Visit mometrix.com/academy and enter code: 308470

A **simile** is a figurative expression similar to a metaphor, though it requires the use of a distancing word like *like* or *as*. Some examples are "The sun was like an orange," "eager as a beaver," and "nimble as a mountain goat." Because a simile includes *like* or *as,* it creates a little space between the description and the thing being described. If an author says that a house was "like a shoebox," the tone is slightly different than if the author said that the house *was* a shoebox. In a simile, the author indicates an awareness that the description is not the same thing as the thing being described. In a metaphor, there is no such distinction, even though one may safely assume that the author is aware of it. This is a subtle difference, but authors will alternately use metaphors and similes depending on their intended tone.

Review Video: Simile
Visit mometrix.com/academy and enter code: 642949

Another type of figurative language is **personification.** This is the description of the nonhuman as if it were human. Literally, the word means the process of making something into a person. There is a wide range of approaches to personification, from common expressions like "whispering wind" to full novels like *Animal Farm*, by George Orwell, in which the Bolshevik Revolution is reenacted by farmyard animals. The general intent of personification is to describe things in a manner that will be comprehensible to readers. When an author states that a tree "groans" in the wind, she of course does not mean that the tree is emitting a low, pained sound from its mouth. Instead, she means that the tree is making a noise similar to a human groan. Of course, this personification establishes a tone of sadness or suffering. A different tone would be established if the author said the tree was "swaying" or "dancing."

Review Video: Personification
Visit mometrix.com/academy and enter code: 260066

Irony is a statement that suggests its opposite. In other words, it is when an author or character says one thing but means another. For example, imagine a man walks in his front door, covered in mud and in tattered clothes. His wife asks him, "How was your day?" and he says "Great!" The man's comment is an example of irony. As in this example, irony often depends on information the reader obtains elsewhere. There is a fine distinction between irony and sarcasm. Irony is any statement in which the literal meaning is opposite from the intended meaning, while **sarcasm** is a statement of this type that is also insulting to the person at whom it is directed. A sarcastic statement suggests that the other person is stupid enough to believe an obviously false statement is true. Irony is a bit more subtle than sarcasm.

Review Video: Irony
Visit mometrix.com/academy and enter code: 374204

The more words a person is exposed to, the greater their **vocabulary** will become. By reading on a regular basis, a person can increase the number of ways they have seen a word in context. Based on experience, a person can recall how a word was used in the past and apply that knowledge to a new context. For example, a person may have seen the word *gull* used to mean a bird that is found near the seashore. However, a *gull* can also be a person who is easily tricked. If the word is used in context in reference to a character, the reader can recognize that the character is being called a bird that is not seen as extremely intelligent. Using what the reader knows about a word can be useful when making comparisons or figuring out the meaning of a new use of a word, as in figurative language, idioms, analogies, and multiple-meaning words.

Verbal Chapter Quiz

1. The doctors were less concerned with Bill's respiration than with the *precipitous* rise in his blood pressure.

Precipitous means:

   a. detached
   b. sordid
   c. encompassed
   d. steep

2. At first, Gerald suspected that he had caught the disease at the office; later, though, he concluded that it was *endogenous.*

Endogenous means:

   a. contagious
   b. painful to the touch
   c. continuous
   d. growing from within

3. Allowing most visitors into the operating room is *incongruous.*

Incongruous means:

   a. forbidden
   b. unacceptable
   c. inappropriate
   d. befitting

4. The patient in room 201 has a *voracious* appetite.

Voracious means:

   a. minimal
   b. gluttonous
   c. hearty
   d. bland

5. Elisabeth visited her sister in the hospital every day despite the latter's *dyspeptic* behavior. *Dyspeptic* means:

   a. sullen
   b. erratic
   c. comatose
   d. ill-tempered

Questions 6-9 pertain to the following passage:

> Protozoa are microscopic, one-celled organisms that can be free-living or parasitic in nature. They are able to multiply in humans, a factor which contributes to their survival and also permits serious infections to develop from just a single organism. Transmission of protozoa that live in the human intestine to another human typically occurs by a fecal-oral route (for example, contaminated food or water, or person-to-person contact). Protozoa that thrive in the blood or tissue of

41

humans are transmitted to their human hosts by an arthropod vector (for example, through the bite of a mosquito or sand fly).

Helminths are large, multicellular organisms that are generally visible to the naked eye in their adult stages. Like protozoa, helminths can be either free-living or parasitic in nature. In their adult form, helminths cannot multiply in humans. There are three main groups of helminths (derived from the Greek word for worms) that are human parasites:

1. Flatworms (platyhelminths) – these include the trematodes (flukes) and cestodes (tapeworms).
2. Thorny-headed worms (acanthocephalins) – the adult forms of these worms reside in the gastrointestinal tract. The acanthocephala are thought to be intermediate between the cestodes and nematodes.
3. Roundworms (nematodes) – the adult forms of these worms can reside in the gastrointestinal tract, blood, lymphatic system or subcutaneous tissues. Alternatively, the immature (larval) states can cause disease through their infection of various body tissues.

6. As used in this passage, the word "parasite" means

a. a person who lives in Paris
b. an organism that live on or in another organism
c. microscopic insects
d. a person who takes advantage of the generosity of others

7. According to the passage, adult Roundworms can live in

a. the arthropod vector
b. fecal matter
c. the subcutaneous tissue of humans
d. contaminated water

8. You can infer from this passage that

a. larval stages of parasites are more dangerous than the adult forms
b. mosquitoes do not transmit parasites
c. worms cannot infect humans
d. clean sanitary conditions will keep you free of protozoa

9. According to the passage, which of the following is true?

I. Protozoa live in the blood or tissue of humans.
II. Adult helminthes cannot reproduce in humans.
III. Adult Thorny-headed worms live in the intestinal tract.

a. I only
b. II only
c. I and II only
d. I, II, and III

10. The hospital auditorium is used for lectures and other events because it is *capacious*.
Capacious means:

   a. grand
   b. remodeled
   c. spacious
   d. retrofitted

Verbal Chapter Quiz Answers

1. D: The word *precipitous* as it is used this sentence means "steep." Doctors will often refer to a precipitous change in blood pressure. In general, precipitous changes are dangerous to the health. The word *detached* means "unconnected or aloof." A common example is a detached retina, a condition in which part of the eye becomes disconnected, and vision is damaged. The word *sordid* means "dirty" or "vile." The word *encompassed* means "surrounded or entirely contained within." For instance, a doctor might describe a treatment protocol as encompassing all aspects of the patient's life.

2. D: The word *endogenous* as it is used in this sentence means "growing from within." Doctors occasionally refer to endogenous cholesterol, which comes from inside the body rather than from the diet. *Contagious* means "capable of spreading from person to person." A person with a contagious disease needs to be kept away from other people. Often, diseases are only contagious for a limited time. *Continuous* means "proceeding on without stopping." If a patient is suffering from continuous back pain, for instance, he or she is experiencing the pain at all times.

3. C: *Inappropriate* is a synonym for *incongruous*, which in this context means "not appropriate for the occasion or situation." Incongruous can also mean "inconsistent." Two of the other words are related terms: (1) *forbidden*, which means "not permitted," and (2) *unacceptable*, which means "falling short of a standard." *Befitting* is an antonym defined as "appropriate for."

4. B: In this sentence, *voracious* is a synonym for gluttonous, which means "very hungry." Voracious can also mean "unusually eager or enthusiastic." *Hearty* is a related term; of its numerous meanings, the closest meaning for this sentence would be "substantial." In this sentence, *minimal* means "very small." In the context of this sentence, *bland* would mean, "lacking flavor," but the term would be more appropriate for defining the person's diet rather than their appetite.

5. D: *Dyspeptic* has the same definition as *ill-tempered*, meaning in this case "possessing or exhibiting a habitually bad temper." Dyspeptic can also mean, "having acid indigestion". *Sullen* is a similar term that as used here signifies, "displaying hostile or resentful silence." *Erratic* has several meanings that could apply here, including "random," "fitful," and "uneven." Comatose literally can mean "in a coma," but it also can be defined as "unable to function."

6. B: As used in this passage, the word "parasite" means an organism that lives on or in another organism, Choice B. Choice A and C are obviously wrong, since the passage mentions nothing of Paris or insects. Choice D is another definition for "parasite," but does not fit the context of the word used in this passage.

7. C: According to the description of Roundworms, they can live in the subcutaneous tissue of humans, Choice C. Choices A, B, and D describe where protozoa live and how they are transmitted.

8. D: According to the first paragraph, protozoa are transmitted through food and water contaminated by fecal matter. It can then be inferred that clean sanitary conditions will prevent the spread of protozoa, Choice D. Choice A is an incorrect inference because the passage discusses both larval and adult forms of parasites that infect humans. Choice B is an incorrect inference, since the first paragraph states that protozoa are transmitted by mosquitoes. Choice C is an incorrect inference because the second paragraph is about worms that infect humans.

9. D: To answer this question, you will need to verify all three statements in the passage. All three of these statements are true and are supported by the passage.

10. C: *Capacious* and *spacious* both mean "more than adequate in terms of capacity." *Grand* has several meanings, but in this sentence the applicable meaning is "large and impressive in size or grandeur." The other words, although unrelated terms, could be inserted. *Remodeled* means "renovated," and *retrofitted* means "modified or installed with new parts."

Mathematics

Math Foundations

THE NUMBER LINE

A number line is a graph to see the distance between numbers. Basically, this graph shows the relationship between numbers. So, a number line may have a point for zero and may show negative numbers on the left side of the line. Also, any positive numbers are placed on the right side of the line.

EXAMPLE

Name each point on the number line below:

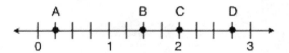

Use the dashed lines on the number line to identify each point. Each dashed line between two whole numbers is $\frac{1}{4}$. The line halfway between two numbers is $\frac{1}{2}$.

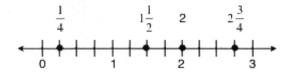

CLASSIFICATIONS OF NUMBERS

Numbers are the basic building blocks of mathematics. Specific features of numbers are identified by the following terms:

- **Integer** – any positive or negative whole number, including zero. Integers do not include fractions $\left(\frac{1}{3}\right)$, decimals (0.56), or mixed numbers $\left(7\frac{3}{4}\right)$.
- **Prime number** – any whole number greater than 1 that has only two factors, itself and 1; that is, a number that can be divided evenly only by 1 and itself.
- **Composite number** – any whole number greater than 1 that has more than two different factors; in other words, any whole number that is not a prime number. For example: The composite number 8 has the factors of 1, 2, 4, and 8.
- **Even number** – any integer that can be divided by 2 without leaving a remainder. For example: 2, 4, 6, 8, and so on.
- **Odd number** – any integer that cannot be divided evenly by 2. For example: 3, 5, 7, 9, and so on.
- **Decimal number** – any number that uses a decimal point to show the part of the number that is less than one. Example: 1.234.

- **Decimal point** – a symbol used to separate the ones place from the tenths place in decimals or dollars from cents in currency.
- **Decimal place** – the position of a number to the right of the decimal point. In the decimal 0.123, the 1 is in the first place to the right of the decimal point, indicating tenths; the 2 is in the second place, indicating hundredths; and the 3 is in the third place, indicating thousandths.
- The **decimal**, or base 10, system is a number system that uses ten different digits (0, 1, 2, 3, 4, 5, 6, 7, 8, 9). An example of a number system that uses something other than ten digits is the **binary**, or base 2, number system, used by computers, which uses only the numbers 0 and 1. It is thought that the decimal system originated because people had only their 10 fingers for counting.
- **Rational numbers** include all integers, decimals, and fractions. Any terminating or repeating decimal number is a rational number.
- **Irrational numbers** cannot be written as fractions or decimals because the number of decimal places is infinite and there is no recurring pattern of digits within the number. For example, pi (π) begins with 3.141592 and continues without terminating or repeating, so pi is an irrational number.
- **Real numbers** are the set of all rational and irrational numbers.

> **Review Video: Numbers and Their Classifications**
> Visit mometrix.com/academy and enter code: 461071

PLACE VALUE

Write the place value of each digit in the following number: 14,059.826

1: ten-thousands
4: thousands
0: hundreds
5: tens
9: ones
8: tenths
2: hundredths
6: thousandths

> **Review Video: Number Place Value**
> Visit mometrix.com/academy and enter code: 205433

ROUNDING AND ESTIMATION

Rounding is reducing the digits in a number while still trying to keep the value similar. The result will be less accurate, but will be in a simpler form, and will be easier to use. Whole numbers can be rounded to the nearest ten, hundred or thousand.

EXAMPLE 1

Round each number:

a. Round each number to the nearest ten: 11, 47, 118
b. Round each number to the nearest hundred: 78, 980, 248
c. Round each number to the nearest thousand: 302, 1274, 3756

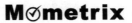

ANSWER

a. Remember, when rounding to the nearest ten, anything ending in 5 or greater rounds up. So, 11 rounds to 10, 47 rounds to 50, and 118 rounds to 120

b. Remember, when rounding to the nearest hundred, anything ending in 50 or greater rounds up. So, 78 rounds to 100, 980 rounds to 1000, and 248 rounds to 200.

c. Remember, when rounding to the nearest thousand, anything ending in 500 or greater rounds up. So, 302 rounds to 0, 1274 rounds to 1000, and 3756 rounds to 4000.

When you are asked for the solution a problem, you may need to provide only an approximate figure or **estimation** for your answer. In this situation, you can round the numbers that will be calculated to a non-zero number. This means that the first digit in the number is not zero, and the following numbers are zeros.

EXAMPLE 2

Estimate the solution to 345,932 + 96,369.

Start by rounding each number to have only one digit as a non-zero number: 345,932 becomes 300,000 and 96,369 becomes 100,000.

Then, add the rounded numbers: 300,000 + 100,000 = 400,000. So, the answer is approximately 400,000.

The exact answer would be 345,932 + 96,369 = 442,301. So, the estimate of 400,000 is a similar value to the exact answer.

EXAMPLE 3

A runner's heart beats 422 times over the course of six minutes. About how many times did the runner's heart beat during each minute?

"About how many" indicates that you need to estimate the solution. In this case, look at the numbers you are given. 422 can be rounded down to 420, which is easily divisible by 6. A good estimate is 420 ÷ 6 = 70 beats per minute. More accurately, the patient's heart rate was just over 70 beats per minute since his heart actually beat a little more than 420 times in six minutes.

> **Review Video: Rounding and Estimation**
> Visit mometrix.com/academy and enter code: 126243

MEAN

The mean, or the **arithmetic mean or average**, of a data set is found by adding all of the values in the set. Then you divide the sum by how many values that you had in a set. For example, a data set has 6 numbers, and the sum of those 6 numbers is 30. So, the mean is 30/6 = 5. When you know the average, you may be asked to find a missing value. Look over the following steps for how this is done.

Example: You are given the values of 5, 10, 12, and 13. Also, you are told that the average is 9.6. So, what is the one missing value?

First: Add the known values together: 5 + 10 + 12 + 13 =40. Now, set up an equation with the sum of the known values in the divisor. Then, put the number of values in the dividend. For this example,

you have 5 values. So, you have $\frac{40+?}{5} = 9.6$. Now, multiply both sides by 5: $5 \times \frac{40+?}{5} = 9.6 \times 5$
Second: You are left with $40+? = 48$. Now, subtract 40 from both sides: $40 - 40+? = 48 - 40$. So, you know that the missing value is 8.

When you know the frequency of a list of values, you may be asked to find the average. Look over the following steps for how this is done.

Example: A group of high school students took a math exam. Their scores are given in the table:

Score Range	Frequency
60-69	6
70-79	10
80-89	14
90-99	5

First: We need an average for each score range. For this example, we will use a rounded number for each average. Now, the average of 60 and 69 is 64.5. So, we will use 65 for this example.

Second: Plug in the numbers for division: $\frac{65 \times 6 + 75 \times 10 + 85 \times 14 + 95 \times 5}{6+10+14+5} = \frac{2805}{35} = 80$.

Thus, the average for the scores on the math exam is 80.

OPERATIONS
There are four basic mathematical operations:

ADDITION AND SUBTRACTION
Addition increases the value of one quantity by the value of another quantity. Example: $2 + 4 = 6; 8 + 9 = 17$. The result is called the **sum**. With addition, the order does not matter. $4 + 2 = 2 + 4$.

Subtraction is the opposite operation to addition; it decreases the value of one quantity by the value of another quantity. Example: $6 - 4 = 2; 17 - 8 = 9$. The result is called the **difference**. Note that with subtraction, the order does matter. $6 - 4 \neq 4 - 6$.

> **Review Video: Addition and Subtraction**
> Visit mometrix.com/academy and enter code: 521157

MULTIPLICATION AND DIVISION
Multiplication can be thought of as repeated addition. One number tells how many times to add the other number to itself. Example: 3×2 (three times two) $= 2 + 2 + 2 = 6$. With multiplication, the order does not matter. $2 \times 3 = 3 \times 2$ or $3 + 3 = 2 + 2 + 2$.

Division is the opposite operation to multiplication; one number tells us how many parts to divide the other number into. Example: $20 \div 4 = 5$; if 20 is split into 4 equal parts, each part is 5. With division, the order of the numbers does matter. $20 \div 4 \neq 4 \div 20$.

> **Review Video: Multiplication and Division**
> Visit mometrix.com/academy and enter code: 643326

ORDER OF OPERATIONS
Order of operations is a set of rules that dictates the order in which we must perform each operation in an expression so that we will evaluate it accurately. If we have an expression that

includes multiple different operations, order of operations tells us which operations to do first. The most common mnemonic for order of operations is **PEMDAS**, or "Please Excuse My Dear Aunt Sally." PEMDAS stands for parentheses, exponents, multiplication, division, addition, and subtraction. It is important to understand that multiplication and division have equal precedence, as do addition and subtraction, so those pairs of operations are simply worked from left to right in order.

EXAMPLE

Evaluate the expression $5 + 20 \div 4 \times (2 + 3) - 6$ using the correct order of operations.

P: Perform the operations inside the parentheses: $(2 + 3) = 5$

E: Simplify the exponents.

The equation now looks like this: $5 + 20 \div 4 \times 5 - 6$

MD: Perform multiplication and division from left to right: $20 \div 4 = 5$; then $5 \times 5 = 25$

The equation now looks like this: $5 + 25 - 6$

AS: Perform addition and subtraction from left to right: $5 + 25 = 30$; then $30 - 6 = 24$

> **Review Video: <u>Order of Operations</u>**
> Visit mometrix.com/academy and enter code: 259675

OPERATIONS WITH POSITIVE AND NEGATIVE NUMBERS

ADDITION

When adding signed numbers, if the signs are the same simply add the absolute values of the addends and apply the original sign to the sum. For example, $(+4) + (+8) = +12$ and $(-4) + (-8) = -12$. When the original signs are different, take the absolute values of the addends and subtract the smaller value from the larger value, then apply the original sign of the larger value to the difference. For instance, $(+4) + (-8) = -4$ and $(-4) + (+8) = +4$.

SUBTRACTION

For subtracting signed numbers, change the sign of the number after the minus symbol and then follow the same rules used for addition. For example, $(+4) - (+8) = (+4) + (-8) = -4$.

MULTIPLICATION

If the signs are the same the product is positive when multiplying signed numbers. For example, $(+4) \times (+8) = +32$ and $(-4) \times (-8) = +32$. If the signs are opposite, the product is negative. For example, $(+4) \times (-8) = -32$ and $(-4) \times (+8) = -32$. When more than two factors are multiplied together, the sign of the product is determined by how many negative factors are present. If there are an odd number of negative factors then the product is negative, whereas an even number of negative factors indicates a positive product. For instance, $(+4) \times (-8) \times (-2) = +64$ and $(-4) \times (-8) \times (-2) = -64$.

DIVISION

The rules for dividing signed numbers are similar to multiplying signed numbers. If the dividend and divisor have the same sign, the quotient is positive. If the dividend and divisor have opposite signs, the quotient is negative. For example, $(-4) \div (+8) = -0.5$.

SUBTRACTION WITH REGROUPING
EXAMPLE 1

Demonstrate how to subtract 189 from 525 using regrouping.

First, set up the subtraction problem:

```
    525
 -  189
```

Notice that the numbers in the ones and tens columns of 525 are smaller than the numbers in the ones and tens columns of 189. This means you will need to use regrouping to perform subtraction.

```
   5   2   5
 - 1   8   9
```

To subtract 9 from 5 in the ones column you will need to borrow from the 2 in the tens columns:

```
   5   1   15
 - 1   8   9
               6
```

Next, to subtract 8 from 1 in the tens column you will need to borrow from the 5 in the hundreds column:

```
   4   11  15
 - 1   8   9
       3   6
```

Last, subtract the 1 from the 4 in the hundreds column:

```
   4   11  15
 - 1   8   9
   3   3   6
```

Example 2

Demonstrate how to subtract 477 from 620 using regrouping.

First, set up the subtraction problem:

```
    620
 -  477
```

Notice that the numbers in the ones and tens columns of 620 are smaller than the numbers in the ones and tens columns of 477. This means you will need to use regrouping to perform subtraction.

```
   6   2   0
 - 4   7   7
```

To subtract 7 from 0 in the ones column you will need to borrow from the 2 in the tens column.

```
  6   1  10
- 4   7   7
          3
```

Next, to subtract 7 from the 1 that's still in the tens column you will need to borrow from the 6 in the hundreds column.

```
  5  11 10
- 4   7   7
      4   3
```

Lastly, subtract 4 from the 5 remaining in the hundreds column to get:

```
  5  11 10
- 4   7   7
  1   4   3
```

EXPONENTS

An exponent is a superscript number placed next to another number at the top right. It indicates how many times the base number is to be multiplied by itself. **Exponents** provide a shorthand way to write what would be a longer mathematical expression. Example: $a^2 = a \times a$; $2^4 = 2 \times 2 \times 2 \times 2$. A number with an exponent of 2 is said to be "squared," while a number with an exponent of 3 is said to be "cubed." The value of a number raised to an exponent is called its **power**. So, 8^4 is read as "8 to the 4th power," or "8 raised to the power of 4." A **negative exponent** is the same as the **reciprocal** of a positive exponent. Example: $a^{-2} = \frac{1}{a^2}$.

> **Review Video: Exponents**
> Visit mometrix.com/academy and enter code: 600998

ROOTS

A root, such as a square root, is another way of writing a fractional exponent. Instead of using a superscript, roots use the radical symbol ($\sqrt{}$) to indicate the operation. A **radical** will have a number underneath the bar, and may sometimes have a number in the upper left: $\sqrt[n]{a}$, read as "the nth root of a." The relationship between radical notation and exponent notation can be described by this equation: $\sqrt[n]{a} = a^{\frac{1}{n}}$. The two special cases of $n = 2$ and $n = 3$ are called square roots and cube roots. If there is no number to the upper left, it is understood to be a square root ($n = 2$). Nearly all of the roots you encounter will be square roots. A square root is the same as a number raised to the one-half power. When we say that a is the square root of b ($a = \sqrt{b}$), we mean that a multiplied by itself equals b: ($a \times a = b$).

> **Review Video: Roots**
> Visit mometrix.com/academy and enter code: 795655
>
> **Review Video: Square Root and Perfect Square**
> Visit mometrix.com/academy and enter code: 648063

A **perfect square** is a number that has an integer for its square root. There are 10 perfect squares from 1 to 100: 1, 4, 9, 16, 25, 36, 49, 64, 81, 100 (the squares of integers 1 through 10).

Parentheses are used to designate which operations should be done first when there are multiple operations. Example: $4-(2+1) = 1$; the parentheses tell us that we must add 2 and 1, and then subtract the sum from 4, rather than subtracting 2 from 4 and then adding 1 (this would give us an answer of 3).

Fractions

A **fraction** is a number that is expressed as one integer written above another integer, with a dividing line between them $\left(\frac{x}{y}\right)$. It represents the **quotient** of the two numbers "x divided by y." It can also be thought of as x out of y equal parts.

The top number of a fraction is called the **numerator**, and it represents the number of parts under consideration. The 1 in $\frac{1}{4}$ means that 1 part out of the whole is being considered in the calculation. The bottom number of a fraction is called the **denominator**, and it represents the total number of equal parts. The 4 in $\frac{1}{4}$ means that the whole consists of 4 equal parts. A fraction cannot have a denominator of zero; this is referred to as "**undefined**."

Fractions can be manipulated, without changing the value of the fraction, by multiplying or dividing (but not adding or subtracting) both the numerator and denominator by the same number. If you divide both numbers by a common factor, you are **reducing** or simplifying the fraction. Two fractions that have the same value but are expressed differently are known as **equivalent fractions**. For example, $\frac{2}{10}, \frac{3}{15}, \frac{4}{20}$, and $\frac{5}{25}$ are all equivalent fractions. They can also all be reduced or simplified to $\frac{1}{5}$.

When two fractions are manipulated so that they have the same denominator, this is known as finding a **common denominator**. The number chosen to be that common denominator should be the least common multiple of the two original denominators. Example: $\frac{3}{4}$ and $\frac{5}{6}$; the least common multiple of 4 and 6 is 12. Manipulating to achieve the common denominator: $\frac{3}{4} = \frac{9}{12}; \frac{5}{6} = \frac{10}{12}$.

PROPER FRACTIONS AND MIXED NUMBERS

A fraction whose denominator is greater than its numerator is known as a **proper fraction**, while a fraction whose numerator is greater than its denominator is known as an **improper fraction**. Proper fractions have values *less than one* and improper fractions have values *greater than one*.

A **mixed number** is a number that contains both an integer and a fraction. Any improper fraction can be rewritten as a mixed number. Example: $\frac{8}{3} = \frac{6}{3} + \frac{2}{3} = 2 + \frac{2}{3} = 2\frac{2}{3}$. Similarly, any mixed number can be rewritten as an improper fraction. Example: $1\frac{3}{5} = 1 + \frac{3}{5} = \frac{5}{5} + \frac{3}{5} = \frac{8}{5}$.

> **Review Video: <u>Proper and Improper Fractions and Mixed Numbers</u>**
> Visit mometrix.com/academy and enter code: 211077
>
> **Review Video: <u>Fractions</u>**
> Visit mometrix.com/academy and enter code: 262335

SIMPLIFY

EXAMPLE 1

How to simplify:

$$\frac{\frac{2}{5}}{\frac{4}{7}}$$

Dividing a fraction by a fraction may appear tricky, but it's not if you write out your steps carefully. Follow these steps to divide a fraction by a fraction.

Step 1: Rewrite the problem as a multiplication problem. Dividing by a fraction is the same as multiplying by its **reciprocal**, also known as its **multiplicative inverse**. The product of a number and its reciprocal is 1. Because $\frac{4}{7}$ times $\frac{7}{4}$ is 1, these numbers are reciprocals. Note that reciprocals can be found by simply interchanging the numerators and denominators. So, rewriting the problem as a multiplication problem gives $\frac{2}{5} \times \frac{7}{4}$.

Step 2: Perform multiplication of the fractions by multiplying the numerators by each other and the denominators by each other. In other words, multiply across the top and then multiply across the bottom.

$$\frac{2}{5} \times \frac{7}{4} = \frac{2 \times 7}{5 \times 4} = \frac{14}{20}$$

Step 3: Make sure the fraction is reduced to lowest terms. Both 14 and 20 can be divided by 2.

$$\frac{14}{20} = \frac{14 \div 2}{20 \div 2} = \frac{7}{10}$$

The answer is $\frac{7}{10}$.

EXAMPLE 2

How to simplify:

$$\frac{1}{4} + \frac{3}{6}$$

Fractions with common denominators can be easily added or subtracted. Recall that the denominator is the bottom number in the fraction and that the numerator is the top number in the fraction.

The denominators of $\frac{1}{4}$ and $\frac{3}{6}$ are 4 and 6, respectively. The lowest common denominator of 4 and 6 is 12 because 12 is the least common multiple of 4 (multiples 4, 8, 12, 16, ...) and 6 (multiples 6, 12, 18, 24, ...). Convert each fraction to its equivalent with the newly found common denominator of 12.

$$\frac{1 \times 3}{4 \times 3} = \frac{3}{12}; \frac{3 \times 2}{6 \times 2} = \frac{6}{12}$$

Now that the fractions have the same denominator, you can add them.

$$\frac{3}{12} + \frac{6}{12} = \frac{9}{12}$$

Be sure to write your answer in lowest terms. Both 9 and 12 can be divided by 3, so the answer is $\frac{3}{4}$.

EXAMPLE 3

How to simplify:

$$\frac{7}{8} - \frac{8}{16}$$

Fractions with common denominators can be easily added or subtracted. Recall that the denominator is the bottom number in the fraction and that the numerator is the top number in the fraction.

The denominators of $\frac{7}{8}$ and $\frac{8}{16}$ are 8 and 16, respectively. The lowest common denominator of 8 and 16 is 16 because 16 is the least common multiple of 8 (multiples 8, 16, 24 ...) and 16 (multiples 16, 32, 48, ...). Convert each fraction to its equivalent with the newly found common denominator of 16.

$$\frac{7 \times 2}{8 \times 2} = \frac{14}{16}; \frac{8 \times 1}{16 \times 1} = \frac{8}{16}$$

Now that the fractions have the same denominator, you can subtract them.

$$\frac{14}{16} - \frac{8}{16} = \frac{6}{16}$$

Be sure to write your answer in lowest terms. Both 6 and 16 can be divided by 2, so the answer is $\frac{3}{8}$.

EXAMPLE 4

How to simplify:

$$\frac{1}{2} + \left(3\left(\frac{3}{4}\right) - 2\right) + 4$$

When simplifying expressions, first perform operations within groups. Within the set of parentheses are multiplication and subtraction operations. Perform the multiplication first to get $\frac{1}{2} + \left(\frac{9}{4} - 2\right) + 4$. Then, subtract two to obtain $\frac{1}{2} + \frac{1}{4} + 4$. Finally, perform addition from left to right:

$$\frac{1}{2} + \frac{1}{4} + 4 = \frac{2}{4} + \frac{1}{4} + \frac{16}{4} = \frac{19}{4}$$

EXAMPLE 5

How to simplify: $0.22 + 0.5 - (5.5 + 3.3 \div 3)$

First, evaluate the terms in the parentheses $(5.5 + 3.3 \div 3)$ using order of operations. $3.3 \div 3 = 1.1$, and $5.5 + 1.1 = 6.6$.

Next, rewrite the problem: $0.22 + 0.5 - 6.6$.

Finally, add and subtract from left to right: $0.22 + 0.5 = 0.72$; $0.72 - 6.6 = -5.88$. The answer is -5.88.

EXAMPLE 6

How to simplify:

$$\frac{3}{2} + (4(0.5) - 0.75) + 2$$

First, simplify within the parentheses:

$$\frac{3}{2} + (2 - 0.75) + 2 =$$

$$\frac{3}{2} + 1.25 + 2$$

Finally, change the fraction to a decimal and perform addition from left to right:

$$1.5 + 1.25 + 2 = 4.75$$

EXAMPLE 7

How to simplify: $1.45 + 1.5 + (6 - 9 \div 2) + 45$

First, evaluate the terms in the parentheses using proper order of operations.

$$1.45 + 1.5 + (6 - 4.5) + 45$$

$$1.45 + 1.5 + 1.5 + 45$$

Finally, add from left to right.

$$1.45 + 1.5 + 1.5 + 45 = 49.45$$

OPERATIONS WITH FRACTIONS

ADDING AND SUBTRACTING FRACTIONS

If two fractions have a common denominator, they can be **added** or **subtracted** simply by adding or subtracting the two numerators and retaining the same denominator. Example: $\frac{1}{2} + \frac{1}{4} = \frac{2}{4} + \frac{1}{4} = \frac{3}{4}$. If the two fractions do not already have the same denominator, one or both of them must be manipulated to achieve a common denominator before they can be added or subtracted.

> **Review Video: Adding and Subtracting Fractions**
> Visit mometrix.com/academy and enter code: 378080

MULTIPLYING FRACTIONS

Two fractions can be **multiplied** by multiplying the two numerators to find the new numerator and the two denominators to find the new denominator. Example: $\frac{1}{3} \times \frac{2}{3} = \frac{1 \times 2}{3 \times 3} = \frac{2}{9}$.

> **Review Video: Multiplying Fractions**
> Visit mometrix.com/academy and enter code: 638849

DIVIDING FRACTIONS

Two fractions can be **divided** by flipping the numerator and denominator of the second fraction and then proceeding as though it were a multiplication. Example: $\frac{2}{3} \div \frac{3}{4} = \frac{2}{3} \times \frac{4}{3} = \frac{8}{9}$.

Review Video: <u>Dividing Fractions</u>
Visit mometrix.com/academy and enter code: 300874

COMMON DENOMINATORS WITH FRACTIONS

When two fractions are manipulated so that they have the same denominator, this is known as finding a **common denominator**. The number chosen to be that common denominator should be the **least common multiple** of the two original denominators. Example: $\frac{3}{4}$ and $\frac{5}{6}$; the least common multiple of 4 and 6 is 12. Manipulating to achieve the common denominator: $\frac{3}{4} = \frac{9}{12}$; $\frac{5}{6} = \frac{10}{12}$.

Decimals

DECIMAL ILLUSTRATION

Use a model to represent the decimal: 0.24. Write 0.24 as a fraction.

The decimal 0.24 is twenty-four hundredths. One possible model to represent this fraction is to draw 100 pennies, since each penny is worth one-hundredth of a dollar. Draw one hundred circles to represent one hundred pennies. Shade 24 of the pennies to represent the decimal twenty-four hundredths.

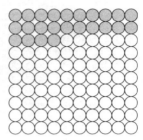

To write the decimal as a fraction, write a fraction: $\frac{\text{\# shaded spaces}}{\text{\# total spaces}}$. The number of shaded spaces is 24, and the total number of spaces is 100, so as a fraction 0.24 equals $\frac{24}{100}$. This fraction can then be reduced to $\frac{6}{25}$.

> **Review Video: Decimals**
> Visit mometrix.com/academy and enter code: 837268

OPERATIONS WITH DECIMALS

ADDING AND SUBTRACTING DECIMALS

When adding and subtracting decimals, the **decimal points** must always be aligned. Adding decimals is just like adding regular whole numbers. Example: $4.5 + 2 = 6.5$.

If the problem-solver does not properly align the decimal points, an incorrect answer of 4.7 may result. An easy way to add decimals is to align all of the decimal points in a vertical column visually. This will allow one to see exactly where the decimal should be placed in the final answer. Begin adding from right to left. Add each column in turn, making sure to carry the number to the left if a column adds up to more than 9. The same rules apply to the subtraction of decimals.

> **Review Video: Adding and Subtracting Decimals**
> Visit mometrix.com/academy and enter code: 381101

MULTIPLYING DECIMALS

A simple multiplication problem has two components: a **multiplicand** and a **multiplier**. When multiplying decimals, work as though the numbers were whole rather than decimals. Once the final product is calculated, count the number of places to the right of the decimal in both the multiplicand and the multiplier. Then, count that number of places from the right of the product and place the decimal in that position.

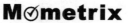

For example, 12.3×2.56 has three places to the right of the respective decimals. Multiply 123×256 to get 31488. Now, beginning on the right, count three places to the left and insert the decimal. The final product will be 31.488.

DIVIDING DECIMALS

Every division problem has a **divisor** and a **dividend**. The dividend is the number that is being divided. In the problem $14 \div 7$, 14 is the dividend and 7 is the divisor. In a division problem with decimals, the divisor must be converted into a whole number. Begin by moving the decimal in the divisor to the right until a whole number is created. Next, move the decimal in the dividend the same number of spaces to the right. For example, 4.9 into 24.5 would become 49 into 245. The decimal was moved one space to the right to create a whole number in the divisor, and then the same was done for the dividend. Once the whole numbers are created, the problem is carried out normally: $245 \div 49 = 5$.

SCIENTIFIC NOTATION

Scientific notation is a way of writing large numbers in a shorter form. The form $a \times 10^n$ is used in scientific notation, where a is greater than or equal to 1, but less than 10, and n is the number of places the decimal must move to get from the original number to a. Example: The number 230,400,000 is cumbersome to write. To write the value in **scientific notation**, place a decimal point between the first and second numbers, and include all digits through the last non-zero digit ($a = 2.304$). To find the appropriate power of 10, count the number of places the decimal point had to move ($n = 8$). The number is positive if the decimal moved to the left, and negative if it moved to the right. We can then write 230,400,000 as 2.304×10^8. If we look instead at the number 0.00002304, we have the same value for a, but this time the decimal moved 5 places to the right ($n = -5$). Thus, 0.00002304 can be written as 2.304×10^{-5}. Using this notation makes it simple to compare very large or very small numbers. By comparing exponents, it is easy to see that 3.28×10^4 is smaller than 1.51×10^5, because 4 is less than 5.

Percentages

Percentages can be thought of as fractions that are based on a whole of 100; that is, one whole is equal to 100%. The word percent means "per hundred." Fractions can be expressed as a percentage by finding equivalent fractions with a denomination of 100. Example: $\frac{7}{10} = \frac{70}{100} = 70\%$; $\frac{1}{4} = \frac{25}{100} = 25\%$.

To express a percentage as a **fraction**, divide the percentage number by 100 and reduce the fraction to its simplest possible terms. Example: $60\% = \frac{60}{100} = \frac{3}{5}$; $96\% = \frac{96}{100} = \frac{24}{25}$.

Review Video: Percentages
Visit mometrix.com/academy and enter code: 141911

REAL WORLD PROBLEMS WITH PERCENTAGES

A percentage problem can be presented three main ways: (1) Find what percentage of some number another number is. Example: What percentage of 40 is 8? (2) Find what number is some percentage of a given number. Example: What number is 20% of 40? (3) Find what number another number is a given percentage of. Example: What number is 8 20% of?

The three components in all of these cases are the same: a **whole** (W), a **part** (P), and a **percentage** (%). These are related by the equation: $P = W \times \%$. This is the form of the equation you would use to solve problems of type (2). To solve types (1) and (3), you would use these two forms:

$$\% = \frac{P}{W} \text{ and } W = \frac{P}{\%}$$

The thing that frequently makes percentage problems difficult is that they are most often also word problems, so a large part of solving them is figuring out which quantities are what. Example: In a school cafeteria, 7 students choose pizza, 9 choose hamburgers, and 4 choose tacos. Find the percentage that chooses tacos. To find the whole, you must first add all of the parts: $7 + 9 + 4 = 20$. The percentage can then be found by dividing the part by the whole ($\% = \frac{P}{W}$): $\frac{4}{20} = \frac{20}{100} = 20\%$.

EXAMPLE 1

What is 30% of 120?

The word "**of**" indicates multiplication, so 30% of 120 is found by multiplying 30% by 120. First, change 30% to a fraction or decimal. Recall that "percent" means per hundred, so $30\% = \frac{30}{100} = 0.30$. 120 times 0.3 is 36.

EXAMPLE 2

What is 150% of 20?

150% of 20 is found by multiplying 150% by 20. First, change 150% to a fraction or decimal. Recall that "percent" means per hundred, so $150\% = \frac{150}{100} = 1.50$. So, $(1.50)(20) = 30$. Notice that 30 is greater than the original number of 20. This makes sense because you are finding a number that is more than 100% of the original number.

EXAMPLE 3

What is 14.5% of 96?

Change 14.5% to a decimal before multiplying. $0.145 \times 96 = 13.92$. Notice that 13.92 is much smaller than the original number of 96. This makes sense because you are finding a small percentage of the original number.

EXAMPLE 4

According to a survey, about 82% of engineers were highly satisfied with their job. If 145 engineers were surveyed, how many reported that they were highly satisfied?

82% of $145 = 0.82 \times 145 = 118.9$. Because you can't have 0.9 of a person, we must round up to say that 119 engineers reported that they were highly satisfied with their jobs.

EXAMPLE 5

On Monday, Lucy spent 5 hours observing sales, 3 hours working on advertising, and 4 hours doing paperwork. On Tuesday, she spent 4 hours observing sales, 6 hours working on advertising, and 2 hours doing paperwork. What was the percent change for time spent on each task between the two days?

The three tasks are observing sales, working on advertising, and doing paperwork. To find the amount of change, compare the first amount with the second amount for each task. Then, write this difference as a percentage compared to the initial amount.

Amount of change for observing sales:

$$5 \text{ hours} - 4 \text{ hours} = 1 \text{ hour}$$

The percent of change is

$$\frac{\text{amount of change}}{\text{original amount}} \times 100\%. \frac{1 \text{ hour}}{5 \text{ hours}} \times 100\% = 20\%.$$

Lucy spent 20% less time observing sales on Tuesday than she did on Monday.

Amount of change for working on advertising:

$$6 \text{ hours} - 3 \text{ hours} = 3 \text{ hours}$$

The percent of change is

$$\frac{\text{amount of change}}{\text{original amount}} \times 100\%. \frac{3 \text{ hours}}{3 \text{ hours}} \times 100\% = 100\%.$$

Lucy spent 100% more time (or twice as much time) working on advertising on Tuesday than she did on Monday.

Amount of change for doing paperwork:

$$4 \text{ hours} - 2 \text{ hours} = 2 \text{ hours}$$

The percent of change is

$$\frac{\text{amount of change}}{\text{original amount}} \times 100\%. \ \frac{2 \text{ hours}}{4 \text{ hours}} \times 100\% = 50\%.$$

Lucy spent 50% less time (or half as much time) working on paperwork on Tuesday than she did on Monday.

EXAMPLE 6

A patient was given 40 mg of a certain medicine. Later, the patient's dosage was increased to 45 mg. What was the percent increase in his medication?

To find the percent increase, first compare the original and increased amounts. The original amount was 40 mg, and the increased amount is 45 mg, so the dosage of medication was increased by 5 mg ($45-40 = 5$). Note, however, that the question asks not by how much the dosage increased but by what percentage it increased. Percent increase $= \frac{\text{new amount} - \text{original amount}}{\text{original amount}} \times 100\%$.

So, $\frac{45 \text{ mg} - 40 \text{ mg}}{40 \text{ mg}} \times 100\% = \frac{5}{40} \times 100\% = 0.125 \times 100\% = 12.5\%$

The percent increase is 12.5%.

EXAMPLE 7

A patient was given 100 mg of a certain medicine. The patient's dosage was later decreased to 88 mg. What was the percent decrease?

The medication was decreased by 12 mg:

$$(100 \text{ mg} - 88 \text{ mg} = 12 \text{ mg})$$

To find by what percent the medication was decreased, this change must be written as a percentage when compared to the original amount.

In other words, $\frac{\text{new amount} - \text{original amount}}{\text{original amount}} \times 100\% = \text{percent change}$

So $\frac{12 \text{ mg}}{100 \text{ mg}} \times 100\% = 0.12 \times 100\% = 12\%$.

The percent decrease is 12%.

EXAMPLE 8

A barista used 125 units of coffee grounds to make a liter of coffee. The barista later reduced the amount of coffee to 100 units. By what percentage was the amount of coffee grounds reduced?

In this problem you must determine which information is necessary to answer the question. The question asks by what percentage the coffee grounds were reduced. Find the two amounts and perform subtraction to find their difference. The first pot of coffee used 125 units. The second time, the barista used 100 units. Therefore, the difference is 125 units − 100 units = 25 units. The percentage reduction can then be calculated as:

$$\frac{\text{change}}{\text{original}} = \frac{25}{125} = \frac{1}{5} = 20\%$$

EXAMPLE 9

In a performance review, an employee received a score of 70 for efficiency and 90 for meeting project deadlines. Six months later, the employee received a score of 65 for efficiency and 96 for meeting project deadlines. What was the percent change for each score on the performance review?

To find the percent change, compare the first amount with the second amount for each score; then, write this difference as a percentage of the initial amount.

Percent change for efficiency score:

$$70 - 65 = 5; \frac{5}{70} \approx 7.1\%$$

The employee's efficiency decreased by about 7.1%.

Percent change for meeting project deadlines score:

$$96 - 90 = 6; \frac{6}{90} \approx 6.7\%$$

The employee increased his ability to meet project deadlines by about 6.7%.

CONVERTING PERCENTAGES, FRACTIONS, AND DECIMALS

Converting decimals to percentages and percentages to decimals is as simple as moving the decimal point. To convert from a decimal to a percentage, move the decimal point **two places to the right**. To convert from a percentage to a decimal, move it **two places to the left**. Example: $0.23 = 23\%$; $5.34 = 534\%$; $0.007 = 0.7\%$; $700\%\ 7.00$; $86\% = 0.86$; $0.15\% = 0.0015$.

It may be helpful to remember that the percentage number will always be larger than the equivalent decimal number.

> **Review Video: <u>Converting Decimals to Fractions and Percentages</u>**
> Visit mometrix.com/academy and enter code: 986765

EXAMPLE 1

Convert 15% to both a fraction and a decimal.

First, write the percentage over 100 because percent means "per one hundred." So, 15% can be written as $\frac{15}{100}$. Fractions should be written in the simplest form, which means that the numbers in the numerator and denominator should be reduced if possible. Both 15 and 100 can be divided by 5:

$$\frac{15 \div 5}{100 \div 5} = \frac{3}{20}$$

As before, write the percentage over 100 because percent means "per one hundred." So, 15% can be written as $\frac{15}{100}$. Dividing a number by a power of ten (10, 100, 1000, etc.) is the same as moving the decimal point to the left by the same number of spaces that there are zeros in the divisor. Since 100 has 2 zeros, move the decimal point two places to the left:

$$15\% = 0.15$$

In other words, when converting from a percentage to a decimal, drop the percent sign and move the decimal point two places to the left.

EXAMPLE 2

Write 24.36% as a fraction and then as a decimal. Explain how you made these conversions.

24.36% written as a fraction is $\frac{24.36}{100}$, or $\frac{2436}{10,000}$, which reduces to $\frac{609}{2500}$. 24.36% written as a decimal is 0.2436. Recall that dividing by 100 moves the decimal two places to the left.

> **Review Video: Converting Percentages to Decimals and Fractions**
> Visit mometrix.com/academy and enter code: 287297

EXAMPLE 3

Convert $\frac{4}{5}$ to a decimal and to a percentage.

To convert a fraction to a decimal, simply divide the numerator by the denominator in the fraction. The numerator is the top number in the fraction and the denominator is the bottom number in a fraction. So $\frac{4}{5} = 4 \div 5 = 0.80 = 0.8$.

Percent means "per hundred." $\frac{4 \times 20}{5 \times 20} = \frac{80}{100} = 80\%$.

EXAMPLE 4

Convert $3\frac{2}{5}$ to a decimal and to a percentage.

The mixed number $3\frac{2}{5}$ has a whole number and a fractional part. The fractional part $\frac{2}{5}$ can be written as a decimal by dividing 5 into 2, which gives 0.4. Adding the whole to the part gives 3.4. Alternatively, note that $3\frac{2}{5} = 3\frac{4}{10} = 3.4$

To change a decimal to a percentage, multiply it by 100.

3.4(100) = 340%. Notice that this percentage is greater than 100%. This makes sense because the original mixed number $3\frac{2}{5}$ is greater than 1.

> **Review Video: Converting Fractions to Percentages and Decimals**
> Visit mometrix.com/academy and enter code: 306233

Rational Number Practice

REAL WORLD ONE OR MULTI-STEP PROBLEMS WITH RATIONAL NUMBERS

EXAMPLE 1

A woman's age is thirteen more than half of 60. How old is the woman?

"More than" indicates addition, and "of" indicates multiplication. The expression can be written as $\frac{1}{2}(60) + 13$. So, the woman's age is equal to $\frac{1}{2}(60) + 13 = 30 + 13 = 43$. The woman is 43 years old.

EXAMPLE 2

A patient was given pain medicine at a dosage of 0.22 grams. The patient's dosage was then increased to 0.80 grams. By how much was the patient's dosage increased?

The first step is to determine what operation (addition, subtraction, multiplication, or division) the problem requires. Notice the keywords and phrases "by how much" and "increased." "Increased" means that you go from a smaller amount to a larger amount. This change can be found by subtracting the smaller amount from the larger amount: 0.80 grams– 0.22 grams = 0.58 grams.

Remember to line up the decimal when subtracting.

$$
\begin{array}{r}
0.80 \\
-\ 0.22 \\
\hline
0.58
\end{array}
$$

EXAMPLE 3

At a hotel, $\frac{3}{4}$ of the 100 rooms are occupied today. Yesterday, $\frac{4}{5}$ of the 100 rooms were occupied. On which day were more of the rooms occupied and by how much more?

First, find the number of rooms occupied each day. To do so, multiply the fraction of rooms occupied by the number of rooms available:

$$\text{Number occupied} = \text{Fraction occupied} \times \text{Total number}$$

Today:

$$\text{Number of rooms occupied} = \frac{3}{4} \times 100 = 75$$

Today, 75 rooms are occupied.

Yesterday:

$$\text{Number of rooms occupied} = \frac{4}{5} \times 100 = 80$$

Yesterday, 80 rooms were occupied.

The difference in the number of rooms occupied is

$$80 - 75 = 5 \text{ rooms}$$

Therefore, five more rooms were occupied yesterday than today.

EXAMPLE 4

At a school, 40% of the teachers teach English. If 20 teachers teach English, how many teachers work at the school?

To answer this problem, first think about the number of teachers that work at the school. Will it be more or less than the number of teachers who work in a specific department such as English? More teachers work at the school, so the number you find to answer this question will be greater than 20.

40% of the teachers are English teachers. "Of" indicates multiplication, and words like "is" and "are" indicate equivalence. Translating the problem into a mathematical sentence gives $40\% \times t = 20$, where t represents the total number of teachers. Solving for t gives $t = \frac{20}{40\%} = \frac{20}{0.40} = 50$. Fifty teachers work at the school.

EXAMPLE 5

A patient was given blood pressure medicine at a dosage of 2 grams. The patient's dosage was then decreased to 0.45 grams. By how much was the patient's dosage decreased?

The decrease is represented by the difference between the two amounts:

$$2 \text{ grams} - 0.45 \text{ grams} = 1.55 \text{ grams}.$$

Remember to line up the decimal point before subtracting.

$$
\begin{array}{r}
2.00 \\
- \ 0.45 \\
\hline
1.55
\end{array}
$$

EXAMPLE 6

Two weeks ago, $\frac{2}{3}$ of the 60 customers at a skate shop were male. Last week, $\frac{3}{6}$ of the 80 customers were male. During which week were there more male customers?

First, you need to find the number of male customers that were in the skate shop each week. You are given this amount in terms of fractions. To find the actual number of male customers, multiply the fraction of male customers by the number of customers in the store.

Actual number of male customers = fraction of male customers × total number of customers.

Two weeks ago: Actual number of male customers $= \frac{2}{3} \times 60$.

$$\frac{2}{3} \times \frac{60}{1} = \frac{2 \times 60}{3 \times 1} = \frac{120}{3} = 40$$

Two weeks ago, 40 of the customers were male.

Last week: Actual number of male customers $= \frac{3}{6} \times 80$.

$$\frac{3}{6} \times \frac{80}{1} = \frac{3 \times 80}{6 \times 1} = \frac{240}{6} = 40$$

Last week, 40 of the patients were customers.

The number of male customers was the same both weeks.

EXAMPLE 7

Jane ate lunch at a local restaurant. She ordered a \$4.99 appetizer, a \$12.50 entrée, and a \$1.25 soda. If she wants to tip her server 20%, how much money will she spend in all?

To find total amount, first find the sum of the items she ordered from the menu and then add 20% of this sum to the total.

In other words:

$$\$4.99 + \$12.50 + \$1.25 = \$18.74$$

Then 20% *of* \$18.74 is $(20\%)(\$18.74) = (0.20)(\$18.74) = \$3.75$.

So, the total she spends is cost of the meal plus the tip or $\$18.74 + \$3.75 = \$22.49$.

Another way to find this sum is to multiply 120% by the cost of the meal.

$$\$18.74(120\%) = \$18.74(1.20) = \$22.49.$$

RATIONAL NUMBERS FROM LEAST TO GREATEST

Order the following rational numbers from least to greatest: 0.55, 17%, $\sqrt{25}$, $\frac{64}{4}$, $\frac{25}{50}$, 3.

Recall that the term **rational** simply means that the number can be expressed as a ratio or fraction. The set of rational numbers includes integers and decimals. Notice that each of the numbers in the problem can be written as a decimal or integer:

$$17\% = 0.1717$$
$$\sqrt{25} = 5$$
$$\frac{64}{4} = 16$$
$$\frac{25}{50} = \frac{1}{2} = 0.5$$

So, the answer is 17%, $\frac{25}{50}$, 0.55, 3, $\sqrt{25}$, $\frac{64}{4}$.

RATIONAL NUMBERS FROM GREATEST TO LEAST

Order the following rational numbers from greatest to least: $0.3, 27\%, \sqrt{100}, \frac{72}{9}, \frac{1}{9}, 4.5$

Recall that the term **rational** simply means that the number can be expressed as a ratio or fraction. The set of rational numbers includes integers and decimals. Notice that each of the numbers in the problem can be written as a decimal or integer:

$$27\% = 0.27$$
$$\sqrt{100} = 10$$
$$\frac{72}{9} = 8$$
$$\frac{1}{9} \approx 0.11$$

So, the answer is $\sqrt{100}, \frac{72}{9}, 4.5, 0.3, 27\%, \frac{1}{9}$.

> **Review Video: Ordering Rational Numbers**
> Visit mometrix.com/academy and enter code: 419578

Proportions and Ratios

PROPORTIONS

A proportion is a relationship between two quantities that dictates how one changes when the other changes. A **direct proportion** describes a relationship in which a quantity increases by a set amount for every increase in the other quantity, or decreases by that same amount for every decrease in the other quantity. Example: Assuming a constant driving speed, the time required for a car trip increases as the distance of the trip increases. The distance to be traveled and the time required to travel are directly proportional.

Inverse proportion is a relationship in which an increase in one quantity is accompanied by a decrease in the other, or vice versa. Example: the time required for a car trip decreases as the speed increases, and increases as the speed decreases, so the time required is inversely proportional to the speed of the car.

> **Review Video: Proportions**
> Visit mometrix.com/academy and enter code: 505355

RATIOS

A ratio is a comparison of two quantities in a particular order. Example: If there are 14 computers in a lab, and the class has 20 students, there is a student to computer ratio of 20 to 14, commonly written as 20:14. Ratios are normally reduced to their smallest whole number representation, so 20:14 would be reduced to 10:7 by dividing both sides by 2.

> **Review Video: Ratios**
> Visit mometrix.com/academy and enter code: 996914

CONSTANT OF PROPORTIONALITY

When two quantities have a proportional relationship, there exists a **constant of proportionality** between the quantities; the product of this constant and one of the quantities is equal to the other quantity. For example, if one lemon costs $0.25, two lemons cost $0.50, and three lemons cost $0.75, there is a proportional relationship between the total cost of lemons and the number of lemons purchased. The constant of proportionality is the **unit price**, namely $0.25/lemon. Notice that the total price of lemons, t, can be found by multiplying the unit price of lemons, p, and the number of lemons, n: $t = pn$.

WORK/UNIT RATE

Unit rate expresses a quantity of one thing in terms of one unit of another. For example, if you travel 30 miles every two hours, a unit rate expresses this comparison in terms of one hour: in one hour you travel 15 miles, so your unit rate is 15 miles per hour. Other examples are how much one ounce of food costs (price per ounce) or figuring out how much one egg costs out of the dozen (price per 1 egg, instead of price per 12 eggs). The denominator of a unit rate is always 1. Unit rates are used to **compare** different situations to solve problems. For example, to make sure you get the best deal when deciding which kind of soda to buy, you can find the unit rate of each. If Soda #1 costs $1.50 for a 1-liter bottle, and soda #2 costs $2.75 for a 2-liter bottle, it would be a better deal to buy Soda #2, because its unit rate is only $1.375 per 1-liter, which is cheaper than Soda #1. Unit rates can also help determine the length of time a given event will take. For example, if you can paint 2 rooms in 4.5 hours, you can determine how long it will take you to paint 5 rooms by solving for the unit rate per room and then multiplying that by 5.

Review Video: Rates and Unit Rates
Visit mometrix.com/academy and enter code: 185363

EXAMPLE 1

Janice made $40 during the first 5 hours she spent babysitting. She will continue to earn money at this rate until she finishes babysitting in 3 more hours. Find how much money Janice earned babysitting and how much she earns per hour.

Janice will earn $64 babysitting in her 8 total hours (adding the first 5 hours to the remaining 3 gives the 8-hour total). This can be found by setting up a proportion comparing money earned to babysitting hours. Since she earns $40 for 5 hours and since the rate is constant, she will earn a proportional amount in 8 hours: $\frac{40}{5} = \frac{x}{8}$. Cross multiplying will yield $5x = 320$, and division by 5 shows that $x = 64$.

Janice earns $8 per hour. This can be found by taking her total amount earned, $64, and dividing it by the total number of hours worked, 8. Since $\frac{64}{8} = 8$, Janice makes $8 in one hour. This can also be found by finding the unit rate, money earned per hour: $\frac{64}{8} = \frac{x}{1}$. Since cross multiplying yields $8x = 64$, and division by 8 shows that $x = 8$, Janice earns $8 per hour.

EXAMPLE 2

The McDonalds are taking a family road trip, driving 300 miles to their cabin. It took them 2 hours to drive the first 120 miles. They will drive at the same speed all the way to their cabin. Find the speed at which the McDonalds are driving and how much longer it will take them to get to their cabin.

The McDonalds are driving 60 miles per hour. This can be found by setting up a proportion to find the unit rate, the number of miles they drive per one hour: $\frac{120}{2} = \frac{x}{1}$. Cross multiplying yields $2x = 120$ and division by 2 shows that $x = 60$.

Since the McDonalds will drive this same speed, it will take them another 3 hours to get to their cabin. This can be found by first finding how many miles the McDonalds have left to drive, which is $300-120 = 180$. The McDonalds are driving at 60 miles per hour, so a proportion can be set up to determine how many hours it will take them to drive 180 miles: $\frac{180}{x} = \frac{60}{1}$. Cross multiplying yields $60x = 180$, and division by 60 shows that $x = 3$. This can also be found by using the formula $D = r \times t$ (or Distance = rate × time), where $180 = 60 \times t$, and division by 60 shows that $t = 3$.

EXAMPLE 3

It takes Andy 10 minutes to read 6 pages of his book. He has already read 150 pages in his book that is 210 pages long. Find how long it takes Andy to read 1 page and also find how long it will take him to finish his book if he continues to read at the same speed.

It takes Andy 1 minute and 40 seconds to read one page in his book. This can be found by finding the unit rate per one page, by dividing the total time it takes him to read 6 pages by 6. Since it takes him 10 minutes to read 6 pages, $\frac{10}{6} = 1\frac{2}{3}$ minutes, which is 1 minute and 40 seconds.

It will take Andy another 100 minutes, or 1 hour and 40 minutes to finish his book. This can be found by first figuring out how many pages Andy has left to read, which is $210-150 = 60$. Since it is now known that it takes him $1\frac{2}{3}$ minutes to read each page, then that rate must be multiplied by however many pages he has left to read (60) to find the time he'll need: $60 \times 1\frac{2}{3} = 100$, so it will take him 100 minutes, or 1 hour and 40 minutes, to read the rest of his book.

REAL WORLD PROBLEMS WITH PROPORTIONS AND RATIOS
EXAMPLE 1

A thermos has a leak and loses 100 mg of hot chocolate every two hours. How much hot chocolate will the thermos lose in five hours?

Using proportional reasoning, since five hours is two and a half times as long as two hours, the thermos will lose two and a half times as much hot chocolate, 2.5×100 mg $= 250$ mg, in five hours. To compute the answer, first write the amount of hot chocolate per 2 hours as a ratio: $\frac{100 \text{ mg}}{2 \text{ hours}}$. Next setup a proportion to relate the time increments of 2 hours and 5 hours: $\frac{100 \text{ mg}}{2 \text{ hours}} = \frac{x \text{ mg}}{5 \text{ hours}}$ where x is the amount of hot chocolate the thermos loses in five hours. Make sure to keep the same units in either the numerator or denominator. In this case the numerator units must be mg for both ratios and the denominator units must be hours for both ratios.

Use cross multiplication and division to solve for x:

$$\frac{100 \text{ mg}}{2 \text{ hours}} = \frac{x \text{ mg}}{5 \text{ hours}}$$

$$100(5) = 2(x)$$
$$500 = 2x$$
$$500 \div 2 = 2x \div 2$$
$$250 = x$$

Therefore, the thermos loses 250 mg every five hours.

EXAMPLE 2

At a school, for every 20 female students there are 15 male students. This same student ratio happens to exist at another school. If there are 100 female students at the second school, how many male students are there?

One way to find the number of male students is to set up and solve a proportion.

$$\frac{\text{number of female students}}{\text{number of male students}} = \frac{20}{15} = \frac{100}{\text{number of male students}}$$

Represent the unknown number of male students as the variable x.

$$\frac{20}{15} = \frac{100}{x}$$

Follow these steps to solve for x:

1. Cross multiply. $20 \times x = 15 \times 100$.

$$20x = 1500$$

2. Divide each side of the equation by 20.

$$x = 75$$

Or, notice that: $\frac{20 \times 5}{15 \times 5} = \frac{100}{75}$, so $x = 75$.

EXAMPLE 3

In a hospital emergency room, there are 4 nurses for every 12 patients. What is the ratio of nurses to patients? If the nurse-to-patient ratio remains constant, how many nurses must be present to care for 24 patients?

The ratio of nurses to patients can be written as 4 to 12, 4:12, or $\frac{4}{12}$. Because four and twelve have a common factor of four, the ratio should be reduced to 1:3, which means that there is one nurse present for every three patients. If this ratio remains constant, there must be eight nurses present to care for 24 patients.

EXAMPLE 4

In a bank, the banker-to-customer ratio is 1:2. If seven bankers are on duty, how many customers are currently in the bank?

Use proportional reasoning or set up a proportion to solve. Because there are twice as many customers as bankers, there must be fourteen customers when seven bankers are on duty. Setting up and solving a proportion gives the same result:

$$\frac{\text{number of bankers}}{\text{number of customers}} = \frac{1}{2} = \frac{7}{\text{number of customers}}$$

Represent the unknown number of patients as the variable x.

$$\frac{1}{2} = \frac{7}{x}$$

To solve for x, cross multiply:

$1 \times x = 7 \times 2$, so $x = 14$.

Algebra

FUNCTION AND RELATION

When expressing functional relationships, the **variables** x and y are typically used. These values are often written as the **coordinates** (x, y). The x-value is the independent variable and the y-value is the dependent variable. A **relation** is a set of data in which there is not a unique y-value for each x-value in the dataset. This means that there can be two of the same x-values assigned to different y-values. A relation is simply a relationship between the x and y-values in each coordinate but does not apply to the relationship between the values of x and y in the data set. A **function** is a relation where one quantity depends on the other. For example, the amount of money that you make depends on the number of hours that you work. In a function, each x-value in the data set has one unique y-value because the y-value depends on the x-value.

> **Review Video: Definition of a Function**
> Visit mometrix.com/academy and enter code: 784611

DETERMINING A FUNCTION

You can determine whether an equation is a **function** by substituting different values into the equation for x. These values are called input values. All possible input values are referred to as the **domain**. The result of substituting these values into the equation is called the output, or **range**. You can display and organize these numbers in a data table. A **data table** contains the values for x and y, which you can also list as coordinates. In order for a function to exist, the table cannot contain any repeating x-values that correspond with different y-values. If each x-coordinate has a unique y-coordinate, the table contains a function. However, there can be repeating y-values that correspond with different x-values. An example of this is when the function contains an exponent. For example, if $x^2 = y$, $2^2 = 4$, and $(-2)^2 = 4$.

> **Review Video: Basics of Functions**
> Visit mometrix.com/academy and enter code: 822500

APPLYING THE BASIC OPERATIONS TO FUNCTIONS

For each of the basic operations, we will use these functions as examples: $f(x) = x^2$ and $g(x) = x$.

To find the **sum** of two functions f and g, assuming the domains are compatible, simply add the two functions together: $(f + g)(x) = f(x) + g(x) = x^2 + x$

To find the **difference** of two functions f and g, assuming the domains are compatible, simply subtract the second function from the first: $(f - g)(x) = f(x) - g(x) = x^2 - x$.

To find the **product** of two functions f and g, assuming the domains are compatible, multiply the two functions together: $(f \cdot g)(x) = f(x) \cdot g(x) = x^2 \cdot x = x^3$.

To find the **quotient** of two functions f and g, assuming the domains are compatible, divide the first function by the second: $\frac{f}{g}(x) = \frac{f(x)}{g(x)} = \frac{x^2}{x} = x \, ; x \neq 0$.

The example given in each case is fairly simple, but on a given problem, if you are looking only for the value of the sum, difference, product or quotient of two functions at a particular x-value, it may be simpler to solve the functions individually and then perform the given operation using those values.

The **composite** of two functions f and g, written as $(f \circ g)(x)$ simply means that the output of the second function is used as the input of the first. This can also be written as $f\big(g(x)\big)$. In general, this can be solved by substituting $g(x)$ for all instances of x in $f(x)$ and simplifying. Using the example functions $f(x) = x^2 - x + 2$ and $g(x) = x + 1$, we can find that $(f \circ g)(x)$ or $f\big(g(x)\big)$ is equal to $f(x + 1) = (x + 1)^2 - (x + 1) + 2$, which simplifies to $x^2 + x + 2$.

It is important to note that $(f \circ g)(x)$ is not necessarily the same as $(g \circ f)(x)$. The process is not commutative like addition or multiplication expressions. If $(f \circ g)(x)$ does equal $(g \circ f)(x)$, the two functions are inverses of each other.

COEFFICIENTS AND THE DISTRIBUTIVE PROPERTY

COEFFICIENTS

A coefficient is a number or symbol that is multiplied by a variable. For example, in the expression 2(ab), the number 2 is the coefficient of (ab). The expression can be written in other ways to have a different coefficient. For example, the expression can be 2a(b). This means that 2a is the coefficient of (b).

DISTRIBUTIVE PROPERTY

The distributive property can be used to multiply each addend in parentheses. Then, the products are added to reach the result. The formula for the distributive property looks like this: a(b+c) = ab+ac.

Example: 6(2+4)

First, multiply 6 and 2. The answer is 12.

Then, multiply 6 and 4. The answer is 24.

Last, we add 12 and 24. So, the final answer is 36.

SIMPLIFYING RATIONAL EXPRESSIONS

To simplify a rational expression, factor the numerator and denominator completely. Factors that are the same and appear in the numerator and denominator have a ratio of 1. The denominator, $(1 - x^2)$, is a difference of squares. It can be factored as $(1 - x)(1 + x)$. The factor $1 - x$ and the numerator $x - 1$ are opposites and have a ratio of -1. Rewrite the numerator as $-1(1 - x)$. So, the rational expression can be simplified as follows:

$$\frac{x - 1}{1 - x^2} = \frac{-1(1 - x)}{(1 - x)(1 + x)} = \frac{-1}{1 + x}$$

(Note that since the original expression is defined for $x \neq \{-1, 1\}$, the simplified expression has the same restrictions.)

SOLVE EQUATIONS IN ONE VARIABLE
MANIPULATING EQUATIONS

Sometimes you will have variables missing in equations. So, you need to find the missing variable. To do this, you need to remember one important thing: *whatever you do to one side of an equation, you need to do to the other side*. If you subtract 100 from one side of an equation, you need to subtract 100 from the other side of the equation. This will allow you to change the form of the equation to find missing values.

EXAMPLE

Ray earns $10 an hour at his job. Write an equation for his earnings as a function of time spent working. Determine how long Ray has to work in order to earn $360.

The number of dollars that Ray earns is dependent on the number of hours he works, so earnings will be represented by the dependent variable y and hours worked will be represented by the independent variable x. He earns 10 dollars per hour worked, so his earning can be calculated as

$$y = 10x$$

To calculate the number of hours Ray must work in order to earn $360, plug in 360 for y and solve for x:

$$360 = 10x$$

$$x = \frac{360}{10} = 36$$

So, Ray must work 36 hours in order to earn $360.

SOLVING ONE VARIABLE LINEAR EQUATIONS

Another way to write an equation is $ax + b = 0$ where $a \neq 0$. This is known as a **one-variable linear equation**. A solution to an equation is called a **root**. Consider the following equation:

$$5x + 10 = 0$$

If we solve for x, the solution is $x = -2$. In other words, the root of the equation is –2.

The first step is to subtract 10 from both sides. This gives $5x = -10$.

Next, divide both sides by the **coefficient** of the variable. For this example, that is 5. So, you should have $x = -2$. You can make sure that you have the correct answer by substituting –2 back into the original equation. So, the equation now looks like this: $(5)(-2) + 10 = -10 + 10 = 0$.

EXAMPLE 1

$\frac{45\%}{12\%} = \frac{15\%}{x}$. Solve for x.

First, cross multiply; then, solve for x: $\frac{45\%}{12\%} = \frac{15\%}{x}$

$$\frac{0.45}{0.12} = \frac{0.15}{x}$$
$$0.45(x) = 0.12(0.15)$$
$$0.45x = 0.0180$$
$$0.45x \div 0.45 = 0.0180 \div 0.45$$
$$x = 0.04 = 4\%$$

Alternatively, notice that $\frac{45\% \div 3}{12\% \div 3} = \frac{15\%}{4\%}$. So, $x = 4\%$.

EXAMPLE 2

How do you solve for x in the proportion $\frac{0.50}{2} = \frac{1.50}{x}$?

First, cross multiply; then, solve for x.

$$\frac{0.50}{2} = \frac{1.50}{x}$$
$$0.50(x) = 2(1.50)$$
$$0.50x = 3$$
$$0.50x \div 0.50 = 3 \div 0.50$$
$$x = 6$$

Or, notice that $\frac{0.50 \times 3}{2 \times 3} = \frac{1.50}{6}$, so $x = 6$.

EXAMPLE 3

$\frac{40}{8} = \frac{x}{24}$. Find x.

One way to solve for x is to first cross multiply.

$$\frac{40}{8} = \frac{x}{24}$$
$$40(24) = 8(x)$$
$$960 = 8x$$
$$960 \div 8 = 8x \div 8$$
$$x = 120$$

Or, notice that:

$$\frac{40 \times 3}{8 \times 3} = \frac{120}{24}, \text{ so } x = 120$$

SYSTEMS OF EQUATIONS

Systems of equations are a set of simultaneous equations that all use the same variables. A solution to a system of equations must be true for each equation in the system. **Consistent systems** are those with at least one solution. **Inconsistent systems** are systems of equations that have no solution.

Review Video: Systems of Equations
Visit mometrix.com/academy and enter code: 658153

SUBSTITUTION

To solve a system of linear equations by **substitution**, start with the easier equation and solve for one of the variables. Express this variable in terms of the other variable. Substitute this expression in the other equation and solve for the other variable. The solution should be expressed in the form (x, y). Substitute the values into both of the original equations to check your answer. Consider the following problem.

Solve the system using substitution:

$$x + 6y = 15$$
$$3x - 12y = 18$$

Solve the first equation for x:

$$x = 15 - 6y$$

Substitute this value in place of x in the second equation, and solve for y:

$$3(15 - 6y) - 12y = 18$$
$$45 - 18y - 12y = 18$$
$$30y = 27$$
$$y = \frac{27}{30} = \frac{9}{10} = 0.9$$

Plug this value for y back into the first equation to solve for x:

$$x = 15 - 6(0.9) = 15 - 5.4 = 9.6$$

Check both equations if you have time:

$$9.6 + 6(0.9) = 9.6 + 5.4 = 15$$
$$3(9.6) - 12(0.9) = 28.8 - 10.8 = 18$$

Therefore, the solution is (9.6, 0.9).

ELIMINATION

To solve a system of equations using **elimination**, begin by rewriting both equations in standard form $Ax + By = C$. Check to see if the coefficients of one pair of like variables add to zero. If not, multiply one or both of the equations by a non-zero number to make one set of like variables add to zero. Add the two equations to solve for one of the variables. Substitute this value into one of the original equations to solve for the other variable. Check your work by substituting into the other equation. Next, we will solve the same problem as above, but using the addition method.

Solve the system using elimination:

$$x + 6y = 15$$
$$3x - 12y = 18$$

76

If we multiply the first equation by 2, we can eliminate the y terms:

$$2x + 12y = 30$$

$$3x - 12y = 18$$

Add the equations together and solve for x:

$$5x = 48$$

$$x = \frac{48}{5} = 9.6$$

Plug the value for x back into either of the original equations and solve for y:

$$9.6 + 6y = 15$$

$$y = \frac{15 - 9.6}{6} = 0.9$$

Check both equations if you have time:

$$9.6 + 6(0.9) = 9.6 + 5.4 = 15$$

$$3(9.6) - 12(0.9) = 28.8 - 10.8 = 18$$

Therefore, the solution is (9.6, 0.9).

GRAPHICALLY

To solve a system of linear equations **graphically**, plot both equations on the same graph. The solution of the equations is the point where both lines cross. If the lines do not cross (are parallel), then there is **no solution**.

For example, consider the following system of equations:

$$y = 2x + 7$$
$$y = -x + 1$$

Since these equations are given in slope-intercept form, they are easy to graph; the y intercepts of the lines are $(0, 7)$ and $(0, 1)$. The respective slopes are 2 and –1, thus the graphs look like this:

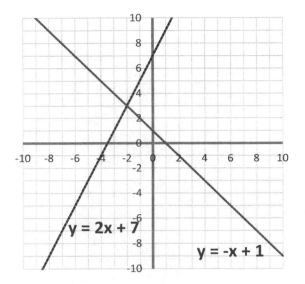

The two lines intersect at the point $(-2, 3)$, thus this is the solution to the system of equations.

Solving a system graphically is generally only practical if both coordinates of the solution are integers; otherwise the intersection will lie between gridlines on the graph and the coordinates will be difficult or impossible to determine exactly. It also helps if, as in this example, the equations are in slope-intercept form or some other form that makes them easy to graph. Otherwise, another method of solution (by substitution or elimination) is likely to be more useful.

SLOPE

On a graph with two points, (x_1, y_1) and (x_2, y_2), the **slope** is found with the formula $m = \frac{y_2 - y_1}{x_2 - x_1}$; where $x_1 \neq x_2$ and m stands for slope. If the value of the slope is **positive**, the line has an *upward direction* from left to right. If the value of the slope is **negative**, the line has a *downward direction* from left to right.

UNIT RATE AS THE SLOPE

A new book goes on sale in bookstores and online stores. In the first month, 5,000 copies of the book are sold. Over time, the book continues to grow in popularity. The data for the number of copies sold is in the table below.

# of Months on Sale	1	2	3	4	5
# of Copies Sold (In Thousands)	5	10	15	20	25

So, the number of copies that are sold and the time that the book is on sale is a proportional relationship. In this example, an equation can be used to show the data: $y = 5x$, where x is the number of months that the book is on sale. Also, y is the number of copies sold. So, the slope is $\frac{\text{rise}}{\text{run}} = \frac{5}{1}$. This can be reduced to 5.

EQUATION USING INDEPENDENT AND DEPENDENT VARIABLES

To write an equation, you must first assign **variables** to the unknown values in the problem and then translate the words and phrases into expressions containing numbers and symbols. For example, if Ray earns $10 an hour, this can be represented by the expression $10x$, where x is equal to the number of hours that Ray works. The value of x represents the number of hours because it is the **independent variable**, or the amount that you choose and can manipulate. To find out how much money he earns in y hours, you would write the equation $10x = y$. The variable y is the **dependent variable** because it depends on x and cannot be manipulated. Once you have the equation for the function, you can choose any number of hours to find the corresponding amount that he earns. For example, if you want to know how much he would earn working 36 hours, you would substitute 36 in for x and multiply to find that he would earn $360.

EQUATIONS AND GRAPHING

When algebraic functions and equations are shown graphically, they are usually shown on a **Cartesian coordinate plane**. The Cartesian coordinate plane consists of two number lines placed perpendicular to each other, and intersecting at the zero point, also known as the origin. The horizontal number line is known as the x-axis, with positive values to the right of the origin, and negative values to the left of the origin. The vertical number line is known as the y-axis, with positive values above the origin, and negative values below the origin. Any point on the plane can be identified by an ordered pair in the form (x,y), called coordinates. The x-value of the coordinate is called the **abscissa**, and the y-value of the coordinate is called the **ordinate**. The two number lines divide the plane into four **quadrants**: I, II, III, and IV.

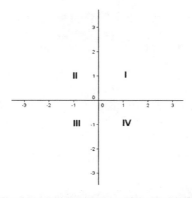

Before learning the different forms in which equations can be written, it is important to understand some terminology. A ratio of the change in the vertical distance to the change in horizontal distance is called the **slope**. On a graph with two points, (x_1, y_1) and (x_2, y_2), the slope is represented by the formula $s = \frac{y_2 - y_1}{x_2 - x_1}$; $x_1 \neq x_2$. If the value of the slope is positive, the line slopes *upward* from left to right. If the value of the slope is negative, the line slopes *downward* from left to right. If the *y*-coordinates are the same for both points, the slope is 0 and the line is a *horizontal* line. If the *x*-coordinates are the same for both points, there is no slope and the line is a *vertical* line. Two or more lines that have equal slopes are *parallel* lines. *Perpendicular* lines have slopes that are negative reciprocals of each other, such as $\frac{a}{b}$ and $\frac{-b}{a}$.

Review Video: Graphs of Functions
Visit mometrix.com/academy and enter code: 492785

Equations are made up of monomials and polynomials. A **monomial** is a single variable or product of constants and variables, such as x, $2x$, or $\frac{2}{x}$. There will never be addition or subtraction symbols in a monomial. Like monomials have like variables, but they may have different coefficients. **Polynomials** are algebraic expressions which use addition and subtraction to combine two or more monomials. Two terms make a binomial; three terms make a trinomial; etc.. The **degree of a monomial** is the sum of the exponents of the variables. The **degree of a polynomial** is the highest degree of any individual term.

As mentioned previously, equations can be written many ways. Below is a list of the many forms equations can take.

- **Standard Form**: $Ax + By = C$; the slope is $\frac{-A}{B}$ and the y-intercept is $\frac{C}{B}$
- **Slope Intercept Form**: $y = mx + b$, where m is the slope and b is the *y*-intercept
- **Point-Slope Form**: $y - y_1 = m(x - x_1)$, where m is the slope and (x_1, y_1) is a point on the line
- **Two-Point Form**: $\frac{y - y_1}{x - x_1} = \frac{y_2 - y_1}{x_2 - x_1}$, where (x_1, y_1) and (x_2, y_2) are two points on the given line
- **Intercept Form**: $\frac{x}{x_1} + \frac{y}{y_1} = 1$, where $(x_1, 0)$ is the point at which a line intersects the *x*-axis, and $(0, y_1)$ is the point at which the same line intersects the *y*-axis

---

Review Video: Slope-Intercept and Point-Slope Forms
Visit mometrix.com/academy and enter code: 113216

Equations can also be written as $ax + b = 0$, where $a \neq 0$. These are referred to as **one variable linear equations**. A solution to such an equation is called a **root**. In the case where we have the equation $5x + 10 = 0$, if we solve for x we get a solution of $x = -2$. In other words, the root of the equation is -2. This is found by first subtracting 10 from both sides, which gives $5x = -10$. Next, simply divide both sides by the coefficient of the variable, in this case 5, to get $x = -2$. This can be checked by plugging -2 back into the original equation $(5)(-2) + 10 = -10 + 10 = 0$.

The **solution set** is the set of all solutions of an equation. In our example, the solution set would simply be -2. If there were more solutions (there usually are in multivariable equations) then they would also be included in the solution set. When an equation has no true solutions, this is referred to as an **empty set**. Equations with identical solution sets are **equivalent equations**. An **identity** is a term whose value or determinant is equal to 1.

MANIPULATION OF FUNCTIONS

Horizontal and vertical shift occur when values are added to or subtracted from the x or y values, respectively.

If a constant is added to the y portion of each point, the graph shifts **up**. If a constant is subtracted from the y portion of each point, the graph shifts **down**. This is represented by the expression $f(x) \pm k$, where k is a constant.

If a constant is added to the x portion of each point, the graph shifts **left**. If a constant is subtracted from the x portion of each point, the graph shifts **right**. This is represented by the expression $f(x \pm k)$, where k is a constant.

Stretch, compression, and reflection occur when different parts of a function are multiplied by different groups of constants. If the function as a whole is multiplied by a real number constant greater than 1, $(k \times f(x))$, the graph is **stretched** vertically. If k in the previous equation is greater than zero but less than 1, the graph is **compressed** vertically. If k is less than zero, the graph is **reflected** about the x-axis, in addition to being either stretched or compressed vertically if k is less than or greater than -1, respectively. If instead, just the x-term is multiplied by a constant greater than 1 $(f(k \times x))$, the graph is compressed horizontally. If k in the previous equation is greater than zero but less than 1, the graph is stretched horizontally. If k is less than zero, the graph is reflected about the y-axis, in addition to being either stretched or compressed horizontally if k is greater than or less than -1, respectively.

CLASSIFICATION OF FUNCTIONS

There are many different ways to classify functions based on their structure or behavior. Listed here are a few common classifications.

Constant functions are given by the equation y=b or $f(x) = b$, where b is a real number. There is no independent variable present in the equation, so the function has a constant value for all x. The graph of a constant function is a horizontal line of slope 0 that is positioned b units from the x-axis. If b is positive, the line is above the x-axis; if b is negative, the line is below the x-axis.

Identity functions are identified by the equation y=x or $f(x) = x$, where every value of y is equal to its corresponding value of x. The only zero is the point (0, 0). The graph is a diagonal line with slope 1.

In **linear functions**, the value of the function changes in direct proportion to x. The rate of change, represented by the slope on its graph, is constant throughout. The standard form of a linear equation is $ax + by = c$, where a, b, and c are real numbers. As a function, this equation is commonly written as $y = mx + b$ or $f(x) = mx + b$. This is known as the slope-intercept form, because the coefficients give the slope of the graphed function (m) and its y-intercept (b). Solve the equation $mx + b = 0$ for x to get $x = -\frac{b}{m}$, which is the only zero of the function. The domain and range are both the set of all real numbers.

> **Review Video: Linear Speed**
> Visit mometrix.com/academy and enter code: 327101

A **polynomial function** is a function with multiple terms and multiple powers of x, such as:

$$f(x) = a_n x^n + a_{n-1} x^{n-1} + a_{n-2} x^{n-2} + \cdots + a_1 x + a_0$$

where n is a non-negative integer that is the highest exponent in the polynomial, and $a_n \neq 0$. The domain of a polynomial function is the set of all real numbers. If the greatest exponent in the polynomial is even, the polynomial is said to be of even degree and the range is the set of real numbers that satisfy the function. If the greatest exponent in the polynomial is odd, the polynomial is said to be odd and the range, like the domain, is the set of all real numbers.

> **Review Video: Simplifying Rational Polynomial Functions**
> Visit mometrix.com/academy and enter code: 351038

A **quadratic function** is a polynomial function that follows the equation pattern $y = ax^2 + bx + c$, or $f(x) = ax^2 + bx + c$, where a, b, and c are real numbers and $a \neq 0$. The domain of a quadratic function is the set of all real numbers. The range is also real numbers, but only those in the subset of the domain that satisfy the equation. The root(s) of any quadratic function can be found by plugging the values of a, b, and c into the **quadratic formula**:

$$x = \frac{-b \pm \sqrt{b^2 - 4ac}}{2a}$$

If the expression $b^2 - 4ac$ is negative, you will instead find complex roots.

A quadratic function has a parabola for its graph. In the equation $f(x) = ax^2 + bx + c$, if a is positive, the parabola will open upward. If a is negative, the parabola will open downward. The axis of symmetry is a vertical line that passes through the vertex. To determine whether or not the parabola will intersect the x-axis, check the number of real roots. An equation with two real roots will cross the x-axis twice. An equation with one real root will have its vertex on the x-axis. An equation with no real roots will not contact the x-axis.

> **Review Video: Deriving the Quadratic Formula**
> Visit mometrix.com/academy and enter code: 317436
>
> **Review Video: Using the Quadratic Formula**
> Visit mometrix.com/academy and enter code: 163102
>
> **Review Video: Changing Constants in Graphs of Functions: Quadratic Equations**
> Visit mometrix.com/academy and enter code: 476276

A **rational function** is a function that can be constructed as a ratio of two polynomial expressions: $f(x) = \frac{p(x)}{q(x)}$, where $p(x)$ and $q(x)$ are both polynomial expressions and $q(x) \neq 0$. The domain is the set of all real numbers, except any values for which $q(x) = 0$. The range is the set of real numbers that satisfies the function when the domain is applied. When you graph a rational function, you will have vertical asymptotes wherever $q(x) = 0$. If the polynomial in the numerator is of lesser degree than the polynomial in the denominator, the x-axis will also be a horizontal asymptote. If the numerator and denominator have equal degrees, there will be a horizontal asymptote not on the x-axis. If the degree of the numerator is exactly one greater than the degree of the denominator, the graph will have an oblique, or diagonal, asymptote. The asymptote will be along the line $y = \frac{p_n}{q_{n-1}} x + \frac{p_{n-1}}{q_{n-1}}$, where p_n and q_{n-1} are the coefficients of the highest degree terms in their respective polynomials.

A **square root function** is a function that contains a radical and is in the format $f(x) = \sqrt{ax + b}$. The domain is the set of all real numbers that yields a positive radicand or a radicand equal to zero. Because square root values are assumed to be positive unless otherwise identified, the range is all real numbers from zero to infinity. To find the zero of a square root function, set the radicand equal to zero and solve for x. The graph of a square root function is always to the right of the zero and always above the x-axis.

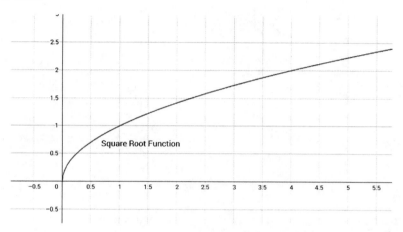

An **absolute value function** is in the format $f(x) = |ax + b|$. Like other functions, the domain is the set of all real numbers. However, because absolute value indicates positive numbers, the range is limited to positive real numbers. To find the zero of an absolute value function, set the portion inside the absolute value sign equal to zero and solve for x.

An absolute value function is also known as a piecewise function because it must be solved in pieces – one for if the value inside the absolute value sign is positive, and one for if the value is negative. The function can be expressed as

$$f(x) = \begin{cases} ax + b \text{ if } ax + b \geq 0 \\ -(ax + b) \text{ if } ax + b < 0 \end{cases}$$

This will allow for an accurate statement of the range.

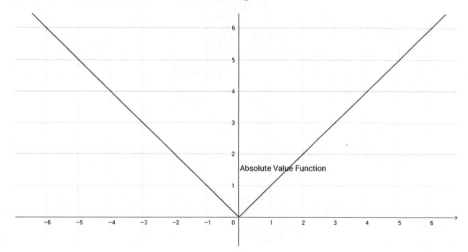

Exponential functions are equations that have the format $y = b^x$, where base $b > 0$ and $b \neq 1$. The exponential function can also be written $f(x) = b^x$.

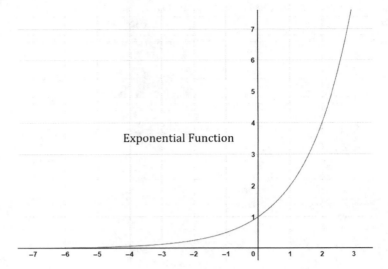

Exponential Function

Logarithmic functions are equations that have the format $y = \log_b x$ or $f(x) = \log_b x$. The base b may be any number except one; however, the most common bases for logarithms are base 10 and base e. The log base e is known the natural logarithm, or ln, expressed by the function $f(x) = \ln x$.

Any logarithm that does not have an assigned value of b is assumed to be base 10: $\log x = \log_{10} x$. Exponential functions and logarithmic functions are related in that one is the inverse of the other. If $f(x) = b^x$, then $f^{-1}(x) = \log_b x$. This can perhaps be expressed more clearly by the two equations: $y = b^x$ and $x = \log_b y$.

The following properties apply to logarithmic expressions:

$$\log_b 1 = 0$$
$$\log_b b = 1$$
$$\log_b b^p = p$$
$$\log_b MN = \log_b M + \log_b N$$
$$\log_b \frac{M}{N} = \log_b M - \log_b N$$
$$\log_b M^p = p \log_b M$$

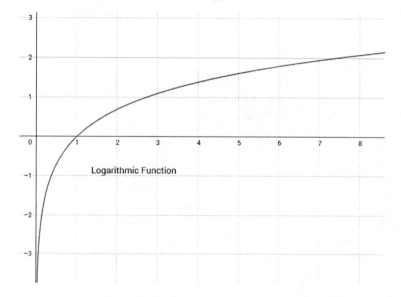

Logarithmic Function

In a **one-to-one function**, each value of x has exactly one value for y (this is the definition of a function) *and* each value of y has exactly one value for x. While the vertical line test will determine if a graph is that of a function, the horizontal line test will determine if a function is a one-to-one function. If a horizontal line drawn at any value of y intersects the graph in more than one place, the graph is not that of a one-to-one function. Do not make the mistake of using the horizontal line test exclusively in determining if a graph is that of a one-to-one function. A one-to-one function must pass both the vertical line test and the horizontal line test. One-to-one functions are also **invertible functions**.

A **monotone function** is a function whose graph either constantly increases or constantly decreases. Examples include the functions $f(x) = x$, $f(x) = -x$, or $f(x) = x^3$.

An **even function** has a graph that is symmetric with respect to the y-axis and satisfies the equation $f(x) = f(-x)$. Examples include the functions $f(x) = x^2$ and $f(x) = ax^n$, where a is any real number and n is a positive even integer.

An **odd function** has a graph that is symmetric with respect to the origin and satisfies the equation $f(x) = -f(-x)$. Examples include the functions $f(x) = x^3$ and $f(x) = ax^n$, where a is any real number and n is a positive odd integer.

Algebraic functions are those that exclusively use polynomials and roots. These would include polynomial functions, rational functions, square root functions, and all combinations of these functions, such as polynomials as the radicand. These combinations may be joined by addition, subtraction, multiplication, or division, but may not include variables as exponents.

85

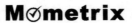

Transcendental functions are all functions that are non-algebraic. Any function that includes logarithms, trigonometric functions, variables as exponents, or any combination that includes any of these is not algebraic in nature, even if the function includes polynomials or roots.

RELATED CONCEPTS

According to the **fundamental theorem of algebra**, every non-constant, single variable polynomial has exactly as many roots as the polynomial's highest exponent. For example, if x^4 is the largest exponent of a term, the polynomial will have exactly 4 roots. However, some of these roots may have multiplicity or be non-real numbers. For instance, in the polynomial function $f(x) = x^4 - 4x + 3$, the only real roots are 1 and -1. The root 1 has multiplicity of 2 and there is one non-real root $(-1 - \sqrt{2}i)$.

The **remainder theorem** is useful for determining the remainder when a polynomial is divided by a binomial. The Remainder Theorem states that if a polynomial function $f(x)$ is divided by a binomial $x - a$, where a is a real number, the remainder of the division will be the value of $f(a)$. If $f(a) = 0$, then a is a root of the polynomial.

The **factor theorem** is related to the Remainder Theorem and states that if $f(a) = 0$ then $(x - a)$ is a factor of the function.

According to the **rational root theorem,** any rational root of a polynomial function $f(x) = a_n x^n + a_{n-1}x^{n-1} + \cdots + a_1 x + a_0$ with integer coefficients will, when reduced to its lowest terms, be a positive or negative fraction such that the numerator is a factor of a_0 and the denominator is a factor of a_n. For instance, if the polynomial function $f(x) = x^3 + 3x^2 - 4$ has any rational roots, the numerators of those roots can only be factors of 4 (1, 2, 4), and the denominators can only be factors of 1 (1). The function in this example has roots of 1 $\left(\text{or } \frac{1}{1}\right)$ and -2 $\left(\text{or } -\frac{2}{1}\right)$.

Variables that vary **directly** are those that either both increase at the same rate or both decrease at the same rate. For example, in the functions $f(x) = kx$ or $f(x) = kx^n$, where k and n are positive, the value of $f(x)$ increases as the value of x increases and decreases as the value of x decreases.

Variables that vary **inversely** are those where one increases while the other decreases. For example, in the functions $f(x) = \frac{k}{x}$ or $f(x) = \frac{k}{x^n}$ where k is a positive constant, the value of y increases as the value of x decreases, and the value of y decreases as the value of x increases.

In both cases, k is the constant of variation.

A **weighted mean**, or weighted average, is a mean that uses "weighted" values. The formula is weighted mean $= \frac{w_1 x_1 + w_2 x_2 + w_3 x_3 \ldots + w_n x_n}{w_1 + w_2 + w_3 + \cdots + w_n}$. Weighted values, such as $w_1, w_2, w_3, \ldots w_n$ are assigned to each member of the set $x_1, x_2, x_3, \ldots x_n$. If calculating weighted mean, make sure a weight value for each member of the set is used.

INEQUALITIES

Commonly in algebra and other upper-level fields of math you find yourself working with mathematical expressions that do not equal each other. The statement comparing such expressions with symbols such as < (less than) or > (greater than) is called an **inequality**. An example of an inequality is $7x > 5$. To solve for x, simply divide both sides by 7 and the solution is shown to be $x > \frac{5}{7}$. Graphs of the solution set of inequalities are represented on a number line. Open circles are used to show that an expression approaches a number but is never quite equal to that number.

Conditional inequalities are those with certain values for the variable that will make the condition true and other values for the variable where the condition will be false. **Absolute inequalities** can have any real number as the value for the variable to make the condition true, while there is no real number value for the variable that will make the condition false. Solving inequalities is done by following the same rules as for solving equations with the exception that when multiplying or dividing by a negative number the direction of the inequality sign must be flipped or reversed. **Double inequalities** are situations where two inequality statements apply to the same variable expression. An example of this is $-c < ax + b < c$.

GRAPHING INEQUALITIES

Graph the inequality $10 > -2x + 4$.

In order to **graph the inequality** $10 > -2x + 4$, you must first solve for x. The opposite of addition is subtraction, so subtract 4 from both sides. This results in $6 > -2x$. Next, the opposite of multiplication is division, so divide both sides by -2. Don't forget to flip the inequality symbol since you are dividing by a negative number. This results in $-3 < x$. You can rewrite this as $x > -3$. To graph an inequality, you create a number line and put a circle around the value that is being compared to x. If you are graphing a greater than or less than inequality, as the one shown, the circle remains open. This represents all of the values excluding -3. If the inequality happens to be a greater than or equal to or less than or equal to, you draw a closed circle around the value. This would represent all of the values including the number. Finally, take a look at the values that the solution represents and shade the number line in the appropriate direction. You are graphing all of the values greater than -3 and since this is all of the numbers to the right of -3, shade this region on the number line.

DETERMINING SOLUTIONS TO INEQUALITIES

Determine whether $(-2, 4)$ is a solution of the inequality $y \geq -2x + 3$.

To determine whether a coordinate is a **solution of an inequality**, you can either use the inequality or its graph. Using $(-2, 4)$ as (x, y), substitute the values into the inequality to see if it makes a true statement. This results in $4 \geq -2(-2) + 3$. Using the integer rules, simplify the right side of the inequality by multiplying and then adding. The result is $4 \geq 7$, which is a false statement. Therefore, the coordinate is not a solution of the inequality. You can also use the **graph** of an inequality to see if a coordinate is a part of the solution. The graph of an inequality is shaded over the section of the coordinate grid that is included in the solution. The graph of $y \geq -2x + 3$ includes the solid line $y = -2x + 3$ and is shaded to the right of the line, representing all of the points greater than and including the points on the line. This excludes the point $(-2, 4)$, so it is not a solution of the inequality.

CALCULATIONS USING POINTS

Sometimes you need to perform calculations using only points on a graph as input data. Using points, you can determine what the **midpoint** and **distance** are. If you know the equation for a line you can calculate the distance between the line and the point.

To find the **midpoint** of two points (x_1, y_1) and (x_2, y_2), average the x-coordinates to get the x-coordinate of the midpoint, and average the y-coordinates to get the y-coordinate of the midpoint. The formula is Midpoint $= \left(\frac{x_1+x_2}{2}, \frac{y_1+y_2}{2}\right)$.

The **distance** between two points is the same as the length of the hypotenuse of a right triangle with the two given points as endpoints, and the two sides of the right triangle parallel to the x-axis and y-axis, respectively. The length of the segment parallel to the x-axis is the difference between the x-coordinates of the two points. The length of the segment parallel to the y-axis is the difference between the y-coordinates of the two points. Use the Pythagorean theorem $a^2 + b^2 = c^2$ or $c = \sqrt{a^2 + b^2}$ to find the distance. The formula is distance $= \sqrt{(x_2 - x_1)^2 + (y_2 - y_1)^2}$.

When a line is in the format $Ax + By + C = 0$, where A, B, and C are coefficients, you can use a point (x_1, y_1) not on the line and apply the formula $d = \frac{|Ax_1 + By_1 + C|}{\sqrt{A^2 + B^2}}$ to find the distance between the line and the point (x_1, y_1).

EXAMPLE

Find the distance and midpoint between points (2, 4) and (8, 6).

MIDPOINT

$$\text{Midpoint} = \left(\frac{x_1 + x_2}{2}, \frac{y_1 + y_2}{2}\right)$$
$$\text{Midpoint} = \left(\frac{2 + 8}{2}, \frac{4 + 6}{2}\right)$$
$$\text{Midpoint} = \left(\frac{10}{2}, \frac{10}{2}\right)$$
$$\text{Midpoint} = (5,5)$$

DISTANCE

$$\text{Distance} = \sqrt{(x_2 - x_1)^2 + (y_2 - y_1)^2}$$
$$\text{Distance} = \sqrt{(8 - 2)^2 + (6 - 4)^2}$$
$$\text{Distance} = \sqrt{(6)^2 + (2)^2}$$
$$\text{Distance} = \sqrt{36 + 4}$$
$$\text{Distance} = \sqrt{40} \text{ or } 2\sqrt{10}$$

LAWS OF EXPONENTS

Multiply $(2x^4)^2(xy)^4 \cdot 4y^3$ using the **laws of exponents**.

According the order of operations, the first step in simplifying expressions is to evaluate within the parentheses. Moving from left to right, the first set of parentheses contains a power raised to a power. The rules of exponents state that when a power is raised to a power, you *multiply* the exponents. Since $4 \times 2 = 8$, $(2x^4)^2$ can be written as $4x^8$. The second set of parentheses raises a product to a power. The **rules of exponents** state that you raise every value within the parentheses to the given power. Therefore, $(xy)^4$ can be written as x^4y^4. Combining these terms with the last term gives you, $4x^8 \cdot x^4y^4 \cdot 4y^3$. In this expression, there are powers with the same base. The rules of exponents state that you *add* powers with the same base, while multiplying the coefficients. You can group the expression as $(4x^8 \cdot x^4) \cdot (y^4 \cdot 4y^3)$ to organize the values with the same base. Then, using this rule add the exponents. The result is $4x^{12} \cdot 4y^7$, or $16y^{12}y^7$.

> **Review Video: Laws of Exponents**
> Visit mometrix.com/academy and enter code: 532558

Measurement and Geometry

MEASUREMENT CONVERSION

When going from a larger unit to a smaller unit, multiply the number of the known amount by the **equivalent amount**. When going from a smaller unit to a larger unit, divide the number of the known amount by the equivalent amount.

Also, you can set up **conversion fractions**. In these fractions, one fraction is the **conversion factor**. The other fraction has the unknown amount in the numerator. So, the known value is placed in the denominator. Sometimes the second fraction has the known value from the problem in the numerator, and the unknown in the denominator. Multiply the two fractions to get the converted measurement.

CONVERSION UNITS

METRIC CONVERSIONS

1000 mcg (microgram)	1 mg
1000 mg (milligram)	1 g
1000 g (gram)	1 kg
1000 kg (kilogram)	1 metric ton
1000 mL (milliliter)	1 L
1000 um (micrometer)	1 mm
1000 mm (millimeter)	1 m
100 cm (centimeter)	1 m
1000 m (meter)	1 km

U.S. AND METRIC EQUIVALENTS

Unit	U.S. equivalent	Metric equivalent
Inch	1 inch	2.54 centimeters
Foot	12 inches	0.305 meters
Yard	3 feet	0.914 meters
Mile	5280 feet	1.609 kilometers

CAPACITY MEASUREMENTS

Unit	U.S. equivalent	Metric equivalent
Ounce	8 drams	29.573 milliliters
Cup	8 ounces	0.237 liter
Pint	16 ounces	0.473 liter
Quart	2 pints	0.946 liter
Gallon	4 quarts	3.785 liters

WEIGHT MEASUREMENTS

Unit	U.S. equivalent	Metric equivalent
Ounce	16 drams	28.35 grams
Pound	16 ounces	453.6 grams
Ton	2,000 pounds	907.2 kilograms

FLUID MEASUREMENTS

Unit	English equivalent	Metric equivalent
1 tsp	1 fluid dram	5 milliliters
3 tsp	4 fluid drams	15 or 16 milliliters
2 tbsp	1 fluid ounce	30 milliliters
1 glass	8 fluid ounces	240 milliliters

MEASUREMENT CONVERSION PRACTICE PROBLEMS

EXAMPLE 1

a. Convert 1.4 meters to centimeters.

b. Convert 218 centimeters to meters.

EXAMPLE 2

a. Convert 42 inches to feet.

b. Convert 15 feet to yards.

EXAMPLE 3

a. How many pounds are in 15 kilograms?

b. How many pounds are in 80 ounces?

EXAMPLE 4

a. How many kilometers are in 2 miles?

b. How many centimeters are in 5 feet?

EXAMPLE 5

a. How many gallons are in 15.14 liters?

b. How many liters are in 8 quarts?

EXAMPLE 6

a. How many grams are in 13.2 pounds?

b. How many pints are in 9 gallons?

MEASUREMENT CONVERSION PRACTICE SOLUTIONS

EXAMPLE 1

Write ratios with the conversion factor $\frac{100 \text{ cm}}{1 \text{ m}}$. Use proportions to convert the given units.

a. $\frac{100 \text{ cm}}{1 \text{ m}} = \frac{x \text{ cm}}{1.4 \text{ m}}$. Cross multiply to get $x = 140$. So, 1.4 m is the same as 140 cm.

b. $\frac{100\text{ cm}}{1\text{ m}} = \frac{218\text{ cm}}{x\text{ m}}$. Cross multiply to get $100x = 218$, or $x = 2.18$. So, 218 cm is the same as 2.18 m.

EXAMPLE 2

Write ratios with the conversion factors $\frac{12\text{ in}}{1\text{ ft}}$ and $\frac{3\text{ ft}}{1\text{ yd}}$. Use proportions to convert the given units.

a. $\frac{12\text{ in}}{1\text{ ft}} = \frac{42\text{ in}}{x\text{ ft}}$. Cross multiply to get $12x = 42$, or $x = 3.5$. So, 42 inches is the same as 3.5 feet.

b. $\frac{3\text{ ft}}{1\text{ yd}} = \frac{15\text{ ft}}{x\text{ yd}}$. Cross multiply to get $3x = 15$, or $x = 5$. So, 15 feet is the same as 5 yards.

EXAMPLE 3

a. 15 kilograms $\times \frac{2.2\text{ pounds}}{1\text{ kilogram}} = 33$ pounds

b. 80 ounces $\times \frac{1\text{ pound}}{16\text{ ounces}} = 5$ pounds

EXAMPLE 4

a. 2 miles $\times \frac{1.609\text{ kilometers}}{1\text{ mile}} = 3.218$ kilometers

b. 5 feet $\times \frac{12\text{ inches}}{1\text{ foot}} \times \frac{2.54\text{ centimeters}}{1\text{ inch}} = 152.4$ centimeters

EXAMPLE 5

a. 15.14 liters $\times \frac{1\text{ gallon}}{3.785\text{ liters}} = 4$ gallons

b. 8 quarts $\times \frac{1\text{ gallon}}{4\text{ quarts}} \times \frac{3.785\text{ liters}}{1\text{ gallon}} = 7.57$ liters

EXAMPLE 6

a. 13.2 pounds $\times \frac{1\text{ kilogram}}{2.2\text{ pounds}} \times \frac{1000\text{ grams}}{1\text{ kilogram}} = 6000$ grams

b. 9 gallons $\times \frac{4\text{ quarts}}{1\text{ gallon}} \times \frac{2\text{ pints}}{1\text{ quarts}} = 72$ pints

LINES AND PLANES

A **point** is a fixed location in space; has no size or dimensions; commonly represented by a dot.

A **line** is a set of points that extends infinitely in two opposite directions. It has length, but no width or depth. A line can be defined by any two distinct points that it contains. A **line segment** is a portion of a line that has definite endpoints. A **ray** is a portion of a line that extends from a single point on that line in one direction along the line. It has a definite beginning, but no ending.

A **plane** is a two-dimensional flat surface defined by three non-collinear points. A plane extends an infinite distance in all directions in those two dimensions. It contains an infinite number of points, parallel lines and segments, intersecting lines and segments, as well as parallel or intersecting rays. A plane will never contain a three-dimensional figure or skew lines. Two given planes will either be parallel or they will intersect to form a line. A plane may intersect a circular conic surface, such as a cone, to form conic sections, such as the parabola, hyperbola, circle or ellipse.

Perpendicular lines are lines that intersect at right angles. They are represented by the symbol ⊥. The shortest distance from a line to a point not on the line is a perpendicular segment from the point to the line.

Parallel lines are lines in the same plane that have no points in common and never meet. It is possible for lines to be in different planes, have no points in common, and never meet, but they are not parallel because they are in different planes.

A **bisector** is a line or line segment that divides another line segment into two equal lengths. A perpendicular bisector of a line segment is composed of points that are equidistant from the endpoints of the segment it is dividing.

Intersecting lines are lines that have exactly one point in common. Concurrent lines are multiple lines that intersect at a single point.

A **transversal** is a line that intersects at least two other lines, which may or may not be parallel to one another. A transversal that intersects parallel lines is a common occurrence in geometry.

REFLECTION OVER A LINE AND REFLECTION IN A POINT

A reflection of a figure over a *line* (a "flip") creates a congruent image that is the same distance from the line as the original figure but on the opposite side. The **line of reflection** is the perpendicular bisector of any line segment drawn from a point on the original figure to its reflected image (unless the point and its reflected image happen to be the same point, which happens when a figure is reflected over one of its own sides).

A reflection of a figure in a *point* is the same as the rotation of the figure 180° about that point. The image of the figure is congruent to the original figure. The **point of reflection** is the midpoint of a line segment which connects a point in the figure to its image (unless the point and its reflected image happen to be the same point, which happens when a figure is reflected in one of its own points).

> **Review Video: Reflection**
> Visit mometrix.com/academy and enter code: 955068

EXAMPLE

Use the coordinate plane of the given image below to reflect the image across the *y*-axis.

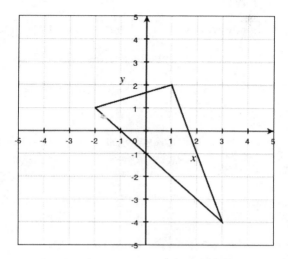

To reflect the image across the *y*-axis, replace each *x*-coordinate of the points that are the vertex of the triangle, *x*, with its negative, −*x*.

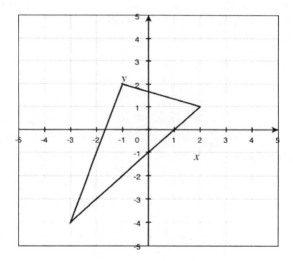

ANGLES

An angle is formed when two lines or line segments meet at a common point. It may be a common starting point for a pair of segments or rays, or it may be the intersection of lines. Angles are represented by the symbol ∠.

The **vertex** is the point at which two segments or rays meet to form an angle. If the angle is formed by intersecting rays, lines, and/or line segments, the vertex is the point at which four angles are formed. The pairs of angles opposite one another are called vertical angles, and their measures are equal.

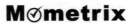

An **acute angle** is an angle with a degree measure less than 90°.

A **right angle** is an angle with a degree measure of exactly 90°.

An **obtuse angle** is an angle with a degree measure greater than 90° but less than 180°.

A **straight angle** is an angle with a degree measure of exactly 180°. This is also a semicircle.

A **reflex angle** is an angle with a degree measure greater than 180° but less than 360°.

A **full angle** is an angle with a degree measure of exactly 360°.

> **Review Video: <u>Geometric Symbols: Angles</u>**
> Visit mometrix.com/academy and enter code: 452738

Two angles whose sum is exactly 90° are said to be **complementary**. The two angles may or may not be adjacent. In a right triangle, the two acute angles are complementary.

Two angles whose sum is exactly 180° are said to be **supplementary**. The two angles may or may not be adjacent. Two intersecting lines always form two pairs of supplementary angles. Adjacent supplementary angles will always form a straight line.

Two angles that have the same vertex and share a side are said to be **adjacent**. Vertical angles are not adjacent because they share a vertex but no common side.

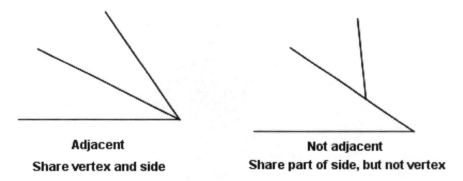

Adjacent
Share vertex and side

Not adjacent
Share part of side, but not vertex

When two parallel lines are cut by a transversal, the angles that are between the two parallel lines are **interior angles**. In the diagram below, angles 3, 4, 5, and 6 are interior angles.

When two parallel lines are cut by a transversal, the angles that are outside the parallel lines are **exterior angles**. In the diagram below, angles 1, 2, 7, and 8 are exterior angles.

When two parallel lines are cut by a transversal, the angles that are in the same position relative to the transversal and a parallel line are **corresponding angles**. The diagram below has four pairs of corresponding angles: angles 1 and 5; angles 2 and 6; angles 3 and 7; and angles 4 and 8. Corresponding angles formed by parallel lines are congruent.

When two parallel lines are cut by a transversal, the two interior angles that are on opposite sides of the transversal are called **alternate interior angles**. In the diagram below, there are two pairs of alternate interior angles: angles 3 and 6, and angles 4 and 5. Alternate interior angles formed by parallel lines are congruent.

When two parallel lines are cut by a transversal, the two exterior angles that are on opposite sides of the transversal are called **alternate exterior angles**.

In the diagram below, there are two pairs of alternate exterior angles: angles 1 and 8, and angles 2 and 7. Alternate exterior angles formed by parallel lines are congruent.

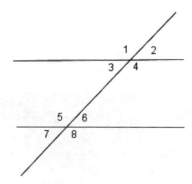

When two lines intersect, four angles are formed. The non-adjacent angles at this vertex are called **vertical angles**. Vertical angles are congruent. In the diagram, $\angle ABD \cong \angle CBE$ and $\angle ABC \cong \angle DBE$.

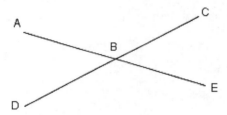

POLYGONS

Each straight line segment of a polygon is called a **side**.

The point at which two sides of a polygon intersect is called the **vertex**. In a polygon, the number of sides is always equal to the number of vertices.

A polygon with all sides congruent and all angles equal is called a **regular polygon**.

A line segment from the center of a polygon perpendicular to a side of the polygon is called the **apothem**. In a regular polygon, the apothem can be used to find the area of the polygon using the formula $A = \frac{1}{2}ap$, where a is the apothem and p is the perimeter.

A line segment from the center of a polygon to a vertex of the polygon is called a **radius**. The radius of a regular polygon is also the radius of a circle that can be circumscribed about the polygon.

Triangle – 3 sides

Quadrilateral – 4 sides

Pentagon – 5 sides

Hexagon – 6 sides

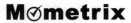

Heptagon – 7 sides

Octagon – 8 sides

Nonagon – 9 sides

Decagon – 10 sides

Dodecagon – 12 sides

More generally, an **n-gon** is a polygon that has *n* angles and *n* sides.

The sum of the interior angles of an *n*-sided polygon is (n – 2)180°. For example, in a triangle $n = 3$, so the sum of the interior angles is $(3 - 2)180° = 180°$. In a quadrilateral, $n = 4$, and the sum of the angles is $(4 - 2)180° = 360°$. The sum of the interior angles of a polygon is equal to the sum of the interior angles of any other polygon with the same number of sides.

A **diagonal** is a line segment that joins two non-adjacent vertices of a polygon.

A **convex polygon** is a polygon whose diagonals all lie within the interior of the polygon.

A **concave polygon** is a polygon with a least one diagonal that lies outside the polygon. In the diagram below, quadrilateral *ABCD* is concave because diagonal $\overline{AC}$ lies outside the polygon.

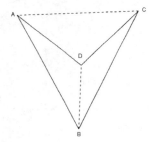

The number of diagonals a polygon has can be found by using the formula: number of diagonals = $\frac{n(n-3)}{2}$, where *n* is the number of sides in the polygon. This formula works for all polygons, not just regular polygons.

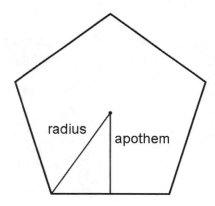

96

Congruent figures are geometric figures that have the same size and shape. All corresponding angles are equal, and all corresponding sides are equal. It is indicated by the symbol ≅.

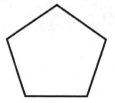 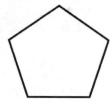

Congruent polygons

Similar figures are geometric figures that have the same shape, but do not necessarily have the same size. All corresponding angles are equal, and all corresponding sides are proportional, but they do not have to be equal. It is indicated by the symbol ~.

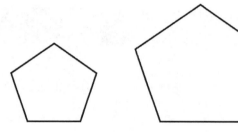

Similar polygons

Note that all congruent figures are also similar, but not all similar figures are congruent.

Review Video: Polygons, Similarity, and Congruence
Visit mometrix.com/academy and enter code: 686174

LINE OF SYMMETRY

A line of symmetry is a line that divides a figure or object into two symmetric parts. Each symmetric half is congruent to the other. An object may have no lines of symmetry, one line of symmetry, or more than one line of symmetry.

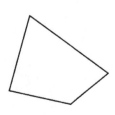 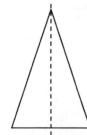 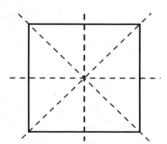

No lines of symmetry   One line of symmetry   Multiple lines of symmetry

97

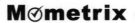

Quadrilateral: A closed two-dimensional geometric figure composed of exactly four straight sides. The sum of the interior angles of any quadrilateral is 360°.

PARALLELOGRAM

A parallelogram is a quadrilateral that has exactly two pairs of opposite parallel sides. The sides that are parallel are also congruent. The opposite interior angles are always congruent, and the consecutive interior angles are supplementary. The diagonals of a parallelogram bisect each other. Each diagonal divides the parallelogram into two congruent triangles.

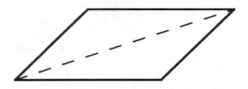

TRAPEZOID

Traditionally, a trapezoid is a quadrilateral that has exactly one pair of parallel sides. Some math texts define trapezoid as a quadrilateral that has at least one pair of parallel sides. Because there are no rules governing the second pair of sides, there are no rules that apply to the properties of the diagonals of a trapezoid.

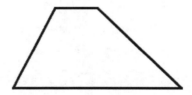

Rectangles, rhombuses, and squares are all special forms of parallelograms.

RECTANGLE

A rectangle is a parallelogram with four right angles. All rectangles are parallelograms, but not all parallelograms are rectangles. The diagonals of a rectangle are congruent.

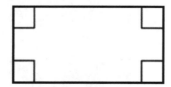

RHOMBUS

A rhombus is a parallelogram with four congruent sides. All rhombuses are parallelograms, but not all parallelograms are rhombuses. The diagonals of a rhombus are perpendicular to each other.

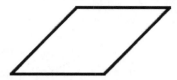

Review Video: Diagonals of Parallelograms, Rectangles, and Rhombi
Visit mometrix.com/academy and enter code: 320040

SQUARE

A square is a parallelogram with four right angles and four congruent sides. All squares are also parallelograms, rhombuses, and rectangles. The diagonals of a square are congruent and perpendicular to each other.

A quadrilateral whose diagonals bisect each other is a **parallelogram**. A quadrilateral whose opposite sides are parallel (2 pairs of parallel sides) is a parallelogram.

A quadrilateral whose diagonals are perpendicular bisectors of each other is a **rhombus**. A quadrilateral whose opposite sides (both pairs) are parallel and congruent is a rhombus.

A parallelogram that has a right angle is a **rectangle**. (Consecutive angles of a parallelogram are supplementary. Therefore, if there is one right angle in a parallelogram, there are four right angles in that parallelogram.)

A rhombus with one right angle is a **square**. Because the rhombus is a special form of a parallelogram, the rules about the angles of a parallelogram also apply to the rhombus.

AREA AND PERIMETER FORMULAS

TRIANGLE

The **perimeter of any triangle** is found by summing the three side lengths; $P = a + b + c$. For an equilateral triangle, this is the same as $P = 3s$, where s is any side length, since all three sides are the same length.

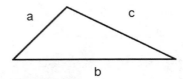

The **area of any triangle** can be found by taking half the product of one side length (base or b) and the perpendicular distance from that side to the opposite vertex (height or h). In equation form, $A = \frac{1}{2}bh$. For many triangles, it may be difficult to calculate h, so using one of the other formulas given here may be easier.

Another formula that works for any triangle is $A = \sqrt{s(s-a)(s-b)(s-c)}$, where A is the area, s is the semiperimeter $s = \frac{a+b+c}{2}$, and a, b, and c are the lengths of the three sides.

The **area of an equilateral triangle** can be found by the formula $A = \frac{\sqrt{3}}{4}s^2$, where A is the area and s is the length of a side. You could use the $30° - 60° - 90°$ ratios to find the height of the triangle and then use the standard triangle area formula, but this is faster.

The **area of an isosceles triangle** can be found by the formula, $A = \frac{1}{2}b\sqrt{a^2 - \frac{b^2}{4}}$, where A is the area, b is the base (the unique side), and a is the length of one of the two congruent sides. If you do not remember this formula, you can use the Pythagorean theorem to find the height so you can use the standard formula for the area of a triangle.

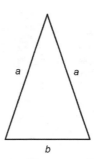

Review Video: Area and Perimeter of a Triangle
Visit mometrix.com/academy and enter code: 853779

SQUARE

The **area of a square** is found by using the formula $A = s^2$, where and s is the length of one side.

The **perimeter of a square** is found by using the formula $P = 4s$, where s is the length of one side. Because all four sides are equal in a square, it is faster to multiply the length of one side by 4 than to add the same number four times. You could use the formulas for rectangles and get the same answer.

RECTANGLE

The **area of a rectangle** is found by the formula $A = lw$, where A is the area of the rectangle, l is the length (usually considered to be the longer side) and w is the width (usually considered to be the shorter side). The numbers for l and w are interchangeable.

The **perimeter of a rectangle** is found by the formula $P = 2l + 2w$ or $P = 2(l + w)$, where l is the length, and w is the width. It may be easier to add the length and width first and then double the result, as in the second formula.

PARALLELOGRAM

The **area of a parallelogram** is found by the formula $A = bh$, where b is the length of the base, and h is the height. Note that the base and height correspond to the length and width in a rectangle, so this formula would apply to rectangles as well. Do not confuse the height of a parallelogram with the length of the second side. The two are only the same measure in the case of a rectangle.

The **perimeter of a parallelogram** is found by the formula $P = 2a + 2b$ or $P = 2(a + b)$, where a and b are the lengths of the two sides.

TRAPEZOID

The **area of a trapezoid** is found by the formula $A = \frac{1}{2}h(b_1 + b_2)$, where h is the height (segment joining and perpendicular to the parallel bases), and b_1 and b_2 are the two parallel sides (bases). Do not use one of the other two sides as the height unless that side is also perpendicular to the parallel bases.

The **perimeter of a trapezoid** is found by the formula $P = a + b_1 + c + b_2$, where a, b_1, c, and b_2 are the four sides of the trapezoid.

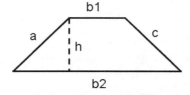

TRIANGLES

An **equilateral triangle** is a triangle with three congruent sides. An equilateral triangle will also have three congruent angles, each 60°. All equilateral triangles are also acute triangles.

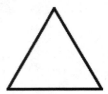

An **isosceles triangle** is a triangle with two congruent sides. An isosceles triangle will also have two congruent angles opposite the two congruent sides.

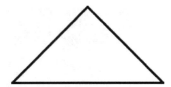

A **scalene triangle** is a triangle with no congruent sides. A scalene triangle will also have three angles of different measures. The angle with the largest measure is opposite the longest side, and the angle with the smallest measure is opposite the shortest side.

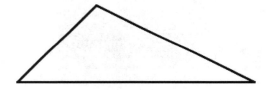

An **acute triangle** is a triangle whose three angles are all less than 90°. If two of the angles are equal, the acute triangle is also an isosceles triangle. If the three angles are all equal, the acute triangle is also an equilateral triangle.

A **right triangle** is a triangle with exactly one angle equal to 90°. All right triangles follow the Pythagorean theorem. A right triangle can never be acute or obtuse.

An **obtuse triangle** is a triangle with exactly one angle greater than 90°. The other two angles may or may not be equal. If the two remaining angles are equal, the obtuse triangle is also an isosceles triangle.

Review Video: Introduction to Types of Triangles
Visit mometrix.com/academy and enter code: 511711

102

ALTITUDE OF A TRIANGLE

A line segment drawn from one vertex perpendicular to the opposite side. In the diagram below, $\overline{BE}$, $\overline{AD}$, and $\overline{CF}$ are altitudes. The three altitudes in a triangle are always concurrent.

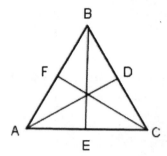

Height of a Triangle

The length of the altitude, although the two terms are often used interchangeably.

Orthocenter of a Triangle

The point of concurrency of the altitudes of a triangle. Note that in an obtuse triangle, the orthocenter will be outside the triangle, and in a right triangle, the orthocenter is the vertex of the right angle.

Median of a Triangle

A line segment drawn from one vertex to the midpoint of the opposite side. This is not the same as the altitude, except the altitude to the base of an isosceles triangle and all three altitudes of an equilateral triangle.

CENTROID OF A TRIANGLE

The point of concurrency of the medians of a triangle. This is the same point as the orthocenter only in an equilateral triangle. Unlike the orthocenter, the centroid is always inside the triangle. The centroid can also be considered the exact center of the triangle. Any shape triangle can be perfectly balanced on a tip placed at the centroid. The centroid is also the point that is two-thirds the distance from the vertex to the opposite side.

PYTHAGOREAN THEOREM

The side of a triangle opposite the right angle is called the **hypotenuse**. The other two sides are called the legs. The Pythagorean theorem states a relationship among the legs and hypotenuse of a right triangle: $a^2 + b^2 = c^2$, where a and b are the lengths of the legs of a right triangle, and c is the length of the hypotenuse. Note that this formula will only work with right triangles.

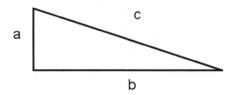

Review Video: Pythagorean Theorem
Visit mometrix.com/academy and enter code: 906576

103

GENERAL RULES

The **triangle inequality theorem** states that the sum of the measures of any two sides of a triangle is always greater than the measure of the third side. If the sum of the measures of two sides were equal to the third side, a triangle would be impossible because the two sides would lie flat across the third side and there would be no vertex. If the sum of the measures of two of the sides was less than the third side, a closed figure would be impossible because the two shortest sides would never meet.

The **sum of the measures of the interior angles** of a triangle is always 180°. Therefore, a triangle can never have more than one angle greater than or equal to 90°.

In any triangle, the angles opposite congruent sides are congruent, and the sides opposite congruent angles are congruent. The largest angle is always opposite the longest side, and the smallest angle is always opposite the shortest side.

The line segment that joins the midpoints of any two sides of a triangle is always parallel to the third side and exactly half the length of the third side.

SIMILARITY AND CONGRUENCE RULES

Similar triangles are triangles whose corresponding angles are equal and whose corresponding sides are proportional. Represented by **AA**. Similar triangles whose corresponding sides are congruent are also congruent triangles.

> **Review Video: Similar Triangles**
> Visit mometrix.com/academy and enter code: 398538

Three sides of one triangle are congruent to the three corresponding sides of the second triangle. Represented as **SSS**.

Two sides and the included angle (the angle formed by those two sides) of one triangle are congruent to the corresponding two sides and included angle of the second triangle. Represented by **SAS**.

Two angles and the included side (the side that joins the two angles) of one triangle are congruent to the corresponding two angles and included side of the second triangle. Represented by **ASA**.

Two angles and a non-included side of one triangle are congruent to the corresponding two angles and non-included side of the second triangle. Represented by **AAS**.

Note that **AAA** is not a form for congruent triangles. This would say that the three angles are congruent, but says nothing about the sides. This meets the requirements for similar triangles, but not congruent triangles.

TRANSFORMATIONS

A **translation** is a transformation which slides a figure from one position in the plane to another position in the plane. The original figure and the translated figure have the same size, shape, and orientation.

> **Review Video: Translation**
> Visit mometrix.com/academy and enter code: 718628

To **rotate** a given figure: 1. Identify the point of rotation. 2. Using tracing paper, geometry software, or by approximation, recreate the figure at a new location around the point of rotation.

To **reflect** a given figure: 1. Identify the line of reflection. 2. By folding the paper, using geometry software, or by approximation, recreate the image at a new location on the other side of the line of reflection.

To **translate** a given figure: 1. Identify the new location. 2. Using graph paper, geometry software, or by approximation, recreate the figure in the new location. If using graph paper, make a chart of the x- and y-values to keep track of the coordinates of all critical points.

A **dilation** is a transformation which proportionally stretches or shrinks a figure by a **scale factor**. The dilated image is the same shape and orientation as the original image but a different size. A polygon and its dilated image are similar.

EXAMPLE 1

Use the coordinate plane to create a dilation of the given image below, where the dilation is the enlargement of the original image.

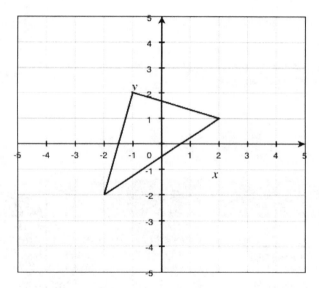

An **enlargement** can be found by multiplying each coordinate of the coordinate pairs located at the triangles vertices by a constant. If the figure is enlarged by a factor of 2, the new image would be:

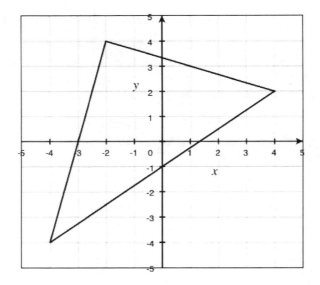

CIRCLES

The **center** is the single point inside the circle that is **equidistant** from every point on the circle. (Point *O* in the diagram below.)

The **radius** is a line segment that joins the center of the circle and any one point on the circle. All radii of a circle are equal. (Segments *OX*, *OY*, and *OZ* in the diagram below.)

The **diameter** is a line segment that passes through the center of the circle and has both endpoints on the circle. The length of the diameter is exactly twice the length of the radius. (Segment *XZ* in the diagram below.)

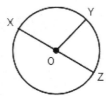

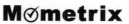

The **area of a circle** is found by the formula $A = \pi r^2$, where r is the length of the radius. If the diameter of the circle is given, remember to divide it in half to get the length of the radius before proceeding.

Review Video: The Diameter, Radius, and Circumference of Circles
Visit mometrix.com/academy and enter code: 448988

The **circumference** of a circle is found by the formula $C = 2\pi r$, where r is the radius. Again, remember to convert the diameter if you are given that measure rather than the radius.

Review Video: Area and Circumference of a Circle
Visit mometrix.com/academy and enter code: 243015

Concentric circles are circles that have the same center, but not the same length of radii. A bulls-eye target is an example of concentric circles.

An **arc** is a portion of a circle. Specifically, an arc is the set of points between and including two points on a circle. An arc does not contain any points inside the circle. When a segment is drawn from the endpoints of an arc to the center of the circle, a sector is formed.

A **central angle** is an angle whose vertex is the center of a circle and whose legs intercept an arc of the circle. Angle *XOY* in the diagram above is a central angle. A minor arc is an arc that has a measure less than 180°. The measure of a central angle is equal to the measure of the minor arc it intercepts. A major arc is an arc having a measure of at least 180°. The measure of the major arc can be found by subtracting the measure of the central angle from 360°.

A **semicircle** is an arc whose endpoints are the endpoints of the diameter of a circle. A semicircle is exactly half of a circle.

An **inscribed angle** is an angle whose vertex lies on a circle and whose legs contain chords of that circle. The portion of the circle intercepted by the legs of the angle is called the intercepted arc. The measure of the intercepted arc is exactly twice the measure of the inscribed angle. In the following diagram, angle *ABC* is an inscribed angle. $\overset{\frown}{AC} = 2(\text{m}\angle ABC)$

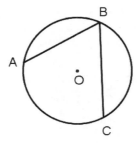

Any angle inscribed in a semicircle is a right angle. The intercepted arc is 180°, making the inscribed angle half that, or 90°. In the diagram below, angle *ABC* is inscribed in semicircle *ABC*, making angle *ABC* equal to 90°.

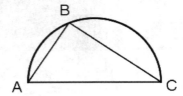

A **chord** is a line segment that has both endpoints on a circle. In the diagram below, $\overline{EB}$ is a chord.

Secant: A line that passes through a circle and contains a chord of that circle. In the diagram below, $\overleftrightarrow{EB}$ is a secant and contains chord $\overline{EB}$.

A **tangent** is a line in the same plane as a circle that touches the circle in exactly one point. While a line segment can be tangent to a circle as part of a line that is tangent, it is improper to say a tangent can be simply a line segment that touches the circle in exactly one point. In the diagram below, $\overleftrightarrow{CD}$ is tangent to circle *A*. Notice that $\overline{FB}$ is not tangent to the circle. $\overline{FB}$ is a line segment that touches the circle in exactly one point, but if the segment were extended, it would touch the circle in a second point. The point at which a tangent touches a circle is called the **point of tangency**. In the diagram below, point *B* is the point of tangency.

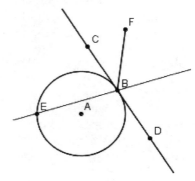

A **secant** is a line that intersects a circle in two points. Two secants may intersect inside the circle, on the circle, or outside the circle. When the two secants intersect on the circle, an inscribed angle is formed.

When two secants intersect inside a circle, the measure of each of two vertical angles is equal to half the sum of the two intercepted arcs. In the diagram below, m∠*AEB* = $\frac{1}{2}(\widehat{AB} + \widehat{CD})$ and m∠*BEC* = $\frac{1}{2}(\widehat{BC} + \widehat{AD})$.

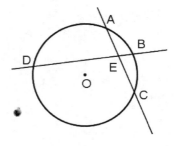

When two secants intersect outside a circle, the measure of the angle formed is equal to half the difference of the two arcs that lie between the two secants. In the diagram below, m$\angle AEB = \frac{1}{2}(\widehat{AB} - \widehat{CD})$.

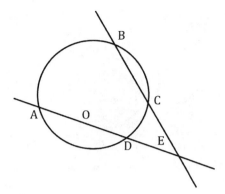

The **arc length** is the length of that portion of the circumference between two points on the circle. The formula for arc length is $s = \frac{\pi r \theta}{180°}$ where s is the arc length, r is the length of the radius, and θ is the angular measure of the arc in degrees, or $s = r\theta$, where θ is the angular measure of the arc in radians (2π radians = 360 degrees).

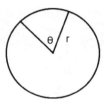

A **sector** is the portion of a circle formed by two radii and their intercepted arc. While the arc length is exclusively the points that are also on the circumference of the circle, the sector is the entire area bounded by the arc and the two radii.

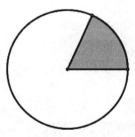

The **area of a sector** of a circle is found by the formula, $A = \frac{\theta r^2}{2}$, where A is the area, θ is the measure of the central angle in radians, and r is the radius. To find the area when the central angle is in degrees, use the formula, $A = \frac{\theta \pi r^2}{360}$, where θ is the measure of the central angle in degrees and r is the radius.

A circle is **inscribed** in a polygon if each of the sides of the polygon is tangent to the circle. A polygon is inscribed in a circle if each of the vertices of the polygon lies on the circle.

A circle is **circumscribed** about a polygon if each of the vertices of the polygon lies on the circle. A polygon is circumscribed about the circle if each of the sides of the polygon is tangent to the circle.

If one figure is inscribed in another, then the other figure is circumscribed about the first figure.

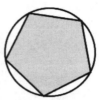

Circle circumscribed about a pentagon
Pentagon inscribed in a circle

SOLIDS

The **surface area** of a solid object is the area of all sides or exterior surfaces. For objects such as prisms and pyramids, a further distinction is made between base surface area (B) and lateral surface area (LA). For a prism, the total surface area (SA) is $SA = LA + 2B$. For a pyramid or cone, the total surface area is $SA = LA + B$.

Review Video: How to Calculate the Volume of 3D Objects
Visit mometrix.com/academy and enter code: 163343

The **surface area of a sphere** can be found by the formula $A = 4\pi r^2$, where r is the radius. The **volume** is given by the formula $V = \frac{4}{3}\pi r^3$, where r is the radius. Both quantities are generally given in terms of π.

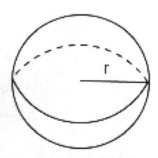

Review Video: Volume and Surface Area of a Sphere
Visit mometrix.com/academy and enter code: 786928

The **volume of any prism** is found by the formula $V = Bh$, where B is the area of the base, and h is the height (perpendicular distance between the bases). The surface area of any prism is the sum of the areas of both bases and all sides. It can be calculated as $SA = 2B + Ph$, where P is the perimeter of the base.

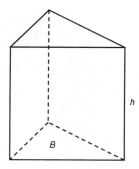

For a **rectangular prism**, the **volume** can be found by the formula $V = lwh$, where V is the volume, l is the length, w is the width, and h is the height. The surface area can be calculated as $SA = 2lw + 2hl + 2wh$ or $SA = 2(lw + hl + wh)$.

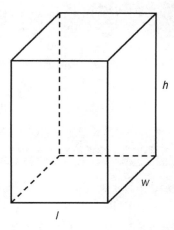

The **volume of a cube** can be found by the formula $V = s^3$, where s is the length of a side. The surface area of a cube is calculated as $SA = 6s^2$, where SA is the total surface area and s is the length of a side. These formulas are the same as the ones used for the volume and surface area of a rectangular prism, but simplified since all three quantities (length, width, and height) are the same.

> **Review Video: <u>Volume and Surface Area of a Cube</u>**
> Visit mometrix.com/academy and enter code: 664455

The **volume of a cylinder** can be calculated by the formula $V = \pi r^2 h$, where r is the radius, and h is the height. The surface area of a cylinder can be found by the formula $SA = 2\pi r^2 + 2\pi r h$. The first term is the base area multiplied by two, and the second term is the perimeter of the base multiplied by the height.

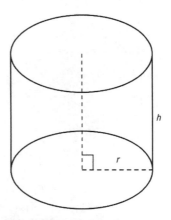

The **volume of a pyramid** is found by the formula $V = \frac{1}{3}Bh$, where B is the area of the base, and h is the height (perpendicular distance from the vertex to the base). Notice this formula is the same as $\frac{1}{3}$ times the volume of a prism. Like a prism, the base of a pyramid can be any shape.

Finding the **surface area of a pyramid** is not as simple as the other shapes we've looked at thus far. If the pyramid is a right pyramid, meaning the base is a regular polygon and the vertex is directly over the center of that polygon, the surface area can be calculated as $SA = B + \frac{1}{2}Ph_s$, where P is the perimeter of the base, and h_s is the slant height (distance from the vertex to the midpoint of one side of the base). If the pyramid is irregular, the area of each triangle side must be calculated individually and then summed, along with the base.

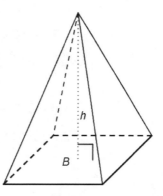

The **volume of a cone** is found by the formula $V = \frac{1}{3}\pi r^2 h$, where r is the radius, and h is the height. Notice this is the same as $\frac{1}{3}$ times the volume of a cylinder. The surface area can be calculated as $SA = \pi r^2 + \pi rs$, where s is the slant height. The slant height can be calculated using the

Pythagorean Thereom to be $\sqrt{r^2 + h^2}$, so the surface area formula can also be written as $SA = \pi r^2 + \pi r \sqrt{r^2 + h^2}$.

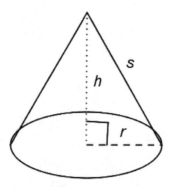

Review Video: <u>Volume and Surface Area of a Right Circular Cone</u>
Visit mometrix.com/academy and enter code: 573574

Mathematics Chapter Quiz

1.

  4,307
+1,864
___

     a. 5,161
     b. 5,271
     c. 6,171
     d. 6,271

2. $7\overline{)917}$

     a. 131
     b. 131 R4
     c. 145
     d. 145 R4

3. 32 is what percent of 80?

     a. 25%
     b. 32%
     c. 40%
     d. 44%

4. Sheila, Janice, and Karen, working together at the same rate, can complete a job in 3 1/3 days. Working at the same rate, how much of the job could Janice and Karen do in one day?

     a. 1/5
     b. 1/4
     c. 1/3
     d. 1/9

5. Which formula shown below is the correct formula for finding the area of the following polygon?

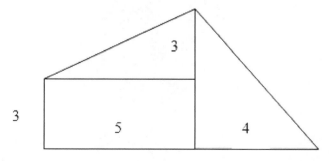

     a. (3 x 5)/2 + (3 x 5) + (4 x 6)/2
     b. 2(3 x 5) + (4 x 6)/2
     c. (3 x 5) + (3 x 6)/x + (4 x 6)
     d. (5 x 6) + (4 x 6)/2

6. The scientific notation for the diameter of a red blood cell is approximately 7.4×10^{-4} centimeters. What is that amount in standard form?

    a. 0.00074
    b. 0.0074
    c. 7.40000
    d. 296

7. A woman wants to stack two small bookcases beneath a window that is 26½ inches from the floor. The larger bookcase is 14½ inches tall. The other bookcase is 8¾ inches tall. How tall will the two bookcases be when they are stacked together?

    a. 12 inches tall
    b. 23¼ inches tall
    c. 35¼ inches tall
    d. 41 inches tall

8. 0.023 as a percentage

    a. 23%
    b. 2.3%
    c. .23%
    d. .023%

9. $2(r + 4) + 8 = (r + 3)4$

    a. $r = -2$
    b. $r = 2$
    c. $r = -4$
    d. $r = 4$

10. Which algebraic expression best represents the following statement: the number of books Brian read over the summer (B) is 2 less than 3 times the number of books his brother Adam read over the summer (A)?

    a. B = 3A – 2
    b. B = 3A + 2
    c. A = 3B – 2
    d. A = 3B + 2

Mathematics Chapter Quiz Answers

1. C: This is a simple addition problem with carrying. Start with the ones column and add 7+4, write down the 1 and add the 1 to the digits in the ten's column. Now add 0+6+1. Write down the 7. Now add 3+8 and write down the 1. Add the 1 to the thousand's column. Add 4+1+1 and write the 6 to get the answer 6171.

$$
\begin{array}{r} 4307 \\ +\ 1864 \\ \hline \end{array}
\qquad
\begin{array}{r} {\scriptstyle +1} \\ 4307 \\ +\ 1864 \\ \hline 1 \end{array}
\qquad
\begin{array}{r} 4307 \\ +\ 1864 \\ \hline 71 \end{array}
\qquad
\begin{array}{r} {\scriptstyle +1} \\ 4307 \\ +\ 1864 \\ \hline 171 \end{array}
\qquad
\begin{array}{r} 4307 \\ +\ 1864 \\ \hline 6171 \end{array}
$$

2. A: This is a simple division problem. Divide the 7 into 9. It goes in 1 time. Write 1 above the 9 and subtract 7 from 9 to get 2. Bring down the 1 and place it beside the 2. Divide 7 into 21. It goes in 3 times. Divide 7 into 7. It goes 1 time.

$$
\begin{array}{r}
131 \\
7\overline{)\ 917} \\
\underline{7} \\
21 \\
\underline{21} \\
07 \\
\underline{07} \\
0
\end{array}
$$

3. C: This problem is solved by finding x in this equation: $32/80 = x/100$.

4. A: If it takes 3 people 3 1/3 days to do the job, then it would take one person 10 days: $3 \times 3\frac{1}{3} = 10$. Thus, it would take 2 people 5 days, and one day of work for two people would complete 1/5 of the job.

5. A: To find the area of the parallelogram, the area of each shape must be determined and then added together. The area of the smaller triangle is (3 x 5)/2. The area of the rectangle is (3 x 5), and the area of the larger triangle is (4 x 6)/2. This leaves only the formula provided in answer choice A.

6. A: To solve, you will need to move the decimal 4 places. Since the scientific notation had a negative power of 10, move the decimal left. If the power of 10 had been positive, you would have needed to move it to the right. In this problem, solve as follows:

7.4 x 10^{-4}

7.4 x 1/10,000

7.4 x 0.0001

0.00074

7. B: Add to solve. The height of the window from the floor is not needed in this equation. It is extra information. You only need to add the heights of the two bookcases. Change the fractions so that they have a common denominator. After you add, simplify the fraction.

$14\frac{1}{2} + 8\frac{3}{4}$

$= 14 \; 2/4 + 8\frac{3}{4}$

$= 22 \; 5/4$

$= 23\frac{1}{4}$

8. B: To change a decimal to a percent, multiply it by 100 by moving the decimal point two spaces to the right.

9. B: To solve, first do the operations in parenthesis, then add/subtract like terms in order to get like terms on opposite sides of the equation: $2r + 8 + 8 = 4r + 12$

$2r + 16 = 4r + 12; \; 4 = 2r; \; r = 2$

10. A: The correct answer is B = 3A - 2.

Biology

Cells: Structure and Function

CELL STRUCTURE

- **Ribosomes**: Ribosomes are involved in synthesizing proteins from amino acids. They are numerous, making up about one quarter of the cell. Some cells contain thousands of ribosomes. Some are mobile and some are embedded in the rough endoplasmic reticulum.
- **Golgi complex** (Golgi apparatus): This is involved in synthesizing materials such as proteins that are transported out of the cell. It is located near the nucleus and consists of layers of membranes.
- **Vacuoles**: These are sacs used for storage, digestion, and waste removal. There is one large vacuole in plant cells. Animal cells have small, sometimes numerous vacuoles.
- **Vesicle**: This is a small organelle within a cell. It has a membrane and performs varying functions, including moving materials within a cell.
- **Cytoskeleton**: This consists of microtubules that help shape and support the cell.
- **Microtubules**: These are part of the cytoskeleton and help support the cell. They are made of protein.
- **Cytosol**: This is the liquid material in the cell. It is mostly water, but also contains some floating molecules.
- **Cytoplasm**: This is a general term that refers to cytosol and the substructures (organelles) found within the plasma membrane, but not within the nucleus.
- **Cell membrane** (plasma membrane): This defines the cell by acting as a barrier. It helps keeps cytoplasm in and substances located outside the cell out. It also determines what is allowed to enter and exit the cell. Some cell membranes are composed of a phospholipid bilayer.
- **Endoplasmic reticulum**: The two types of endoplasmic reticulum are rough (has ribosomes on the surface) and smooth (does not have ribosomes on the surface). It is a tubular network that comprises the transport system of a cell. It is fused to the nuclear membrane and extends through the cytoplasm to the cell membrane.
- **Mitochondrion** (pl. mitochondria): These cell structures vary in terms of size and quantity. Some cells may have one mitochondrion, while others have thousands. This structure performs various functions such as generating ATP, and is also involved in cell growth and death. Mitochondria contain their own DNA that is separate from that contained in the nucleus.

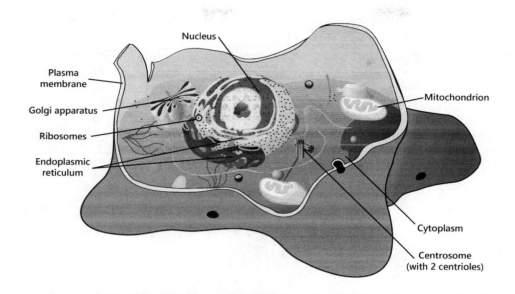

Review Video: <u>Mitochondria</u>
Visit mometrix.com/academy and enter code: 444287

NUCLEAR PARTS OF A CELL

- **Nucleus** (pl. nuclei): This is a small structure that contains the chromosomes and regulates the DNA of a cell. The nucleus is the defining structure of eukaryotic cells, and all eukaryotic cells have a nucleus. The nucleus is responsible for the passing on of genetic traits between generations. The nucleus contains a nuclear envelope, nucleoplasm, a nucleolus, nuclear pores, chromatin, and ribosomes.
- **Chromosomes**: These are highly condensed, threadlike rods of DNA. Short for deoxyribonucleic acid, DNA is the genetic material that stores information.
- **Chromatin**: This consists of the DNA and protein that make up chromosomes.
- **Nucleolus** (nucleole): This structure contained within the nucleus consists of protein. It is small, round, does not have a membrane, is involved in protein synthesis, and synthesizes and stores RNA (ribonucleic acid).
- **Nuclear envelope**: This encloses the structures of the nucleus. It consists of inner and outer membranes made of lipids.

- **Nuclear pores**: These are involved in the exchange of material between the nucleus and the cytoplasm.
- **Nucleoplasm**: This is the liquid within the nucleus, and is similar to cytoplasm.

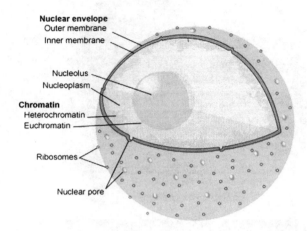

PLANT CELL STRUCTURE

- **Cell wall**: Made of cellulose and composed of numerous layers, the cell wall provides plants with a sturdy barrier that can hold fluid within the cell. The cell wall surrounds the cell membrane.
- **Chloroplast**: This is a specialized organelle that plant cells use for photosynthesis, which is the process plants use to create food energy from sunlight. Chloroplasts contain **chlorophyll**, which has a green color.

- **Plastid**: This is a membrane-bound organelle found in plant cells that is used to make chemical compounds and store food. It can also contain pigments used during photosynthesis. Plastids can develop into more specialized structures such as chloroplasts, chromoplasts (make and hold yellow and orange pigments), amyloplasts (store starch), and leucoplasts (lack pigments, but can become differentiated).
- **Plasmodesmata** (sing. plasmodesma): These are channels between the cell walls of plant cells that allow for transport between cells.

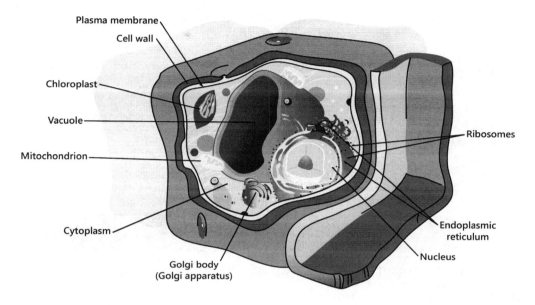

ANIMAL CELL STRUCTURE

- **Centrosome**: This is comprised of the pair of centrioles located at right angles to each other and surrounded by protein. The centrosome is involved in mitosis and the cell cycle.
- **Centriole**: These are cylinder-shaped structures near the nucleus that are involved in cellular division. Each cylinder consists of nine groups of three microtubules. Centrioles occur in pairs.
- **Lysosome**: This digests proteins, lipids, and carbohydrates, and also transports undigested substances to the cell membrane so they can be removed. The shape of a lysosome depends on the material being transported.
- **Cilia** (singular: cilium): These are appendages extending from the surface of the cell, the movement of which causes the cell to move. They can also result in fluid being moved by the cell.
- **Flagella**: These are tail-like structures on cells that use whip-like movements to help the cell move. They are similar to cilia, but are usually longer and not as numerous. A cell usually only has one or a few flagella.

PROKARYOTIC AND EUKARYOTIC CELLS

Cells can be broadly characterized as prokaryotic and eukaryotic. The main difference is that **eukaryotic cells** have a nucleus and **prokaryotic cells** do not. In eukaryotic cells, DNA is mostly contained in chromosomes in the nucleus, although there is some DNA in mitochondria and chloroplasts. In prokaryotic cells, the genetic material aggregates in the cytoplasm in a nucleoid.

There are other differences. Eukaryotic cells are considered more complex than prokaryotic cells. Eukaryotic cells have membrane-bound organelles that perform various functions and contribute to the complexity of these types of cells. Prokaryotic cells do not contain membrane-bound organelles. Prokaryotic cells usually divide by binary fission and are haploid. Eukaryotic cells divide by mitosis and are diploid.

Plant and animal cells are eukaryotic. **Bacteria** are prokaryotic.

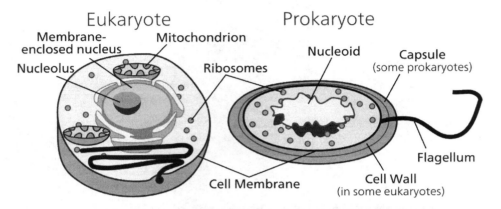

LIPIDS, ORGANELLES, RNA, POLYMERS, MONOMERS, NUCLEOTIDES, AND NUCLEOIDS

- **Lipids**: molecules that are hydrophobic or amphiphilic (having hydrophilic and hydrophobic properties) in nature. Examples include fats, triglycerides, steroids, and waxes. Lipids take many forms and have varying functions, such as storing energy and acting as a building block of cell membranes. Lipids are produced by anabolysis.
- **Organelle**: This is a general term that refers to an organ or smaller structure within a cell. Membrane-bound organelles are found in eukaryotic cells.
- **RNA**: RNA is short for ribonucleic acid, which is a type of molecule that consists of a long chain (polymer) of nucleotide units.
- **Polymer**: This is a compound of large molecules formed by repeating monomers.
- **Monomer**: A monomer is a small molecule. It is a single compound that forms chemical bonds with other monomers to make a polymer.
- **Nucleotides**: These are molecules that combine to form DNA and RNA.
- **Nucleoid**: This is the nucleus-like, irregularly-shaped mass of DNA that contains the chromatin in a prokaryotic cell.

MITOCHONDRIA FUNCTIONS

Four functions of **mitochondria** are: the production of cell energy, cell signaling (how communications are carried out within a cell, cellular differentiation (the process whereby a non-differentiated cell becomes transformed into a cell with a more specialized purpose), and cell cycle and growth regulation (the process whereby the cell gets ready to reproduce and reproduces). Mitochondria are numerous in eukaryotic cells. There may be hundreds or even thousands of mitochondria in a single cell. Mitochondria can be involved in many functions, their main one being supplying the cell with **energy**. Mitochondria consist of an inner and outer membrane. The inner membrane encloses the matrix, which contains the mitochondrial DNA (mtDNA) and ribosomes. Between the inner and outer membranes are folds (cristae). Chemical reactions occur here that release energy, control water levels in cells, and recycle and create proteins and fats. Aerobic respiration also occurs in the mitochondria.

CELL CYCLE

The term **cell cycle** refers to the process by which a cell reproduces, which involves cell growth, the duplication of genetic material, and cell division. Complex organisms with many cells use the cell cycle to replace cells as they lose their functionality and wear out. The entire cell cycle in animal cells can take 24 hours. The time required varies among different cell types. Human skin cells, for example, are constantly reproducing. Some other cells only divide infrequently. Once neurons are mature, they do not grow or divide. The two ways that cells can reproduce are through meiosis and mitosis. When cells replicate through **mitosis**, the "daughter cell" is an exact replica of the parent cell. When cells divide through **meiosis**, the daughter cells have different genetic coding than the parent cell. Meiosis only happens in specialized reproductive cells called gametes.

BIOLOGICAL IMPORTANCE OF CHEMICALS

Water molecules are important for many reasons, including:

- Water is a strong solvent for ionic compounds such as salts
- Water acts as a transport medium for polar solutes
- Metabolic reactions happen in solutions that contain water
- Water can act as a temperature buffer for enzyme-catalyzed reactions
- Water is used in photosynthesis
- Water molecules are used or formed in oxidation and reduction reactions

Carbon dioxide is used by plants during photosynthesis, which produces oxygen. Oxygen is used by organisms during respiration. Nitrogen is also used by organisms. Nitrogen is a nutrient for plants, and is also used in the formation of proteins and nucleic acids.

CELL DIVISION

- **Cell division** is performed in organisms so they can grow and replace cells that are old, worn out, or damaged.
- **Chromatids**: During cell division, the DNA is replicated, and chromatids are the two identical replicated pieces of chromosome that are joined at the centromere to form an "X."
- **Gametes**: These are cells used by organisms to reproduce sexually. Gametes in humans are haploid, meaning they contain only half of the organism's genetic information (23 chromosomes). Other human cells contain all 46 chromosomes.
- **Haploid**: Haploid means there is one set of chromosomes.
- **Diploid**: Diploid means there are two sets of chromosomes (one set from each parent).

MITOSIS

- **Interphase**: The cell prepares for division by replicating its genetic and cytoplasmic material. Interphase can be further divided into G_1, S, and G_2.
- **Prophase**: The chromatin thickens into chromosomes and the nuclear membrane begins to disintegrate. Pairs of centrioles move to opposite sides of the cell and spindle fibers begin to form. The mitotic spindle, formed from cytoskeleton parts, moves chromosomes around within the cell.

- **Metaphase**: The spindle moves to the center of the cell and chromosome pairs align along the center of the spindle structure.
- **Anaphase**: The pairs of chromosomes, called sisters, begin to pull apart, and may bend. When they are separated, they are called daughter chromosomes. Grooves appear in the cell membrane.
- **Telophase**: The spindle disintegrates, the nuclear membranes reform, and the chromosomes revert to chromatin. In animal cells, the membrane is pinched. In plant cells, a new cell wall begins to form.
- **Cytokinesis**: This is the physical splitting of the cell (including the cytoplasm) into two cells. Cytokinesis begins during anaphase, as the cell begins to furrow, and is completed following telophase.

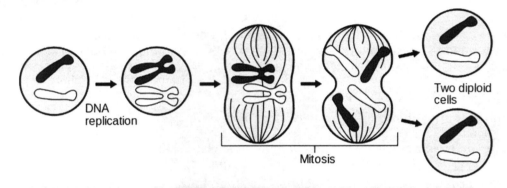

DNA replication

Mitosis

Two diploid cells

Review Video: Mitosis
Visit mometrix.com/academy and enter code: 849894

MEIOSIS

Meiosis has the same phases as mitosis, but they happen **twice**. In addition, different events occur during some phases of meiosis than mitosis. The events that occur during the first phase of meiosis are interphase (I), prophase (I), metaphase (I), anaphase (I), telophase (I), and cytokinesis (I). During this first phase of meiosis, chromosomes cross over, genetic material is exchanged, and tetrads of four chromatids are formed. The nuclear membrane dissolves. Homologous pairs of chromatids are separated and travel to different poles. At this point, there has been one cell division resulting in two cells. Each cell goes through a second cell division, which consists of prophase (II), metaphase (II), anaphase (II), telophase (II), and cytokinesis (II). The result is four daughter cells with different sets of chromosomes. The daughter cells are **haploid**, which means they contain half the genetic material of the parent cell. The second phase of meiosis is similar to the process of mitosis. Meiosis encourages **genetic diversity**.

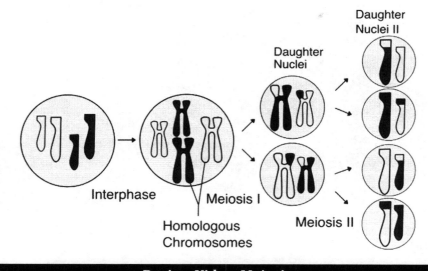

Diffusion and Osmosis

CELL TRANSPORT MECHANISMS

Active transport mechanisms include exocytosis and endocytosis. Active transport involves transferring substances from areas of lower concentration to areas of higher concentration. Active transport requires energy in the form of ATP. **Endocytosis** is the ingestion of large particles into a cell, and can be categorized as phagocytosis (ingestion of a particle), pinocytosis (ingestion of a liquid), or receptor mediated. Endocytosis occurs when a substance is too large to cross a cell membrane. Endocytosis is a process by which eukaryotes ingest food particles. During phagocytosis, cell-eating vesicles used during ingestion are quickly formed and unformed. **Exocytosis** is the opposite of endocytosis. It is the expulsion or discharge of substances from a cell. A lysosome digests particles with enzymes, and can be expelled through exocytosis. A vacuole containing the substance to be expelled attaches to the cell membrane and expels the substance.

Endocytosis

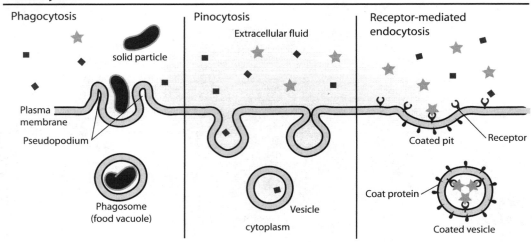

PASSIVE TRANSPORT MECHANISMS

Transport mechanisms allow for the movement of substances through membranes. **Passive transport mechanisms** include simple and facilitated diffusion and osmosis. They do not require energy from the cell. **Diffusion** is when particles are transported from areas of higher concentration to areas of lower concentration. When equilibrium is reached, diffusion stops. Examples are gas exchange (carbon dioxide and oxygen) during photosynthesis and the transport of oxygen from air to blood and from blood to tissue. **Facilitated diffusion** is when specific molecules are transported by a specific carrier protein. Carrier proteins vary in terms of size, shape, and charge. Glucose and amino acids are examples of substances transported by carrier proteins. Osmosis is the diffusion of water through a semi-permeable membrane from an area of higher concentration to one of lower concentration. Examples of osmosis include the absorption of water by plant roots and the alimentary canal. Plants lose and gain water through osmosis. A plant cell that swells because of water retention is said to be **turgid**.

> **Review Video: Passive Transport: Diffusion and Osmosis**
> Visit mometrix.com/academy and enter code: 642038

CHEMIOSMOSIS AND ENZYMES

Chemiosmosis is a process by which energy is made available for ADP to form ATP. When electrons move down the electron transport chain, the energy pumps protons to one side of a membrane. The equilibrium is disrupted at this point because the concentration gradient where the protons have gathered is greater than the concentration gradient on the other side of the membrane. The protons diffuse through the membrane as a result. The energy of this process fuels **phosphorylation**.

Enzymes act as catalysts by lowering the activation energy necessary for a reaction. They are **proteins**, have specific functions, are often globular and 3-D in form, and have names that end in "-ase." An enzyme has an active site where a substrate attaches and products are formed and released. Most enzymes also need a non-protein **coenzyme** that attaches to the enzyme to form the active site.

Tissue Organization

ANIMAL TISSUE TYPES

Epithelial tissue is found on body surfaces (like skin) and lining body cavities (like the stomach). Functions include protection, secretion of chemicals, absorption of chemicals, and responding to external stimuli. Epithelial cells move substances in, around, and out of the body. They can also have protective and secretory functions. Because these cells contain no blood vessels they must receive nourishment from underlying tissue. The three types of epithelial tissue are squamous (flattened), cuboidal (cube-shaped), and columnar (elongated). They can be further classified as simple (a single layer) or stratified (more than one layer). Glands comprised of epithelial tissue can be unicellular or multicellular.

Connective tissue is used to bind, support, protect, store fat, and fill space. The two kinds of connective tissue are loose and fibrous. In the human body, cartilage, bone, tendons, ligaments, blood, and protective layers are types of connective tissue.

The three types of **muscle tissue** are skeletal (striated), smooth, and cardiac.

Bone is a dense, rigid tissue that protects organs, produces blood cells, and provides structural support to the body.

MUSCLE IN MAMMALS

Skeletal muscle is strong, quick, and capable of voluntary contraction. Skeletal muscle fibers are striated and cylinder shaped. They have about 25 nuclei that are located to the side of the cell. Skeletal muscle consists of myofibrils that contain two types of filaments (myofilaments) made of proteins. The two types of filaments are actin and myosin. These filaments are aligned, giving the appearance of striation. During contraction, they slide against each other and become more overlapped. Smooth muscle is weak, slow, and usually contracts involuntarily. Examples in humans can be found in the gastrointestinal tract, blood vessels, bladder, uterus, hair follicles, and parts of the eye.

Smooth muscle fibers are not striated, but spindle shaped. They are somewhat long and a little wider in the center. Each cell contains one nucleus that is centrally located. Smooth muscle cells also contain myofibrils, but they are not aligned.

Cardiac muscle is strong, quick, and continuously contracts involuntarily. It is found in the myocardium of the heart. Cardiac muscle is more akin to skeletal muscle than smooth muscle.

Cardiac dysfunction is a response (a compensatory mechanism) to the heart trying to maintain normal heart function. Eventually, this causes the cardiac system to weaken. When the heart muscle contracts to pump blood out, it is referred to as **systolic blood flow**. When the heart muscle relaxes and blood flows back in, it is referred to as **diastolic blood flow**. If there are problems related to systolic and/or diastolic blood flow, the amount of blood output can be lessened. The ventricle can become stiffer and will not completely fill. Dysfunction can cause the heart to try to compensate and maintain normalcy by pumping harder.

Theory of Evolution and Classification of Organisms

ORIGIN OF LIFE ON EARTH

One theory of how life originated on Earth is that life developed from nonliving materials. The first stage of this transformation happened when **abiotic (nonliving) synthesis** took place, which is the formation of **monomers** like amino acids and nucleotides. Next, monomers joined together to create **polymers** such as proteins and nucleic acids. These polymers are then believed to have formed into protobionts. The last stage was the development of the process of **heredity**. Supporters of this theory believe that RNA was the first genetic material. Another theory postulates that hereditary systems came about before the origination of nucleic acids. Another theory is that life, or the precursors for it, were transported to Earth from a meteorite or other object from space. There is no real evidence to support this theory.

ABIOTIC SYNTHESIS AND ENDOSYMBIOTIC THEORY

The Earth's age is estimated to be 4.5 billion years.

Abiotic synthesis: This is related to the commonly accepted theory that life originated from inorganic matter. It refers to the making of organic molecules outside of a living body, and is believed to have been the first step in the development of life on Earth. The theory was tested by **Stanley Miller**. He combined the inorganic molecules water, hydrogen, methane, and ammonia in a closed, sterile flask and applied an electric discharge. His ingredients started as a clear mixture. After a week, he had a cloudy soup that contained amino acids and organic compounds.

Endosymbiotic theory: This is the belief that **eukaryotes** (cells with nuclei) developed from **prokaryotic cells** (those without nuclei). The theory is that chloroplasts in plant cells and mitochondria in animal cells evolved from smaller prokaryotes living within larger prokaryotes.

CONTRIBUTORS TO THE THEORY OF EVOLUTION

- **Georges Cuvier (1744-1829)** - Cuvier was a French naturalist who used the fossil record (paleontology) to compare the anatomies of extinct species and existing species to make conclusions about extinction. He believed in the catastrophism theory more strongly than the theory of evolution.
- **Jean-Baptise Lamarck (1769-1832)** - Lamarck was a French naturalist who believed in the idea of evolution and thought it was a natural occurrence influenced by the environment. Lamarck put forth a theory of evolution by inheritance of acquired characteristics. He theorized that organisms became more complex by moving up a ladder of progress.
- **Charles Robert Darwin (1809-1882)** - Darwin was an English naturalist known for his belief that evolution occurred by natural selection. He believed that species descend from common ancestors.
- **Alfred Russell Wallace (1823-1913)** - He was a British naturalist who independently developed a theory of evolution by natural selection. He believed in the transmutation of species (that one species develops into another).

THEORY OF EVOLUTION

Scientific evidence supporting the **theory of evolution** can be found in biogeography, comparative anatomy and embryology, the fossil record, and molecular evidence. **Biogeography** studies the geographical distribution of animals and plants. Evidence of evolution related to the area of biogeography includes species that are well suited for extreme environments. The **fossil record** shows that species lived only for a short time period before becoming extinct. The fossil record can also show the succession of plants and animals. Living fossils are existing species that have not changed much morphologically and are very similar to ancient examples in the fossil record. Examples include the horseshoe crab and ginkgo. **Comparative embryology** studies how species are similar in the embryonic stage, but become increasingly specialized and diverse as they age. Vestigial organs are those that still exist, but become nonfunctional. Examples include the hind limbs of whales and the wings of birds that can no longer fly, such as ostriches.

NATURAL SELECTION, GRADUALISM, AND PUNCTUATED EQUILIBRIUM

Natural selection: This theory developed by Darwin states that traits that help give a species a survival advantage are passed on to subsequent generations. Members of a species that do not have the advantageous trait die before they reproduce. Darwin's four principles are:

- from generation to generation, there are various individuals within a species
- genes determine variations
- more individuals are born than survive to maturation
- specific genes enable an organism to better survive

Gradualism: It is an idea that evolution proceeds at a steady pace and does not include sudden developments of new species or features from one generation to the next. This can be contrasted with punctuated equilibrium.

Punctuated equilibrium: This can be contrasted with gradualism. It is the idea in evolutionary biology that states that evolution involves long time periods of no change (stasis) accompanied by relatively brief periods (hundreds of thousands of years) of rapid change.

SPECIATION

- **Spatial**: This refers to species that are separated by a distance that prevents them from mating.
- **Geographical**: This is when species are physically separated by a barrier. A barrier can divide a population, which is known as vicariance. If a population crosses a barrier to create two species, it is known as dispersal.
- **Habitat**: This refers to species that live in different habitats in the same area.
- **Temporal**: This refers to the fact that species reach sexual maturity at different times. An example is plants that flower at different times of the year.
- **Behavioral**: This refers to the fact that mating rituals distinguish interaction between sexes. For example, many species of crickets are morphologically (structurally) the same, yet a female of one species will only respond to the mating rituals of males within her species.
- **Mechanical**: This refers to physiological structural differences that prevent mating or the transfer of gametes.
- **Gametic isolation**: This refers to the fact that fertilization may not occur when gametes of different species are not compatible.

CLASSIFICATION

The most widely accepted system for taxonomy is the **three-domain classification system**; sometimes called the six-kingdom classification system. The three domains are **Archaea**, **Bacteria**, and **Eukarya**. Both Archaea and Bacteria are made of prokaryotic cells, while Eukarya are made of eukaryotic cells. The domains of Bacteria and Archaea each have a single kingdom **Eubacteria** and **Archaebacteria**, respectively. The domain Eukarya has four kingdoms: Protista, Fungi, Plantae, and Animalia. **Kingdom Protista** includes about 250,000 species of unicellular protozoans and unicellular and multicellular algae. **Kingdom Fungi** includes about 100,000 species. **Kingdom Plantae** includes about 320,000 species. **Kingdom Animalia** is estimated to include more than 1,500,000 species. The groupings in this system, in descending order from broadest to most specific, are: domain, kingdom, phylum/division, class, order, family, genus, and species. A memory aid for this is: Dear King Philip Came Over For Good Soup. According to the three-domain classification system, **humans** are: domain Eukarya, kingdom Animalia, phylum Chordata, subphylum Vertebrata, class Mammalia, order Primate, family Hominidae, genus Homo, and species Sapiens.

Biological Organization
Domain (one or more kingdom)
Kingdom (one or more phyla)
Phylum (one or more classes)
Class (one or more orders)
Order (one or more classes)
Family (one or more genera)
Genus (one or more species)
Species (a distinct kind or unit)

Review Video: Biological Classification Systems
Visit mometrix.com/academy and enter code: 736052

Ecology and Plants

FOOD CHAINS AND BIOMAGNIFICATION

A food chain is a linking of organisms in a community that is based on how they use each other as food sources. Each link in the chain consumes the link above it and is consumed by the link below it. The exceptions are the organism at the top of the **food chain** and the organism at the bottom.

Biomagnification (bioamplification) refers to an increase in concentration of a substance within a food chain. Examples are pesticides or mercury. Mercury is emitted from coal-fired power plants and gets into the water supply, where it is eaten by a fish. A larger fish eats smaller fish, and humans eat fish. The concentration of mercury in humans has now risen. Biomagnification is affected by the persistence of a chemical, whether it can be broken down and negated, food chain energetics, and whether organisms can reduce or negate the substance.

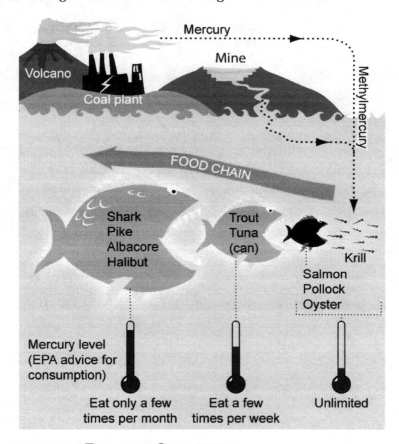

ECOSYSTEM STABILITY AND ECOLOGIC SUCCESSION

Ecosystem stability: This is a concept that states that a stable ecosystem is perfectly efficient. Seasonal changes or expected climate fluctuations are balanced by **homeostasis**. It also states that interspecies interactions are part of the balance of the system. Four principles of ecosystem stability are that waste disposal and nutrient replenishment by recycling is complete, the system uses sunlight as an energy source, biodiversity remains, and populations are stable in that they do not over consume resources.

Ecologic succession: This is the concept that states that there is an orderly progression of change within a community. An example of **primary succession** is that over hundreds of years bare rock

131

decomposes to sand, which eventually leads to soil formation, which eventually leads to the growth of grasses and trees. **Secondary succession** occurs after a disturbance or major event that greatly affects a community, such as a wild fire or construction of a dam.

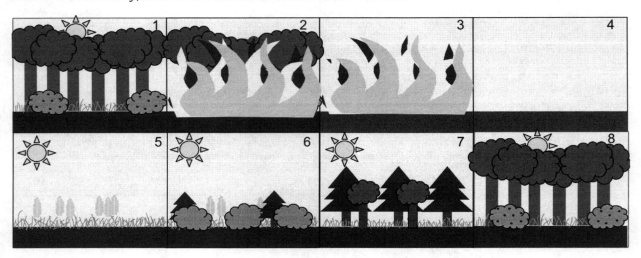

FOOD WEBS

A food web consists of interconnected food chains in a community. The organisms can be linked to show the direction of energy flow. **Energy flow** in this sense is used to refer to the actual caloric flow through a system from trophic level to trophic level. **Trophic level** refers to a link in a food chain or a level of nutrition. The 10% rule is that from trophic level to level, about 90% of the energy is lost (in the form of heat, for example). The lowest trophic level consists of primary producers (usually plants), then primary consumers, then secondary consumers, and finally tertiary consumers (large carnivores). The final link is decomposers, which break down the consumers at the top. Food chains usually do not contain more than six links. These links may also be referred to as **ecological pyramids**.

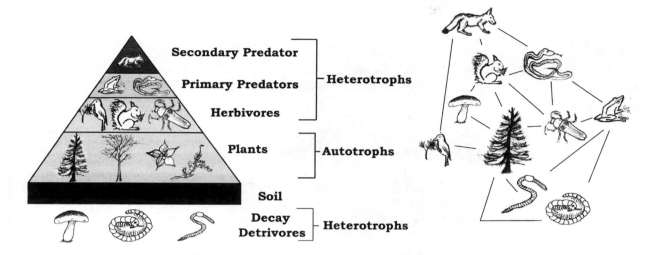

SOCIAL BEHAVIORS

- **Territoriality**: This refers to members of a species protecting areas from other members of their species and from other species. Species members claim specific areas as their own.
- **Dominance**: This refers to the species in a community that is the most populous.
- **Altruism**: This is when a species or individual in a community exhibits behaviors that benefit another individual at a cost to itself. In biology, altruism does not have to be a conscious sacrifice.
- **Threat display**: This refers to behavior by an organism that is intended to intimidate or frighten away members of its own or another species.
- **Competitive exclusion**: This principle states that if there are limited or insufficient resources and species are competing for them, these species will not be able to co-exist. The result is that one of the species will become extinct or be forced to undergo a behavioral or evolutionary change. Another way to say this is that "complete competitors cannot coexist."

POPULATION

- **Population** is a measure of how many individuals exist in a specific area. It can be used to measure the size of human, plant, or animal groups.
- **Population growth** depends on many factors. Factors that can limit the number of individuals in a population include lack of resources such as food and water, space, habitat destruction, competition, disease, and predators.
- **Exponential growth** refers to an unlimited rising growth rate. This kind of growth can be plotted on a chart in the shape of a J.
- **Carrying capacity** is the population size that can be sustained. The world's population is about 6.8 billion and growing. The human population has not yet reached its carrying capacity.

- **Population dynamics** refers to how a population changes over time and the factors that cause changes. An S-shaped curve shows that population growth has leveled off.
- **Biotic potential** refers to the maximum reproductive capacity of a population given ideal environmental conditions.

COMMUNITY

A community is any number of species interacting within a given area. A **niche** is the role of a species within a community. **Species diversity** refers to the number of species within a community and their populations.

- **Biome**: an area in which species are associated because of climate. The six major biomes in North America are desert, tropical rain forest, grassland, coniferous forest, deciduous forest, and tundra.
- **Biotic factors**: the living factors, such as other organisms, that affect a community or population.
- **Abiotic factors**: the nonliving factors that affect a community or population, such as facets of the environment.
- **Ecology**: the study of plants, animals, their environments, and how they interact.
- **Ecosystem**: a community of species and all of the environmental factors that affect them.

RELATIONSHIPS BETWEEN AND WITHIN SPECIES

- **Intraspecific relationships**: relationships among members of a species.
- **Interspecific relationships**: relationships between members of different species.
- **Predation**: relationship in which one individual feeds on another (the prey), causing the prey to die.
- **Parasitism**: relationship in which one organism benefits and the other is harmed.
- **Commensalism**: interspecific relationships in which one of the organisms benefits.
- **Mutualism**: relationship in which both organisms benefit.
- **Competition**: relationship in which both organisms are harmed.
- **Biomass**: the mass of one or all of the species (species biomass) in an ecosystem or area.

> **Review Video: Mutualism, Commensalism, and Parasitism**
> Visit mometrix.com/academy and enter code: 757249

BIOCHEMICAL CYCLES

Biochemical cycles are how chemical elements required by living organisms cycle between living and nonliving organisms. Elements that are frequently required are phosphorus, sulfur, oxygen, carbon, gaseous nitrogen, and water. Elements can go through gas cycles, sedimentary cycles, or both. Elements circulate through the air in a gas cycle and from land to water in a sedimentary one.

MIMICRY

Mimicry is an adaptation developed as a response to predation. It refers to an organism that has a similar appearance to another species, which is meant to fool the predator into thinking the organism is more dangerous than it really is. Two examples are the drone fly and the io moth. The fly looks like a bee but cannot sting. The io moth has markings on its wings that make it look like an owl. The moth can startle predators and gain time to escape. Predators can also use mimicry to lure their prey.

PROCESSES AND SYSTEMS OF PLANTS

Plants are **autotrophs**, which mean they make their own food. in a sense, they are self sufficient. Three major processes used by plants are photosynthesis, transpiration, and respiration. **Photosynthesis** involves using sunlight to make food for plants. **Transpiration** evaporates water out of plants. **Respiration** is the utilization of food that was produced during photosynthesis.

Two major systems in plants are the shoot and the root system. The **shoot system** includes leaves, buds, and stems. It also includes the flowers and fruits in flowering plants. The shoot system is located above the ground. The **root system** is the component of the plant that is underground, and includes roots, tubers, and rhizomes.

PHOTOSYNTHESIS

Photosynthesis is the conversion of sunlight into energy in plant cells, and also occurs in some types of bacteria and protists. Carbon dioxide and water are converted into glucose during photosynthesis, and light is required during this process. Cyanobacteria are thought to be the descendants of the first organisms to use photosynthesis about 3.5 billion years ago. Photosynthesis is a form of **cellular respiration**. It occurs in chloroplasts that use thylakoids, which are structures in the membrane that contain light reaction chemicals. **Chlorophyll** is a pigment that absorbs light. During the process, water is used and oxygen is released. The equation for the chemical reaction that occurs during photosynthesis is $6H_2O + 6CO_2 \rightarrow C_6H_{12}O_6 + 6O_2$. During photosynthesis, six molecules of water and six molecules of carbon dioxide react to form one molecule of sugar and six molecules of oxygen.

> **Review Video: Photosynthesis in Biology**
> Visit mometrix.com/academy and enter code: 402602

PLANT TRANSPIRATION

The rate of **transpiration** is affected by light, temperature, humidity, wind, and the saturation of the soil. Leaves contain structures called **stomata** that regulate gas exchange. Light causes stomata to open, and water is lost more quickly than in the dark. Since water evaporates quicker in higher temperatures, the rate of transpiration increases as the temperature increases. If an area is humid, the rate of transpiration is decreased. The opposite is true for areas of lower humidity. This is explained by the principle of **diffusion**. The greater the difference in humidity or concentrations of substances in two regions, the greater the rate of diffusion between them will be. Water in the soil replaces water that has been lost through transpiration. If water in the soil is not replaced, the rate of transpiration decreases. Photosynthesis also slows, the stomata close, and the plant wilts when it loses turgor as water is lost from cells.

TRANSPIRATION, RESPIRATION, AND PHYLOGENETIC

- **Transpiration** is the movement of water through a vascular plant. It is also the method by which water is evaporated out of plants. Transpiration mainly happens during the process of photosynthesis, when water and minerals travel up through the xylem and water is released through stomata. During transpiration, water is drawn up a plant. This process also helps cool leaves.

- **Respiration**: This refers to the process of metabolizing sugars to provide plants with the energy they need for growth and reproduction. The chemical equation is $C_6H_{12}O_6 + 6O_2 \rightarrow 6CO_2 + 6H_2O +$ energy. During the process of respiration, sugars are burned, energy is released, oxygen is used, and water and carbon dioxide are produced. Respiration can occur as a light or dark reaction.
- **Phylogenetic**: This refers to organisms that are related because of their evolutionary history.

REPRODUCTION IN FLOWERING PLANTS

There are at least 230,000 species of flowering plants. They represent about 90 percent of all plants. **Angiosperms** have a sexual reproduction phase that includes flowering. When growing plants, one may think they develop in the following order: seeds, growth, flowers, and fruit. The reproductive cycle has the following order: flowers, fruit, and seeds. in other words, **seeds** are the products of successful reproduction. The colors and scents of flowers serve to attract pollinators. Flowers and other plants can also be pollinated by wind. When a pollen grain meets the ovule and is successfully fertilized, the ovule develops into a seed. A seed consists of three parts: the embryo, the endosperm, and a seed coat. The **embryo** is a small plant that has started to develop, but this development is paused. Germination is when the embryo starts to grow again. The **endosperm** consists of proteins, carbohydrates, or fats. It typically serves as a food source for the embryo. The **seed coat** provides protection from disease, insects, and water.

SEXUAL PARTS OF FLOWERING PLANTS

Flowering plants can be categorized sexually according to which organs they have. Flowers can be bisexual or unisexual. Species can be **dioecious**, which means male and female flowers are contained on different individual plants. **Monoecious** means that both male and female flowers are on one individual. **Bisexual** flowers are those that have all of the following: sepal, petal, stamen, and pistil. If they have all of these parts, they are considered complete. They have both the male stamen and the female counterpart, the pistil. **Unisexual** flowers only have a pistil or a stamen, not both. Incomplete flowers do not have all four parts. The flower rests upon a pedicel and is contained with the receptacle. The carpal is made up of the stigma at the tip, a style, and the ovary at the base. The ovary contains the ovules (eggs). Carpels are sometimes formed as a single pistil. The stamen includes the anther and the filament, and produces the male pollen.

POLLINATION IN FLOWERING PLANTS

The anthers of the stamens (male parts) have microsporangia that form into a **pollen** grain, which consists of a small germ cell within a larger cell. The pollen grain is released and lands on a **stigma** (female) portion of the pistil. It grows a pollen tube the length of the style and ends up at the **ovule**. The pollen grain releases the sperm and fertilization occurs. in double fertilization, one of the sperm joins with the egg to become a diploid zygote. The other sperm becomes the endosperm nucleus. Seeds are formed. One cotyledon (**monocot**) or two cotyledons (**dicot**) also form to store food and surround the embryo. Correspondingly, monocots produce one seed leaf, while dicots produce two. The seed matures and becomes dormant, and fruits typically form.

FRUITS IN FLOWERING PLANTS

The three main types of **fruits** in flowering plants are simple fruits, aggregate fruits, and multiple fruits.

- **Simple fruits** are formed from one ovary. Simple fruits that develop from one flower are called botanical fruits. Simple fruits can also have fruits that are dry.
- **Aggregate fruits** are produced by many ovaries in one flower. Each ovary is separately fertilized and forms the aggregate fruit. Examples of these are raspberries, blackberries, and strawberries.
- **Multiple fruits** are produced by many flowers on a single structure. Examples are pineapples and figs.

Seeds can be located within the fruit (i.e., tomatoes, cherries, and apples) or on the outside of the fruit (i.e., corn and strawberries).

> **Review Video: Fruits in Flowering Plants**
> Visit mometrix.com/academy and enter code: 867090

REPRODUCTION IN SEEDLESS PLANTS

Bryophytes are seedless plants. They include liverworts, hornworts, and mosses. They use spores that form into gametophytes to reproduce. Sperm are flagellated, meaning they require at least some water to swim to the egg. Some bryophytes are plants that are one sex or the other, but other bryophytes have both sexes on the same plant.

Ferns also have flagellated sperm and require water for the same reason as bryophytes. Both ferns and bryophytes undergo alternation of generations. These plants spend about half of their reproductive cycles as sporophytes, making haploid spores through meiosis during this stage. The other half of the cycle is spent as a haploid gametophyte. At this point, male and female gametes join to form one zygote.

Genetics, DNA, and Lab Work

MENDEL'S LAWS

Mendel's laws are the law of segregation (first law) and the law of independent assortment (second law). The **law of segregation** states that there are two alleles and that half of the total number of alleles are contributed by each parent organism. The **law of independent assortment** states that traits are passed on randomly and are not influenced by other traits. The exception to this is linked traits. A **Punnett square** can illustrate how alleles combine from the contributing genes to form various phenotypes. One set of a parent's genes are put in columns, while the genes from the other parent are placed in rows. The allele combinations are shown in each cell. When two different alleles are present in a pair, the dominant one is expressed. A Punnett square can be used to predict the outcome of crosses.

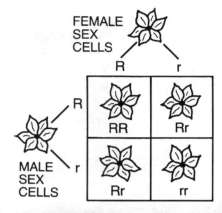

GENE, GENOTYPE, PHENOTYPE, AND ALLELE

A gene is a portion of DNA that identifies how traits are expressed and passed on in an organism. A **gene** is part of the genetic code. Collectively, all genes form the **genotype** of an individual. The genotype includes genes that may not be expressed, such as recessive genes. The **phenotype** is the physical, visual manifestation of genes. It is determined by the basic genetic information and how genes have been affected by their environment.

An **allele** is a variation of a gene. Also known as a trait, it determines the manifestation of a gene. This manifestation results in a specific physical appearance of some facet of an organism, such as eye color or height. The genetic information for eye color is a gene. The gene variations responsible for blue, green, brown, or black eyes are called alleles. **Locus** (pl. loci) refers to the location of a gene or alleles.

DOMINANT AND RECESSIVE GENES

Gene traits are represented in pairs with an uppercase letter for the **dominant trait** (A) and a lowercase letter for the **recessive trait** (a). Genes occur in pairs (AA, Aa, or aa). There is one gene on each chromosome half supplied by each parent organism. Since half the genetic material is from each parent, the offspring's traits are represented as a combination of these. A dominant trait only requires one gene of a gene pair for it to be expressed in a phenotype, whereas a recessive requires both genes in order to be manifested. For example, if the mother's genotype is Dd and the father's is dd, the possible combinations are Dd and dd. The dominant trait will be manifested if the genotype is DD or Dd. The recessive trait will be manifested if the genotype is dd. Both DD and dd are **homozygous** pairs. Dd is **heterozygous**.

ALLELE FREQUENCY

The **gene pool** refers to all alleles of a gene and their combinations. The **Hardy-Weinberg principle** (or Castle-Hardy-Weinberg principle) postulates that the **allele frequency** for dominant and recessive alleles will remain the same in a population through successive generations if certain conditions exist. These conditions are: no mutations, large populations, random mating, no migration, and equal genotypes. Changes in the frequency and types of alleles in a gene pool can be caused by gene flow, random mutation, nonrandom mating, and genetic drift. In organisms that reproduce by sexual reproduction, **reproduction isolation** is defined as something that acts as a barrier to two species reproducing. These barriers are classified as **prezygotic** and **postzygotic**.

MONOHYBRID AND HYBRID CROSSES

Genetic crosses are the possible combinations of alleles, and can be represented using Punnett squares. A **monohybrid cross** refers to a cross involving only one trait. Typically, the ratio is 3:1 (DD, Dd, Dd, dd), which is the ratio of dominant gene manifestation to recessive gene manifestation. This ratio occurs when both parents have a pair of dominant and recessive genes. If one parent has a pair of dominant genes (DD) and the other has a pair of recessive (dd) genes, the recessive trait cannot be expressed in the next generation because the resulting crosses all have the Dd genotype. A **dihybrid cross** refers to one involving more than one trait, which means more combinations are possible. The ratio of genotypes for a dihybrid cross is 9:3:3:1 when the traits are not linked. The ratio for incomplete dominance is 1:2:1, which corresponds to dominant, mixed, and recessive phenotypes.

CROSSING OVER, GAMETES, PEDIGREE ANALYSIS, AND PROBABILITY ANALYSIS

- **Crossing over**: This refers to the swapping of genetic material between homologous chromosomes. This leads to different combinations of genes showing up in a phenotype. This is part of gene recombination, which is when genes are reassembled.
- **Gametes**: These are cells that fuse with one another during sexual reproduction. Each gamete contains half the genetic information of the parent. They are haploid (having 23 chromosome pairs in humans). The resulting zygote, which is formed when the two gametes become one cell, is **diploid** (46 chromosome pairs in humans).
- **Pedigree analysis**: This involves isolating a trait in an organism and tracing its manifestation. Pedigree charts are often used for this type of analysis. A family pedigree shows how a trait can be seen throughout generations.
- **Probability analysis**: This calculates the chances of a particular trait or combination of traits being expressed in an organism.

GENETIC LINKAGE

Genetic linkage is the tendency for genes that are close to one another to be inherited together. Linkage is the exception to independent assortment. **Sex-linked traits** are those that occur on a sex chromosome. **Autosomal** refers to non-sex chromosomes. In humans, there are 22 autosomal pairs of chromosomes and a pair of sex chromosomes. Depending on the sex, pairs are either XX (female) or XY (male). Since females don't have Y chromosomes, alleles on this gene are only manifested in males. Males can only pass on sex-linked traits on the X chromosome to their daughters since sons would not receive an X from them. **Hemizygous** means there is only one copy of a gene. Color blindness occurs more in males than females because it is a sex-linked trait on the X chromosome. Since it is recessive, females have a better chance of expressing the dominant characteristic of non-color blindness.

COMMON GENETIC DISORDERS

- **Cystic fibrosis**: recessive genetic disorder resulting in respiratory disorders
- **Huntington's disease**: autosomal dominant disorder resulting in the degeneration of nerve cells
- **Down syndrome**: caused by an extra copy of chromosome 21

- **Sickle cell anemia**: recessive genetic disorder resulting in deformed blood cells that can cause respiratory and circulation issues
- **Color blindness**: an X-linked recessive inheritance. Because it is X-linked recessive, it is more common in males than females.

BASIC PRINCIPLES OF GENETICS

Humans have 23 pairs of **chromosomes** (bundles of DNA and genes) in the nucleus of body cells, with half of each pair coming from each parent. The chromosomes in each cell contain 35,000 or more **genes**, which carry instructions for producing proteins. Chromosomes carry the blueprint for the individual, including traits inherited from the parents. There are two types of chromosomes:

- **Autosomal**: Pairs 1 to 22, ranked in size according to the number of base pairs they each contain with 1 being the largest and 22 being the smallest.
- **Allosomal** (Sex): Pair 23. XX for female and XY for male.

Genetic disorders occur when there is a **mutation** (spontaneous or transmitted) in one or more genes. Diseases are classified as **autosomal recessive** if both parents must carry the defective autosomal gene in order to pass it on to offspring, and they are classified as **autosomal dominant** if only one parent must carry the defective gene. Genetic disorders may also be X-linked recessive or dominant and Y-linked.

> **Review Video: Chromosomes**
> Visit mometrix.com/academy and enter code: 132083

EMBRYONIC DEVELOPMENT

The stages of **embryonic development** are the zygote, morula, blastula, and gastrula.

- **Zygote**: diploid cell formed by the fusion two gametes during fertilization
- **Morula**: ball-like mass of 16–32 cells formed by mitotic divisions (cleavages) of the zygote
- **Blastula**: hollow, ball-like structure formed when morula cells begin to secrete fluid into the center of the morula; this is the structure that attaches to the lining of the uterus (endometrium)
- **Gastrula**: formed when cells migrate to the center of the blastula to form germ layers that differentiate to form tissues and organs

Roughly two weeks after fertilization, the embryo starts to form a yolk sac that will make blood cells, an embryonic disc, and a chorion (the placenta). By week three, the beginnings of the spinal cord, brain, muscles, bones, and face appear. After that, cardiac cells begin to beat.

FACTORS THAT CAN AFFECT HEREDITY

Inheritance is complex. In some cases, a disorder is directly inherited through transmission of defective **genes**, such as with sickle cell disease; however, in other cases, people may inherit a defective gene that increases risk but does not necessarily result in disease. These include the BRCA1 and BRCA2 gene mutations that increase risk of breast and ovarian cancer as well as the HER2 gene mutation associated with estrogen-progesterone-positive breast cancers. Many **environmental factors** may spur the development of diseases with a genetic component or may cause genetic mutations. Most **sporadic genetic mutations** are harmless, but some result in disease. Environmental factors that may affect outcomes include stress, smoking, poor diet, exposure to second-hand smoke, exposure to ultraviolet (UV) radiation, excessive drinking, poor air quality, some viruses, and exposure to toxic substances. Researchers have theorized that there may be a genetic component to many common disorders.

CONTRIBUTING INDIVIDUALS TO THE STRUCTURE OF DNA

- **James Watson and Francis Crick (1952)** - Formulated the double-helix model of DNA and speculated about its importance in carrying and transferring genetic information.
- **Rosalind Franklin (1952)** - Took the x-ray diffraction image that was used by James Watson and Francis Crick to develop their double-helix model of DNA.

NUCLEOTIDES

A nucleotide, whether DNA or RNA, contains three components: a phosphate group, a ringed, five-carbon sugar (deoxyribose in DNA, ribose in RNA), and a nitrogenous base. The **phosphate group** binds to one side of the **ringed, five-carbon sugar**. The **nitrogenous base** binds to the opposite side of the ringed, five-carbon sugar.

The five bases in DNA and RNA can be categorized as either pyrimidine or purine according to their structure. The **pyrimidine bases** include cytosine (C), thymine (T), and uracil (U). They are six-sided and have a single ring shape. The **purine bases** are adenine (A) and guanine (G), which consist of two attached rings.

DNA contains the bases A, T, C, and G. **RNA** contains the bases A, U, C, and G. In forming higher-order nucleotide structures, A pairs with T or U and C pairs with G.

NUCLEOSIDES

A nucleoside is a nitrogenous base bound only to a sugar (no phosphate group). When combined with a sugar, any of the five bases in DNA and RNA become nucleosides. Nucleosides formed from **purine bases** end in "osine" and those formed from **pyrimidine bases** end in "idine." Adenosine and thymidine are examples of nucleosides.

DNA STRUCTURE AND REPLICATION

DNA has a right-handed, double-helix shape, resembles a twisted ladder, and is compact. It consists of **nucleotides**. Nucleotides consist of a five-carbon sugar (pentose), a phosphate group, and a nitrogenous base. Two bases pair up to form the rungs of the ladder. The "side rails" or backbone consists of the covalently bonded sugar and phosphate. The bases are attached to each other with hydrogen bonds, which are easily dismantled so replication can occur. Each base is attached to a phosphate and to a sugar. There are four types of **nitrogenous bases**: adenine (A), guanine (G), cytosine (C), and thymine (T). There are about 3 billion bases in human DNA. The bases are mostly the same in everybody, but their order is different. It is the order of these bases that creates diversity in people. Adenine (A) pairs with thymine (T), and cytosine (C) pairs with guanine (G).

Pairs of chromosomes are composed of DNA, which is tightly wound to conserve space. When **replication** starts, it unwinds. The steps in DNA replication are controlled by **enzymes**. The enzyme helicase instigates the deforming of hydrogen bonds between the bases to split the two strands. The splitting starts at the A-T bases (adenine and thymine) as there are only two hydrogen bonds. The cytosine-guanine base pair has three bonds. The term **"origin of replication"** is used to refer to where the splitting starts. The portion of the DNA that is unwound to be replicated is called the replication fork. Each strand of DNA is transcribed by an mRNA. It copies the DNA onto itself, base by base, in a complementary manner. The exception is that uracil replaces thymine.

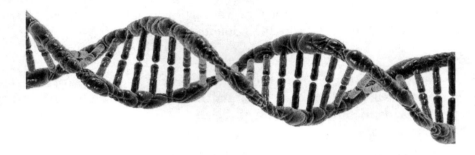

HOMEOSTASIS, GENE EXPRESSION, TRANSCRIPTION, TRANSLATION, AND CELLULAR DIFFERENTIATION

- **Homeostasis**: This describes the ability and tendency of an organism, cell, or body to adjust to environmental changes to maintain equilibrium.
- **Gene expression**: This refers to the use of information in a gene to make a protein or nucleic acid product. Examples of nucleic acid products are tRNA or rRNA.
- **Transcription**: This refers to the synthesis of RNA from DNA.
- **Translation**: Synthesizing a protein from an mRNA strand.
- **Cellular differentiation**: This is the process by which a cell changes to a new cell type.

FUNCTION OF PROTEINS IN DNA REPLICATION

Many proteins are involved in the replication of DNA, and each has a specific function. **Helicase** is a protein that facilitates the unwinding of the double helix structure of DNA. Single-strand binding (SSB) proteins attach themselves to each strand to prevent the DNA strands from joining back together. After DNA is unwound, there are leading and lagging strands. The **leading strand** is synthesized continuously and the **lagging strand** is synthesized in short fragments that are referred to as Okazaki fragments. **Primase**, an RNA polymerase (catalyzing enzyme), acts as a starting point for replication by forming short strands, or primers, of RNA. The DNA clamp, or sliding clamp, helps prevent DNA polymerase from coming apart from the strand. DNA polymerase helps form the DNA strand by linking nucleotides. As the process progresses, **RNase H** removes the primers. **DNA ligase** then links the existing shorter strands into a longer strand.

TYPES OF RNA

Types of RNA include ribosomal RNA (rRNA), transfer RNA (tRNA), and messenger RNA (mRNA).

- **rRNA**: forms the RNA component of the ribosome. It is evolutionarily conserved, which means it can be used to study relationships in organisms.
- **mRNA**: used by the ribosome to generate proteins (translation). The mRNA contains a series of three-nucleotide "codons" that code for the amino acids in a protein sequence.
- **tRNA**: functions in translation by carrying an amino acid to the corresponding codon on the mRNA strand.

> **Review Video: RNA**
> Visit mometrix.com/academy and enter code: 888852

DIFFERENCES BETWEEN RNA AND DNA

RNA and DNA differ in terms of structure and function. **RNA** contains ribose sugars, while **DNA** contains deoxyribose sugars. Uracil is found only in RNA and thymine in found only in DNA. RNA supports the functions carried out by DNA. It aids in gene expression, replication, and transportation.

CODONS

Codons are groups of three nucleotides on the messenger RNA. A **codon** has the code for a single **amino acid**. There are 64 codons but 20 amino acids. More than one combination, or triplet, can be used to synthesize the necessary amino acids. For example, AAA (adenine-adenine-adenine) or AAG (adenine-adenine-guanine) can serve as codons for lysine. These groups of three occur in strings and might be thought of as frames. For example, AAAUCUUCGU, if read in groups of three from the beginning, would be AAA, UCU, UCG. If the same sequence was read in groups of three starting from the second position, the groups would be AAU, CUU, and so on. The resulting protein sequences would be completely different. For this reason, there are **start and stop codons** that indicate the beginning and ending of a sequence (or frame). AUG (methionine) is the start codon. UAA, UGA, and UAG are stop codons.

> **Review Video: Codons**
> Visit mometrix.com/academy and enter code: 978172

TRANSLATION AND tRNA MOLECULES

A tRNA molecule contains a three-nucleotide anticodon region that is complimentary to the mRNA codons. For example, a codon that is AAA on the mRNA would be associated with the anticodon UUU on the tRNA. Each tRNA molecule is bound to the amino acid specified by its anticodon.

The **ribosome** has three tRNA binding sites—A, P, and E. Translation initiates when the *A-site* becomes occupied by the tRNA molecule corresponding to the mRNA start codon. The ribosome then moves the first tRNA from the *A-site* to the *P-site*. The *A-site* is then occupied by the tRNA molecule corresponding to the second mRNA codon. The ribosome then transfers the amino acid on the *P-site* tRNA to the amino acid on the *A-site* tRNA. The first tRNA, which now has no amino acid, is moved from the *P-site* the *E-site*. The second tRNA, complexed to a chain of two amino acids, is moved from the *A-site* to the *P-site*. The *A-site* is then occupied by the tRNA corresponding to the third mRNA codon. The *P-site* amino acid chain is transferred to the amino acid bound to the *A-site* tRNA. The first tRNA then exits from the *E-site* and the second and third tRNA molecules shift, opening the *A-site* for the next tRNA. The growing amino acid chain continues to be transferred from the *P-site* to the *A-site* until translation is complete.

MICROSCOPES

There are different kinds of microscopes, but **optical** or **light microscopes** are the most commonly used in lab settings. Light and lenses are used to magnify and view samples. A specimen or sample is placed on a slide and the slide is placed on a stage with a hole in it. Light passes through the hole and illuminates the sample. The sample is magnified by lenses and viewed through the eyepiece. A simple microscope has one lens, while a typical compound microscope has three lenses. The light source can be room light redirected by a mirror or the microscope can have its own independent light source that passes through a condenser. In this case, there are diaphragms and filters to allow light intensity to be controlled. Optical microscopes also have coarse and fine adjustment knobs.

Other types of microscopes include **digital microscopes**, which use a camera and a monitor to allow viewing of the sample. **Scanning electron microscopes (SEMs)** provide greater detail of a sample in terms of the surface topography and can produce magnifications much greater than those possible with optical microscopes. The technology of an SEM is quite different from an optical microscope in that it does not rely on lenses to magnify objects, but uses samples placed in a chamber. In one type of SEM, a beam of electrons from an electron gun scans and actually interacts with the sample to produce an image.

Wet mount slides designed for use with a light microscope typically require a thin portion of the specimen to be placed on a standard glass slide. A drop of water is added and a cover slip or cover glass is placed on top. Air bubbles and fingerprints can make viewing difficult. Placing the cover slip at a 45-degree angle and allowing it to drop into place can help avoid the problem of air bubbles. A **cover slip** should always be used when viewing wet mount slides. The viewer should start with the objective in its lowest position and then fine focus. The microscope should be carried with two hands and stored with the low-power objective in the down position. **Lenses** should be cleaned with lens paper only. A **graticule slide** is marked with a grid line, and is useful for counting or estimating a quantity.

COMPONENTS OF SCIENTIFIC EXPERIMENTATION

- A **hypothesis** is a tentative supposition about a phenomenon (or a fact or set of facts) made in order to examine and test its logical or empirical consequences through investigation or methodological experimentation.
- A **theory** is a scientifically proven, general principle offered to explain phenomena. A theory is derived from a hypothesis and verified by experimentation and research.
- A **scientific law** is a generally accepted conclusion about a body of observations to which no exceptions have been found. Scientific laws explain things, but do not describe them.
- A **control** is a normal, unchanged situation used for comparison against experimental data.
- **Constants** are factors in an experiment that remain the same.
- **Independent variables** are factors, traits, or conditions that are changed in an experiment. A good experiment has only one independent variable so that the scientist can track one thing at a time. The independent variable changes from experiment to experiment.
- **Dependent variables** are changes that result from variations in the independent variable.

Review Video: Experimental Science
Visit mometrix.com/academy and enter code: 283092

Review Video: Experimental Science Project
Visit mometrix.com/academy and enter code: 584444

GRAPHS AND CHARTS

Graphs and charts are effective ways to present scientific data such as observations, statistical analyses, and comparisons between dependent variables and independent variables. On a line chart, the **independent variable** (the one that is being manipulated for the experiment) is represented on the horizontal axis (the x-axis). Any **dependent variables** (the ones that may change as the independent variable changes) are represented on the y-axis. The points are charted and a line is drawn to connect the points. An **XY** or **scatter plot** is often used to plot many points. A "best fit" line is drawn, which allows outliers to be identified more easily. Charts and their axes should have titles. The x and y interval units should be evenly spaced and labeled. Other types of charts are **bar charts** and **histograms**, which can be used to compare differences between the data collected for two variables. A **pie chart** can graphically show the relation of parts to a whole.

PRESENTATION OF DATA

Data collected during a science lab can be organized and **presented** in any number of ways. While **straight narrative** is a suitable method for presenting some lab results, it is not a suitable way to present numbers and quantitative measurements. These types of observations can often be better presented with **tables** and **graphs**. Data that is presented in tables and organized in rows and columns may also be used to make graphs quite easily. Other methods of presenting data include illustrations, photographs, video, and even audio formats. In a **formal report**, tables and figures are labeled and referred to by their labels. For example, a picture of a bubbly solution might be labeled Figure 1, Bubbly Solution. It would be referred to in the text in the following way: "The reaction created bubbles 10 mm in size, as shown in Figure 1, Bubbly Solution." Graphs are also labeled as figures. Tables are labeled in a different way. Examples include: Table 1, Results of Statistical Analysis, or Table 2, Data from Lab 2.

Human Anatomy and Physiology

Digestive System

Most digestive systems function by the following means:

- **Movement** - Movement mixes and passes nutrients through the system and eliminates waste.
- **Secretion** - Enzymes, hormones, and other substances necessary for digestion are secreted into the digestive tract.
- **Digestion** - Includes the chemical breakdown of nutrients into smaller units that enter the internal environment.
- **Absorption** - The passage of nutrients through plasma membranes into the blood or lymph and then to the body.

The **human digestive system** consists of the mouth, pharynx, esophagus, stomach, small and large intestine, rectum, and anus. Enzymes and other secretions are infused into the digestive system to assist the absorption and processing of nutrients. The **nervous and endocrine systems** control the digestive system. Smooth muscle moves the food by peristalsis, contracting and relaxing to move nutrients along.

> **Review Video: Gastrointestinal System**
> Visit mometrix.com/academy and enter code: 378740

MOUTH AND STOMACH

Digestion begins in the mouth with the chewing and mixing of nutrients with **saliva**. Only humans and other mammals actually chew their food. **Salivary glands** are stimulated and secrete saliva. Saliva contains **enzymes** that initiate the breakdown of starch in digestion. Once swallowed, the food moves down the **pharynx** into the **esophagus** en route to the stomach.

The **stomach** is a flexible, muscular sac. It has three main functions:

- Mixing and storing food
- Dissolving and degrading food via secretions
- Controlling passage of food into the small intestine

Protein digestion begins in the stomach. Stomach acidity helps break down the food and make nutrients available for absorption. Smooth muscle contractions move nutrients into the small intestine where the **absorption** process begins.

LIVER

The liver is the largest solid organ of the body. It is also the largest gland. It weighs about three pounds and is located below the diaphragm on the right side of the chest. The liver is made up of four **lobes**. They are called the *right, left, quadrate, and caudate lobes*. The liver is secured to the diaphragm and abdominal walls by five **ligaments**. They are called the *falciform* (that forms a membrane-like barrier between the right and left lobes), *coronary, right triangular, left triangular, and round ligaments*. Nutrient-rich blood is supplied to the liver via the **hepatic portal vein**. The **hepatic artery** supplies oxygen-rich blood. Blood leaves the liver through the **hepatic veins**. The liver's functional units are called **lobules** (made up of layers of liver cells). Blood enters the lobules

146

through branches of the portal vein and hepatic artery. The blood then flows through small channels called **sinusoids**.

The liver is responsible for performing many vital functions in the body including:

- Production of **bile**
- Production of certain **blood plasma proteins**
- Production of **cholesterol** (and certain proteins needed to carry fats)
- Storage of excess glucose in the form of **glycogen** (that can be converted back to glucose when needed)
- Regulation of **amino acids**
- Processing of **hemoglobin** (to store iron)
- Conversion of ammonia (that is poisonous to the body) to **urea** (a waste product excreted in urine)
- **Purification** of the blood (clears out drugs and other toxins)
- Regulation of **blood clotting**
- Controlling infections by boosting **immune factors** and removing bacteria.

The liver processes all of the blood that passes through the digestive system. The nutrients (and drugs) that pass through the liver are converted into forms that are appropriate for the body to use.

SMALL INTESTINE

In the digestive process, most nutrients are absorbed in the **small intestine**. Enzymes from the pancreas, liver, and stomach are transported to the small intestine to aid digestion. These enzymes act on *fats, carbohydrates, nucleic acids, and proteins*. **Bile** is a secretion of the liver and is particularly useful in breaking down fats. It is stored in the **gall bladder** between meals.

By the time food reaches the lining of the small intestine, it has been reduced to small molecules. The lining of the small intestine is covered with **villi**, tiny absorptive structures that greatly increase the surface area for interaction with **chime** (the semi-liquid mass of partially digested food). Epithelial cells at the surface of the villi, called **microvilli**, further increase the ability of the small intestine to serve as the main absorption organ of the digestive tract.

LARGE INTESTINE

Also called the **colon**, the large intestine concentrates, mixes, and stores waste material. A little over a meter in length, the colon ascends on the right side of the abdominal cavity, cuts across transversely to the left side, then descends and attaches to the **rectum**, a short tube for waste disposal.

When the rectal wall is distended by waste material, the nervous system triggers an impulse in the body to expel the waste from the rectum. A muscle **sphincter** at the end of the **anus** is stimulated to facilitate the expelling of waste matter.

The speed at which waste moves through the colon is influenced by the volume of fiber and other undigested material present. Without adequate bulk in the diet, it takes longer to move waste along, sometimes with negative effects. Lack of bulk in the diet has been linked to a number of disorders.

PANCREAS

The pancreas is six to ten inches long and located at the back of the abdomen behind the stomach. It is a long, tapered organ. The wider (right) side is called the **head** and the narrower (left) side is called the **tail**. The head lies near the **duodenum** (the first part of the small intestine) and the tail ends near the **spleen**. The body of the pancreas lies between the head and the tail. The pancreas is made up of exocrine and endocrine tissues. The **exocrine tissue** secretes digestive enzymes from a series of ducts that collectively form the main pancreatic duct (that runs the length of the pancreas). The **main pancreatic duct** connects to the common bile duct near the duodenum. The **endocrine tissue** secretes hormones (such as insulin) into the bloodstream. Blood is supplied to the pancreas from the *splenic artery, gastroduodenal artery, and the superior mesenteric artery.*

DIGESTIVE ROLE OF THE PANCREAS

The pancreas assists in the digestion of foods by secreting **enzymes** (to the small intestine) that help to break down many foods, especially fats and proteins. The precursors to these enzymes (called **zymogens**) are produced by groups of exocrine cells (called **acini**). They are converted, through a chemical reaction in the gut, to the active enzymes (such as **pancreatic lipase** and **amylase**) once they enter the small intestine. The pancreas also secretes large amounts of **sodium bicarbonate** to neutralize the stomach acid that reaches the small intestine. The **exocrine** functions of the pancreas are controlled by hormones released by the stomach and small intestine (duodenum) when food is present. The exocrine secretions of the pancreas flow into the main pancreatic duct (**Wirsung's duct**) and are delivered to the duodenum through the pancreatic duct.

ENZYMES

Enzymes can be divided into six classes: oxidoreductase, transferase, hydrolase, lyase, isomerase, and ligase. These classes end with the suffix "ase," which is true of most enzymes. Each enzyme catalyzes a chemical reaction. **Oxidoreductase enzymes** catalyze oxidation reduction (redox) reactions, during which hydrogen and oxygen are gained or lost. Examples include cytochrome oxidase, lactate, and dehydrogenase. **Transferase enzymes** catalyze the transfer of functional groups, such as the amino or phosphate group. Examples include acetate kinase and alanine deaminase. **Hydrolase enzymes** break chemical bonds by using water. Examples include lipase and sucrase. **Lyase enzymes** break chemical bonds or remove groups of atoms without using water. Examples include oxalate decarboxylase and isocitrate lyase. **Isomerase enzymes** catalyze the rearrangement of atoms within a molecule. Examples include glucose-phosphate isomerase and alanine racemase. **Ligase enzymes** join two molecules by forming a bond between atoms. Examples of ligases are acetyl-CoA synthetase and DNA ligase.

> **Review Video: Enzymes**
> Visit mometrix.com/academy and enter code: 656995

METABOLISM, MACROMOLECULES, METABOLIC PATHWAYS, AND ANABOLIC AND CATABOLIC REACTIONS

Metabolism is all of the chemical reactions that take place within a living organism. These chemical changes convert nutrients to energy and macromolecules. **Macromolecules** are large and complex, and play an important role in cell structure and function. **Metabolic pathways** refer to a series of reactions in which the product of one reaction is the substrate for the next. These pathways are dependent upon enzymes that act as catalysts. An **anabolic reaction** is one that builds larger and more complex molecules (macromolecules) from smaller ones. **Catabolic reactions** are the opposite. Larger molecules are broken down into smaller, simpler molecules. Catabolic reactions release energy, while anabolic ones require energy. The four basic organic macromolecules produced by anabolic reactions are carbohydrates (polysaccharides), nucleic acids, proteins, and lipids. The four basic building blocks involved in catabolic reactions are monosaccharides (i.e. glucose), amino acids, fatty acids (i.e. glycerol), and nucleotides.

AMINO ACIDS

Amino acids are the building blocks of proteins. Structurally, **amino acids** consist of a central carbon atom that is bound to an amino group (-NH₃), a carboxylic acid group (-COOH), a side chain ("R" group), and a hydrogen atom (H).

Each amino acid contains a different **side chain**. Amino acid side chains may be charged, polar, or hydrophobic.

> **Review Video: Amino Acids**
> Visit mometrix.com/academy and enter code: 190385

PROTEINS

Proteins are made up of amino acids that are linked together into a polypeptide chain that folds into a particular structure. The peptide connections are the result of condensation reactions. A condensation reaction results in a loss of water when two molecules are joined together.

Proteins have four levels of structure: primary, secondary, tertiary, and quaternary. **Primary structure** is the amino acid sequence. **Secondary structure** consists of sub-structures called alpha helices and beta sheets. These structures are formed by hydrogen bonding between polar groups in the protein background and may be stabilized by the side chains. Examples of secondary structure are alpha helices and beta sheets. **Tertiary structure** is the interaction between different elements of secondary structure to form a folded geometric shape. **Quaternary structure** is the interaction of one or more folded polypeptide chains to form a multi-subunit protein.

> **Review Video: Proteins**
> Visit mometrix.com/academy and enter code: 903713

LIPIDS

Lipids are molecules that are hydrophobic or amphiphilic (having hydrophilic and hydrophobic properties) in nature. In this way, they are similar to hydrocarbons (substances consisting only of carbon and hydrogen). The major roles of **lipids** include energy storage and structural functions. Examples of these molecules include fats, triglycerides, steroids, and waxes. Lipids have numerous C-H bonds.

Fats are made of long chains of fatty acids (three fatty acids bound to a glycerol). **Fatty acids** are chains with reduced carbon at one end and a carboxylic acid group at the other. An example is soap, which contains the sodium salts of free fatty acids. **Phospholipids** are lipids that have a phosphate group rather than a fatty acid. **Glycerides** are another type of lipid. Examples of glycerides are fats and oils. Glycerides are formed from fatty acids and glycerol (a type of alcohol).

Unlike carbohydrates, amino acids, and nucleic acids, individual lipids will not covalently bond together to form long **polymers**. But the hydrophobic portions of phospholipids may sequester together to form lipid bilayers in cells.

> **Review Video: Lipids**
> Visit mometrix.com/academy and enter code: 269746

GLYCOLYSIS

In glycolysis, glucose is converted into pyruvate and energy stored in ATP bonds is released. Glycolysis can involve various pathways. Various intermediates are produced that are used in other processes, and the **pyruvic acid** produced by glycolysis can be further used for respiration by the Krebs cycle or in fermentation. Glycolysis occurs in both aerobic and anaerobic organisms. Oxidation of molecules produces **reduced coenzymes**, such as NADH. The coenzymes relocate hydrogens to the electron transport chain. The proton is transported through the cell membrane and the electron is transported down the chain by proteins. At the end of the chain, **water** is formed when the final acceptor releases two electrons that combine with oxygen. The protons are pumped back into the cell or organelle by the ATP synthase enzyme, which uses energy produced to add a phosphate to ADP to form **ATP**. The proton motive force is produced by the protons being moved across the membrane.

> **Review Video: Glycolysis**
> Visit mometrix.com/academy and enter code: 466815

MONOSACCHARIDES, DISACCHARIDES, AND STARCHES

The simple sugars can be grouped into monosaccharides (glucose, fructose, and sucrose) and disaccharides. These are all types of carbohydrates. **Monosaccharides** have one monomer of sugar and **disaccharides** have two. Monosaccharides have a carbon:hydrogen:oxygen ratio of 1:2:1. Aldose and ketose are monosaccharides with a carbonyl functional group (oxygen atom and carbon atom joined by a double bond). The difference between aldose and ketose is that the carbonyl group in aldose is connected at an end carbon and the carbonyl group in ketose is connected at a middle carbon. Glucose is a monosaccharide containing six carbons, making it a hexose and an aldose. A disaccharide is formed from two monosaccharides with a glycosidic link. Examples include two glucoses forming a maltose, a glucose and a galactose forming a lactose, and a glucose and a fructose forming a sucrose. A **starch** is a polysaccharide consisting only of glucose monomers. Examples are amylose, amylopectin, and glycogen.

Cardiovascular System

CIRCULATORY SYSTEM

The circulatory system is responsible for the internal transport of substances to and from the cells. The circulatory system usually consists of the following three parts:

- **Blood** - Blood is composed of water, solutes, and other elements in a fluid connective tissue.
- **Blood Vessels** - Tubules of different sizes that transport blood.
- **Heart** - The heart is a muscular pump providing the pressure necessary to keep blood flowing.

Circulatory systems can be either **open** or **closed**. Most animals have closed systems, where the heart and blood vessels are continually connected. As the blood moves through the system from larger tubules through smaller ones, the rate slows down. The flow of blood in the **capillary beds**, the smallest tubules, is quite slow.

A supplementary system, the **lymph vascular system**, cleans up excess fluids and proteins and returns them to the circulatory system.

BLOOD

Blood helps maintain a **healthy internal environment** in animals by carrying raw materials to cells and removing waste products. It helps stabilize internal pH and hosts various kinds of infection fighters.

An adult human has about five quarts of blood. Blood is composed of **red and white blood cells**, **platelets**, and **plasma**. Plasma constitutes over half of the blood volume. It is mostly water and serves as a solvent. Plasma contains plasma proteins, ions, glucose, amino acids, hormones, and dissolved gases.

Red blood cells transport **oxygen** to cells. Red blood cells form in the bone marrow and can live for about four months. These cells are constantly being replaced by fresh ones, keeping the total number relatively stable.

White blood cells defend the body against **infection** and remove various wastes. The types of white blood cells include lymphocytes, neutrophils, monocytes, eosinophils, and basophils. **Platelets** are fragments of stem cells and serve an important function in blood clotting.

BLOOD PRESSURE

Blood pressure is the fluid pressure generated by the cardiac cycle.

Arterial blood pressure functions by transporting oxygen-poor blood into the lungs and oxygen-rich blood to the body tissues. **Arteries** branch into smaller arterioles which contract and expand based on signals from the body. **Arterioles** are where adjustments are made in blood delivery to specific areas based on complex communication from body systems.

Capillary beds are diffusion sites for exchanges between blood and interstitial fluid. A capillary has the thinnest wall of any blood vessel, consisting of a single layer of **endothelial cells**.

Capillaries merge into venules which in turn merge with larger diameter tubules called **veins**. Veins transport blood from body tissues back to the heart. Valves inside the veins facilitate this transport. The walls of veins are thin and contain smooth muscle and also function as blood volume reserves.

BLOOD TYPES

There are four possible **blood types**: A, B, AB, and O. These types are produced by combinations of the three **alleles**. AA and AO lead to type A blood. BB and BO lead to type B blood. AB leads to type AB blood because the alleles are co-dominant. AB has both A antigens and B antigens. The O allele is recessive. OO leads to blood type O, which lacks proteins and blood-surface antigens. Blood donors with an O blood type are known as universal donors because they do not have the type of antigens that can trigger immune system responses. Blood donors with type AB blood are known as universal recipients because they do not have the antibodies that will attack A and B antigen molecules. If parents have AB and O blood, offspring have a 50% chance of having type A blood and a 0% chance of having type O blood.

Antigens trigger a response in the immune system to help repel foreign substances. Matching blood types during medical procedures is important since the human immune system can detect and attack blood that is a different type. Specific blood types are used in transfusions, and blood types are determined based on the **proteins** (or lack of proteins) contained in the blood.

HEART

The heart is a muscular pump made of **cardiac muscle tissue**. It has four chambers; each half contains both an **atrium** and a **ventricle**, and the halves are separated by a valve, known as the AV valve. It is located between the ventricle and the artery leading away from the heart. Valves keep blood moving in a single direction and prevent any backwash into the chambers.

The heart has its own circulatory system with its own **coronary arteries**. The heart functions by contracting and relaxing. **Atrial contraction** fills the ventricles and **ventricular contraction** empties them, forcing circulation. This sequence is called the **cardiac cycle**. Cardiac muscles are attached to each other and signals for contractions spread rapidly. A complex electrical system controls the heartbeat as cardiac muscle cells produce and conduct electric signals. These muscles are said to be **self-exciting**, needing no external stimuli.

> **Review Video: The Heart**
> Visit mometrix.com/academy and enter Code: 451399

CARDIAC CYCLE

The cardiac cycle consists of **diastole** and **systole** phases, which can be further divided into the first and second phases to describe the events of the right and left sides of the heart. However, these events are simultaneously occurring. During the first diastole phase, blood flows through the **superior** and **inferior venae cavae**. Because the heart is relaxed, blood flows passively from the atrium through the open **atrioventricular valve** (tricuspid valve) to the right ventricle. The **sinoatrial (SA) node**, the cardiac pacemaker located in the wall of the right atrium, generates electrical signals, which are carried by the **Purkinje fibers** to the rest of the atrium, stimulating it to contract and fill the right ventricle with blood. The impulse from the SA node is transmitted to the ventricle through the atrioventricular (AV) node, signaling the right ventricle to contract and initiating the first systole phase. The tricuspid valve closes, and the **pulmonary semilunar valve** opens. Blood is pumped out the **pulmonary arteries** to the lungs. Blood returning from the lungs fills the left atrium as part of the second diastole phase. The SA node triggers the **mitral valve** to open, and blood fills the left ventricle. During the second systole phase, the mitral valve closes and the **aortic semilunar valve** opens. The left ventricle contracts, and blood is pumped out of the aorta to the rest of the body.

TYPES OF CIRCULATION

The **circulatory system** includes coronary circulation, pulmonary circulation, and systemic circulation. **Coronary circulation** is the flow of blood to the heart tissue. Blood enters the **coronary arteries**, which branch off the aorta, supplying major arteries, which enter the heart with oxygenated blood. The deoxygenated blood returns to the right atrium through the **cardiac veins**, which empty into the **coronary sinus**. **Pulmonary circulation** is the flow of blood between the heart and the lungs. Deoxygenated blood flows from the right ventricle to the lungs through **pulmonary arteries**. Oxygenated blood flows back to the left atrium through the **pulmonary veins**. **Systemic circulation** is the flow of blood to the entire body with the exception of coronary circulation and pulmonary circulation. Blood exits the left ventricle through the aorta, which branches into the carotid arteries, subclavian arteries, common iliac arteries, and the renal artery. Blood returns to the heart through the jugular veins, subclavian veins, common iliac veins, and renal veins, which empty into the **superior** and **inferior venae cavae**. Included in systemic circulation is **portal circulation**, which is the flow of blood from the digestive system to the liver and then to the heart, and **renal circulation**, which is the flow of blood between the heart and the kidneys.

Lymphatic System

The main function of the lymphatic system is to *return excess tissue fluid to the bloodstream*. This system consists of transport vessels and lymphoid organs. The lymph vascular system consists of **lymph capillaries**, **lymph vessels**, and **lymph ducts**. The major functions of the lymph vascular system are:

- The return of excess fluid to the blood.
- The return of protein from the capillaries.
- The transport of fats from the digestive tract.
- The disposal of debris and cellular waste.

Lymphoid organs include the lymph nodes, spleen, appendix, adenoids, thymus, tonsils, and small patches of tissue in the small intestine. **Lymph nodes** are located at intervals throughout the lymph vessel system. Each node contains **lymphocytes** and **plasma cells**. The **spleen** stores macrophages which help to filter red blood cells. The **thymus** secretes hormones and is the major site of lymphocyte production.

SPLEEN

The spleen is in the upper left of the abdomen. It is located behind the stomach and immediately below the diaphragm. It is about the size of a thick paperback book and weighs just over half a pound. It is made up of **lymphoid tissue**. The blood vessels are connected to the spleen by **splenic sinuses** (modified capillaries). The following **peritoneal ligaments** support the spleen:

- The **gastrolienal ligament** that connects the stomach to the spleen.
- The **lienorenal ligament** that connects the kidney to the spleen.
- The middle section of the **phrenicocolic ligament** (connects the left colic flexure to the thoracic diaphragm).

The main functions of the spleen are to *filter unwanted materials* from the blood (including old red blood cells) and to help *fight infections*. Up to ten percent of the population has one or more accessory spleens that tend to form at the **hilum** of the original spleen.

IMMUNE SYSTEM

The body's general immune defenses include:

- **Skin** - An intact epidermis and dermis form a formidable barrier against bacteria.
- **Ciliated Mucous Membranes** - Cilia sweep pathogens out of the respiratory tract.
- **Glandular Secretions** - Secretions from exocrine glands destroy bacteria.
- **Gastric Secretions** - Gastric acid destroys pathogens.
- **Normal Bacterial Populations** - Compete with pathogens in the gut and vagina.

In addition, **phagocytes** and **inflammation responses** mobilize white blood cells and chemical reactions to stop infection. These responses include localized redness, tissue repair, and fluid-seeping healing agents. Additionally, **plasma proteins** act as the complement system to repel bacteria and pathogens.

Three types of white blood cells form the foundation of the body's immune system. They are:

- **Macrophages** - Phagocytes that alert T cells to the presence of foreign substances.
- **T Lymphocytes** - These directly attack cells infected by viruses and bacteria.
- **B Lymphocytes** - These cells target specific bacteria for destruction.

Memory cells, **suppressor T cells**, and **helper T cells** also contribute to the body's defense. Immune responses can be **anti-body mediated** when the response is to an antigen, or **cell-mediated** when the response is to already infected cells. These responses are controlled and measured counter-attacks that recede when the foreign agents are destroyed. Once an invader has attacked the body, if it returns it is immediately recognized and a secondary immune response occurs. This secondary response is rapid and powerful, much more so than the original response. These memory lymphocytes circulate throughout the body for years, alert to a possible new attack.

> **Review Video: Immune System**
> Visit mometrix.com/academy and enter code: 622899

ACTIVE AND PASSIVE IMMUNITY

At birth, an **innate immune system** protects an individual from pathogens. When an individual encounters infection or has an immunization, the individual develops an **adaptive immunity** that reacts to pathogens. So, this adaptive immunity is acquired. Active and passive immunities can be acquired naturally or artificially.

A **naturally acquired active immunity** is natural because the individual is exposed and builds immunity to a pathogen without an immunization. An **artificially acquired active immunity** is artificial because the individual is exposed and builds immunity to a pathogen by a vaccine.

A **naturally acquired passive immunity** is natural because it happens during pregnancy as antibodies move from the mother's bloodstream to the bloodstream of the fetus. The antibodies can also be transferred from a mother's breast milk. During infancy, these antibodies provide temporary protection until childhood. An **artificially acquired passive immunity** is an immunization that is given in recent outbreaks or emergency situations. This immunization provides quick and short-lived protection to disease by the use of antibodies that can come from another person or animal.

Respiratory System

STRUCTURE

The respiratory system can be divided into the upper and lower respiratory system. The **upper respiratory system** includes the nose, nasal cavity, mouth, pharynx, and larynx. The **lower respiratory system** includes the trachea, lungs, and bronchial tree. Alternatively, the components of the respiratory system can be categorized as part of the airway, the lungs, or the respiratory muscles. The **airway** includes the nose, nasal cavity, mouth, pharynx, (throat), larynx (voice box), trachea (windpipe), bronchi, and bronchial network. The airway is lined with **cilia** that trap microbes and debris and sweep them back toward the mouth. The **lungs** are structures that house the **bronchi** and bronchial network, which extend into the lungs and terminate in millions of **alveoli** (air sacs). The walls of the alveoli are only one cell thick, allowing for the exchange of gases with the blood capillaries that surround them. The right lung has three lobes. The left lung only has two lobes, leaving room for the heart on the left side of the body. The lungs are surrounded by a **pleural membrane**, which reduces friction between surfaces when breathing. The respiratory muscles include the **diaphragm** and the **intercostal muscles**. The diaphragm is a dome-shaped muscle that separates the thoracic and abdominal cavities. The intercostal muscles are located between the ribs.

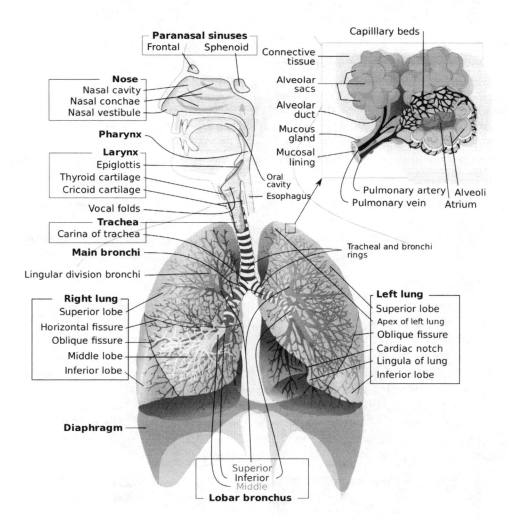

155

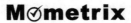

FUNCTION

The main function of the respiratory system is to supply the body with **oxygen** and rid the body of **carbon dioxide**. This exchange of gases occurs in millions of tiny **alveoli**, which are surrounded by blood capillaries.

The respiratory system also filters air. Air is warmed, moistened, and filtered as it passes through the nasal passages before it reaches the lungs.

The respiratory system is responsible for speech. As air passes through the throat, it moves through the **larynx** (voice box), which vibrates and produces sound, before it enters the **trachea** (windpipe). The respiratory system is vital in cough production. Foreign particles entering the nasal passages or airways are expelled from the body by the respiratory system.

The respiratory system functions in the sense of smell. **Chemoreceptors** that are located in the nasal cavity respond to airborne chemicals. The respiratory system also helps the body maintain acid-base **homeostasis**. Hyperventilation can increase blood pH during **acidosis** (low pH). Slowing breathing during **alkalosis** (high pH) helps to lower blood pH.

> **Review Video: Respiratory System**
> Visit mometrix.com/academy and enter code: 783075

BREATHING PROCESS

During the breathing process, the **diaphragm** and the **intercostal muscles** contract to expand the lungs.

During **inspiration** or inhalation, the diaphragm contracts and moves down, increasing the size of the chest cavity. The intercostal muscles contract and the ribs expand, increasing the size of the **chest cavity**. As the volume of the chest cavity increases, the pressure inside the chest cavity decreases. Because the outside air is under a greater amount of pressure than the air inside the lungs, air rushes into the lungs.

When the diaphragm and intercostal muscles relax, the size of the chest cavity decreases, forcing air out of the lungs (**expiration** or exhalation). The breathing process is controlled by the portion of the brain stem called the **medulla oblongata**. The medulla oblongata monitors the level of carbon dioxide in the blood and signals the breathing rate to increase when these levels are too high.

CELLULAR RESPIRATION

Cellular respiration refers to a set of metabolic reactions that convert chemical bonds into energy stored in the form of ATP. Respiration includes many oxidation and reduction reactions that occur thanks to the electron transport system within the cell. Oxidation is a loss of electrons and reduction is a gain of electrons. Electrons in C-H (carbon/hydrogen) and C-C (carbon/carbon) bonds of molecules such as carbohydrates are donated to oxygen atoms. Processes involved in cellular respiration include glycolysis, the Krebs cycle, the electron transport chain, and chemiosmosis. The two forms of respiration are aerobic and anaerobic. **Aerobic respiration** is very common, and oxygen is the final electron acceptor. In **anaerobic respiration**, the final electron acceptor is not oxygen. Aerobic respiration results in more ATP than anaerobic respiration. **Fermentation** is another process by which energy is converted.

> **Review Video: Aerobic Respiration**
> Visit mometrix.com/academy and enter code: 770290

Nervous System

NERVE CELLS

Neurons are nerve cells that transmit nerve impulses throughout the central and peripheral nervous systems for the brain to interpret. The neuron includes the cell body or soma, the dendrites, and the axons. The **soma** contains the nucleus. The **nucleus** contains the chromosomes. The dendrite extends from the cell body and resembles the branches of a tree. The dendrite receives chemical messages from other cells across the synapse, a small gap. The **axon** is a thread-like extension of the cell body, up to 3 feet long in spinal nerves. The axon transmits an electro-chemical message along its length to another cell. Axons of neurons in the **peripheral nervous system (PNS)** that deal with muscles are myelinated with fat to speed up the transmission of messages. Neurons in the PNS that deal with pain are unmyelinated because transmission does not have to be fast. Some neurons in the **central nervous system (CNS)** are myelinated by oligodendrocytes.

NERVOUS SYSTEM

The human nervous system senses, interprets, and issues commands as a response to conditions in the body's environment. This process is made possible by a very complex communication system organized as a grid of **neurons**.

Messages are sent across the plasma membrane of neurons through a process called **action potential**. These messages occur when a neuron is stimulated past a necessary threshold. These stimulations occur in a sequence from the stimulation point of one neuron to its contact with another neuron. At the point of contact, called a **chemical synapse**, a substance is released that stimulates or inhibits the action of the adjoining cell. This network fans out across the body and forms the framework for the nervous system. The direction the information flows depends on the specific organizations of nerve circuits and pathways.

> **Review Video: The Nervous System**
> Visit mometrix.com/academy and enter Code: 708428

CENTRAL NERVOUS SYSTEM

There are two primary components of the central nervous system:

SPINAL CORD

The spinal cord is encased in the bony structure of the **vertebrae**, which protects and supports it. Its nervous tissue functions mainly with respect to limb movement and internal organ activity. Major nerve tracts ascend and descend from the spinal cord to the brain.

BRAIN

The brain consists of the **hindbrain**, which includes the medulla oblongata, cerebellum, and pons. The **midbrain** integrates sensory signals and orchestrates responses to these signals. The **forebrain** includes the cerebrum, thalamus, and hypothalamus. The **cerebral cortex** is a thin layer of gray matter covering the cerebrum. The brain is divided into two **hemispheres**, with each responsible for multiple functions.

The brain is divided into four main **lobes**, the frontal lobe, the parietal lobe, the occipital lobe, and the temporal lobes. The **frontal lobe** located in the front of the brain is responsible for a short term and working memory and information processing as well as decision-making, planning, and judgment. The **parietal lobe** is located slightly toward the back of the brain and the top of the head and is responsible for sensory input as well as spatial positioning of the body. The **occipital lobe** is located at the back of the head just above the brain stem. This lobe is responsible for visual input, processing, and output; specifically nerves from the eyes enter directly into this lobe. Finally, the **temporal lobes** are located at the left and right sides of the brain. These lobes are responsible for all auditory input, processing, and output.

The **cerebellum** plays a role in the processing and storing of *implicit memories*. Specifically, for those memories developed during classical conditioning learning techniques. The role of the cerebellum was discovered by exploring the memory of individuals with damaged cerebellums. These individuals were unable to develop stimulus responses when presented via a classical conditioning technique. Researcher found that this was also the case for automatic responses. For example, when these individuals where presented with a puff or air into their eyes, they did not blink, which would have been the naturally occurring and automatic response in an individual with no brain damage.

The posterior area of the brain that is connected to the spinal cord is known as the **brain stem**. The **midbrain**, the **pons**, and the **medulla oblongata** are the three parts of the brain stem. Information from the body is sent to the brain through the brain stem, and information from the brain is sent to the body through the brain stem. The brain stem is an important part of respiratory, digestive, and circulatory functions.

The **midbrain** lies above the pons and the medulla oblongata. The parts of the midbrain include the **tectum**, the **tegmentum**, and the **ventral tegmentum**. The midbrain is an important part of vision and hearing. The pons comes between the midbrain and the medulla oblongata. Information is sent across the pons from the cerebrum to the medulla and the cerebellum. The **medulla oblongata** (or medulla) is beneath the midbrain and the pons. The medulla oblongata is the piece of the brain stem that connects the spinal cord to the brain. So, it has an important role with the autonomous nervous system in the circulatory and respiratory system.

In addition, the **peripheral nervous system** consists of the nerves and ganglia throughout the body and includes **sympathetic nerves** which trigger the "fight or flight" response, and the **parasympathetic nerves** which control basic body function.

AUTONOMIC NERVOUS SYSTEM

The autonomic nervous system (**ANS**) maintains **homeostasis** within the body. In general, the ANS controls the functions of the internal organs, blood vessels, smooth muscle tissues, and glands. This is accomplished through the direction of the **hypothalamus**, which is located above the midbrain. The hypothalamus controls the ANS through the brain stem. With this direction from the hypothalamus, the ANS helps maintain a stable body environment (homeostasis) by regulating numerous factors including heart rate, breathing rate, body temperature, and blood pH. The ANS consists of two divisions: the sympathetic nervous system and the parasympathetic nervous system. The **sympathetic nervous system** controls the body's reaction to extreme, stressful, and emergency situations. For example, the sympathetic nervous system increases the heart rate, signals the adrenal glands to secrete adrenaline, triggers the dilation of the pupils, and slows digestion. The **parasympathetic nervous system** counteracts the effects of the sympathetic nervous system. For example, the parasympathetic nervous system decreases heart rate, signals the adrenal glands to stop secreting adrenaline, constricts the pupils, and returns the digestion process to normal.

SOMATIC NERVOUS SYSTEM AND REFLEX ARC

The somatic nervous system (**SNS**) controls the five senses and the voluntary movement of skeletal muscle. So, this system has all of the neurons that are connected to sense organs. Efferent (motor) and afferent (sensory) nerves help the somatic nervous system operate the senses and the movement of skeletal muscle. **Efferent nerves** bring signals from the central nervous system to the sensory organs and the muscles. **Afferent nerves** bring signals from the sensory organs and the muscles to the central nervous system. The somatic nervous system also performs involuntary movements which are known as reflex arcs.

A **reflex**, the simplest act of the nervous system, is an automatic response without any conscious thought to a stimulus via the reflex arc. The **reflex arc** is the simplest nerve pathway, which bypasses the brain and is controlled by the spinal cord. For example, in the classic knee-jerk response (patellar tendon reflex), the stimulus is the reflex hammer hitting the tendon, and the response is the muscle contracting, which jerks the foot upward. The stimulus is detected by sensory receptors, and a message is sent along a **sensory** (afferent) neuron to one or more **interneurons** in the spinal cord. The interneuron(s) transmit this message to a **motor** (efferent) neuron, which carries the message to the correct **effector** (muscle).

SENSE OF SIGHT
STRUCTURES OF THE EYE

The eye is composed of many parts that work together to send visual information to the brain through the **optic nerve**, translating the stimuli into images. The front of the eye is clear and called the **cornea**. This is where light travels through and into the pupil, which is the dark center of the iris. The **iris** is the color of the eye, such as brown, blue, or green, and filters the light that comes in. The clear, inside structure of the eye is called the **lens**, and it is responsible for focusing light on the retina. The **retina** is a layer of nerve cells, or photoreceptors, that respond to light stimuli. The **ciliary muscles** help focus this light by manipulating the shape of the lens. Lastly, the middle of the eye is filled with clear fluid known as **vitreous**.

VISUAL PATHWAY IN THE BRAIN

In order to process vision, eyes must send the information they receive to the brain. The **photoreceptors** in the retina capture the visual image and send nerve impulses through the **optic nerve**. Each eye sends its own messages that meet up at the **optic chiasm** and then split up on the way to the brain. Half of the left and right optic nerve travel to the left side of the brain, while the other half of each travel to the right side.

PARALLEL PROCESSING AND FEATURE DETECTION

Parallel processing is when the brain is presented with different stimuli and must process these stimuli at the same time. An example of this would be when the brain is sent an image and it must determine the color, size, texture, and movement simultaneously. **Feature detection** is a theory that explains the reasons why seeing certain images or words may elicit different parts of the brain. It asserts that the nervous system is able to distinguish between significant features of the environment and irrelevant information in the background.

SENSE OF HEARING
STRUCTURE AND FUNCTION OF THE EAR

The three main parts of the ear are classified as the external ear, the middle ear, and the inner ear. The ear canal, which is what sound travels through, and the outside of the ear drum, or tympanic membrane, are in the **external ear**. The bulk of the ear drum resides within the **middle ear** and is what sound bounces off on its way to the brain. Also in the middle ear are the malleus, incus, and stapes or stirrup bones. These bones respond to sound waves by vibrating together, amplifying the sound and creating a wave in the fluid of the ear. This fluid is housed in the cochlea, the structure shaped like a snail containing hair cells that is located in the **inner ear**. The hair cells of the cochlea then send the auditory signals to the brain where they are then processed.

HAIR CELLS

Hair cells are located in the cochlea of the ear and are auditory and vestibular sensory receptors. In response to movement, the hair cells bend and prompt a discharge of neurotransmitters that send signals to the brain. In humans, hair cells are unable to regenerate, so when they are damaged, hearing loss can occur.

AUDITORY PROCESSING AND AUDITORY PATHWAYS IN THE BRAIN

Auditory processing is when sound enters through the ear and is delivered to the brain for interpretation. This sound passes through the ear canal and rebounds off the ear drum, creating vibrations in the cochlea, and is then transmitted via the auditory nerve. The message is sent to the brainstem where it can be translated into information regarding frequency, intensity, and position, and is then passed on through the temporal lobe, specifically the thalamus and auditory cortex. The auditory message is then interpreted to create a comprehensible meaning.

SENSE OF TASTE

Taste receptors pick up signals from specific tastes, which are sent to the brain and translated into flavors. These different tastes include salty, sweet, bitter, sour, and "umami," also known as savory. Taste occurs through **taste buds**, which are spherical-shaped growths on the tongue and are linked to taste receptors. Certain chemicals in food are related to these different tastes, and if present in food, allow the brain to recognize the flavors via the taste hairs covering the taste buds. For a food to be sensed as sweet, it would contain sugar, while umami foods are meaty. Both can be detected by **T1R2** and **T1R3 receptors**. Salt would be present and detected via **sodium channels** to be distinguished as salty. For bitter foods, basic chemicals such as quinine are present, and for sour foods, acidic chemicals would be present. Bitter taste is transmitted through the **T2R receptors** and sour taste through the **transient receptor potential (TRP) channel**.

SENSE OF SMELL

Within the nasal cavity, olfactory cells detect smell, called **olfaction**. These cells are **chemoreceptors** and pick up on specific chemical stimuli in order to deliver messages to the brain about smell.

OLFACTORY PATHWAYS IN THE BRAIN

When a person is exposed to something with a particular smell, this smell enters the **nasal cavity**. Inside the nasal cavity is the **olfactory epithelium**, close in proximity to the brain. Between the brain and the olfactory epithelium are the olfactory bulb and cribriform plate. The **olfactory bulb** has thousands of nerves and these nerves extend through the **cribriform plate** and into the olfactory epithelium. When a smell enters the olfactory epithelium, the cells at the end of these nerves detect the scent and send a message to the brain to interpret the particular smell.

Endocrine System

HORMONES AND GLANDS

Hormones in animals regulate many processes, including growth, metabolism, reproduction, and fluid balance. The names of hormones tend to end in "-one." **Endocrine hormones** are proteins or steroids. **Steroid hormones** (anabolic steroids) help control the manufacture of protein in muscles and bones.

Pancreas: secretes insulin (promotes absorption of glucose) and glucagon (elevates glucose concentration in blood).

Pineal glands: secrete melatonin, which acts as a biological clock.

Pituitary gland: secretes growth hormone (stimulates tissue growth), thyroid stimulating hormone (signals the body to produce thyroxin), adrenocorticotropic hormone (signals the adrenal gland to produce cortisol), follicle-stimulating hormone (signals ovarian follicles to mature in females; helps regulate sperm cell production in males), luteinizing hormone (stimulates the production of estrogens and starts ovulation; stimulates production of testosterone), melanocyte-stimulating hormone (skin tone), and prolactin (stimulates milk let-down).

Thyroid: secretes thyroxine, triiodothyronine, and calcitonin. These are involved with brain development, reproductive tract functions, and metabolism regulation.

Thymus: secretes thymosin.

> **Review Video: Endocrine System**
> Visit mometrix.com/academy and enter code: 678939

HOMEOSTASIS AND FEEDBACK LOOPS

Homeostasis is the ability and tendency of an organism, cell, or body to adjust to environmental changes to maintain equilibrium. One way an organism can maintain homeostasis is through the release of **hormones**. Some hormones work in pairs. When a condition reaches an upper limit, a hormone is released to correct the condition. When a condition reaches the other end of the spectrum, another hormone is released. Hormones that work in this way are termed **antagonistic**. Insulin and glucagon are hormones that help regulate the level of glucagon in the blood. **Positive feedback loops** actually tend to destabilize systems by increasing changes. A **negative feedback loop** acts to make a system more stable by buffering changes.

EXAMPLES OF HOMEOSTASIS

The hormones insulin and glucagon are involved in **negative feedback loops** in the liver's control of blood sugar levels. Alpha cells secrete **glucagon** when the concentration of blood glucose decreases. Glucagon is broken down and fatty acids and amino acids are converted to glucose. Once there is more glucose, glucagon secretion is reduced. Beta cells secrete **insulin** when the concentration of blood glucose increases. This leads to the liver absorbing glucose. Glucose is converted to glycogen, and fat and the concentration of glucose decrease. Insulin production is then reduced.

Hormones work in other ways aside from **antagonistically**. For example, follicle stimulating hormone (FSH) increases the production of estrogen. Once estrogen reaches a certain level, it suppresses FSH production. In some cases, a single hormone can increase or decrease the level of a substance.

161

ENDOCRINE SYSTEM FUNCTION

The endocrine system is responsible for secreting the **hormones** and other molecules that help regulate the entire body in both the short and the long term. There is a close working relationship between the endocrine system and the nervous system. The **hypothalamus** and the **pituitary gland** coordinate to serve as a **neuroendocrine control center**.

Hormone secretion is triggered by a variety of signals, including hormonal signs, chemical reactions, and environmental cues. Only cells with particular **receptors** can benefit from hormonal influence. This is the "key in the lock" model for hormonal action. **Steroid hormones** trigger gene activation and protein synthesis in some target cells. **Protein hormones** change the activity of existing enzymes in target cells. Hormones such as **insulin** work quickly when the body signals an urgent need. Slower acting hormones afford longer, gradual, and sometimes permanent changes in the body.

The eight major endocrine glands and their functions are:

- **Adrenal cortex** - Monitors blood sugar level; helps in lipid and protein metabolism.
- **Adrenal medulla** - Controls cardiac function; raises blood sugar and controls the size of blood vessels.
- **Thyroid gland** - Helps regulate metabolism and functions in growth and development.
- **Parathyroid** - Regulates calcium levels in the blood.
- **Pancreas islets** - Raises and lowers blood sugar; active in carbohydrate metabolism.
- **Thymus gland** - Plays a role in immune responses.
- **Pineal gland** - Has an influence on daily biorhythms and sexual activity.
- **Pituitary gland** - Plays an important role in growth and development.

Endocrine glands are intimately involved in a myriad of reactions, functions, and secretions that are crucial to the well-being of the body.

ENDOCRINE FUNCTIONS OF THE PANCREAS

Located amongst the groupings of **exocrine cells** (acini) are groups of **endocrine cells** (called islets of Langerhans). The **islets of Langerhans** are primarily made up of insulin-producing **beta cells** (fifty to eighty percent of the total) and glucagon-releasing **alpha cells**. The major hormones produced by the pancreas are insulin and glucagon. The body uses **insulin** to control carbohydrate metabolism by lowering the amount of sugar (**glucose**) in the blood. Insulin also affects fat metabolism and can change the liver's ability to release stored fat. The body also uses **glucagon** to control carbohydrate metabolism. Glucagon has the opposite effect of insulin in that the body uses it to increase blood sugar (glucose) levels. The levels of insulin and glucagon are balanced to maintain the optimum level of blood sugar (glucose) throughout the day.

THYROID AND PARATHYROID GLANDS

The thyroid and parathyroid glands are located in the neck just below the larynx. The parathyroid glands are four small glands that are embedded on the posterior side of the thyroid gland. The basic function of the **thyroid gland** is to regulate metabolism. The thyroid gland secretes the hormones thyroxine, triiodothyronine, and calcitonin. **Thyroxine** and **triiodothyronine** increase metabolism, and calcitonin decreases blood calcium by storing calcium in bone tissue. The **hypothalamus** directs the pituitary gland to secrete **thyroid-stimulating hormone (TSH)**, which stimulates the thyroid gland to release these hormones as needed via a negative-feedback mechanism. The **parathyroid glands** secrete **parathyroid hormone**, which can increase blood calcium by moving calcium from the bone to the blood.

Musculoskeletal System

SKELETAL SYSTEM

The skeletal system has an important role in the following body functions:

- **Movement** - The action of skeletal muscles on bones moves the body.
- **Mineral Storage** - Bones serve as storage facilities for essential mineral ions.
- **Support** - Bones act as a framework and support system for the organs.
- **Protection** - Bones surround and protect key organs in the body.
- **Blood Cell Formation** - Red blood cells are produced in the marrow of certain bones.

Bones are classified as either long, short, flat, or irregular. They are a connective tissue with a base of pulp containing **collagen** and living cells. Red marrow, an important site of red blood cell production, fills the spongy tissue of many bones. Bone tissue is constantly regenerating itself as the mineral composition changes. This allows for special needs during growth periods and maintains calcium levels for the body. Bone regeneration can deteriorate in old age, particularly among women, leading to **osteoporosis**.

The skeletal structure in humans contains both **bones** and **cartilage**. There are 206 bones in the human body, divided into two parts:

- **Axial skeleton** - Includes the skull, sternum, ribs, and vertebral column (the spine).
- **Appendicular skeleton** - Includes the bones of the arms, feet, hands, legs, hips, and shoulders.

The flexible and curved **backbone** is supported by muscles and ligaments. **Intervertebral discs** are stacked one above another and provide cushioning for the backbone. Trauma or shock may cause these discs to **herniate** and cause pain. The sensitive **spinal cord** is enclosed in a cavity which is well protected by the bones of the vertebrae.

Joints are areas of contact adjacent to bones. **Synovial joints** are the most common, and are freely moveable. These may be found at the shoulders and knees. **Cartilaginous joints** fill the spaces between some bones and restrict movement. Examples of cartilaginous joints are those between vertebrae. **Fibrous joints** have fibrous tissue connecting bones and no cavity is present.

> **Review Video: Skeletal System**
> Visit mometrix.com/academy and enter code: 256447

HUMAN SKELETON

The human adult skeleton has 206 bones forming a framework that protect and support the internal organs, and work with the muscles to effect movement. The skeleton has two parts: the **axial skeleton**, containing the skull bones, hyoid bone, spinal vertebrae, ribs, and sternum; and the **appendicular skeleton**, containing the pectoral girdle bones, pelvic girdle bones, and extremities, i.e., upper and lower limbs. The **cranial** (skull) bones include the frontal (front), parietal (side), occipital (back), sphenoid (middle) and ethmoid (between the eyes, above the nose) bones. The **facial** bones include the zygomatic (cheekbone), lacrimal (inner eye near the tear duct), and maxilla (several fused upper jaw) and mandible (lower jaw) bones. The **vertebral** bones include the atlas, or first cervical vertebra, supporting the skull; the axis, or second cervical vertebra; the third through seventh cervical vertebrae, i.e., the back bones at the neck level; the 12 thoracic vertebrae, i.e., the back bones at the upper back level; the five lumbar vertebrae, i.e., the back bones at the lower back level; and the sacrum or five sacral vertebrae, the back bones at the level of the pelvis and hips; and three to five small, often fused bones comprising the coccyx or tailbone.

UPPER AND LOWER LIMBS

Bones of the human **upper limbs** include the clavicle, or collarbone; scapula, or shoulder blade; humerus, or upper arm bone; radius and ulna, or forearm bones; carpal or wrist bones; metacarpal or hand bones; and phalanges, or finger bones. The bones of the human **lower limbs** include the os coxa or hip bone, composed of the ilium at the top, pubis at the lower front, and ischium at the lower back, which are fused together. The left and right os coxae form the pelvic girdle. The pelvis is made up of the os coxae, sacrum, and coccyx or tailbone. The femur is the thigh bone, which includes a head, neck, greater trochanter, and shaft. The patella is the knee bone, including a base, medial and lateral facets that articulate (connect) with the femur, and apex. The tibia is the shinbone, to which the thinner fibula (pin) is connected; they connect to the femur. The metatarsal and tarsal bones are the ankle and foot bones; the calcaneus is the heel bone.

MUSCULAR SYSTEM

There are three types of muscle tissue: skeletal, cardiac, and smooth. There are over 600 muscles in the human body. All muscles have these three properties in common:

- **Excitability** - All muscle tissues have an *electric gradient* which can reverse when stimulated.
- **Contraction** - All muscle tissues have the ability to *contract*, or shorten.
- **Elongate** – All muscle tissues share the capacity to *elongate*, or relax.

Only **skeletal muscle** interacts with the skeleton to move the body. When they contract, the muscles transmit force to the attached bones. Working together, the muscles and bones act as a system of levers which move around the joints. A small contraction of a muscle can produce a large movement. A limb can be extended and rotated around a joint due to the way the muscles are arranged.

> **Review Video: Muscular System**
> Visit mometrix.com/academy and enter code: 967216

HEAD, NECK, SHOULDERS, AND CHEST

The **head and neck** include the epicranius frontalis at the cranium's front; epicranius occipitalis at its back; orbicularis oculi around the eye; orbicularis oris around the mouth; buccinator in the cheek; zygomaticus in the cheekbone; platysma in the neck; masseter in the side of the face, connecting and controlling the jaws in chewing; temporalis in the side of the head (also used in chewing); sternocleidomastoid, running from the sternum (chest) along the side of the neck to behind the ear (mastoid) at the base of the skull; splenius capitis in the back of the neck, connecting to the skull's base; and semispinalis capitis in the upper back neck between shoulder and head, rotating the neck. **Shoulders and chest** include the trapezius, a triangle covering the neck, shoulder, and back; rhomboideus major connecting the shoulder blade (scapula) to the vertebrae; levator scapulae; serratus anterior; pectoralis major and minor in the chest; teres major and minor in the shoulder, connecting the upper arm (humerus) to the scapula; latissimus dorsi in the outer sides of the back, connecting to the arms; supraspinatus, a rotator cuff muscle in the shoulder; infraspinatus, a lower-shoulder abductor/external rotator; and deltoid on shoulder top/upper arm.

ABDOMEN, ARMS, THIGHS AND HIPS, AND LOWER LEGS

Abdominal muscles include, outer-to-inner, external (downward/forward) and internal (upward/forward) oblique, transversus abdominis (horizontal/forward), and rectus abdominis. The **arms** contain the biceps brachii (upper-arm front); triceps brachii (upper-arm back); forearm brachioradialis, flexing at the elbow; forearm flexor carpi radialis and flexor carpi ulnaris, flexing and respectively abducting and adducting the hand; extensor carpi ulnaris, extending and adducting the wrist; and extensor digitorum, controlling the middle four fingers. The **thighs and hips** include the rectus femoris, vastus medialis, vastus lateralis, and vastus intermedius, the four quadriceps (front thigh) muscles; sartorius, the body's longest muscle running from the spine along the thigh to the knee; gracilis, running along the inner thigh from pubic bone to tibia; adductor longus, a hip muscle in the inner thigh controlling inward and sideways movement; gluteus maximus, medius, and minimus, three of four buttock muscles—gluteus maximus being the body's largest, strongest muscle; tensor fasciae latae, the fourth, smallest buttock muscle, to the front and side of the others in the thigh; and biceps femoris, semitendinosus, and semimembranosus, the hamstring muscles in the back thigh. The **lower leg** includes the gastrocnemius, plantaris, and soleus in the calf; and tibialis anterior, a dorsal foot flexor.

INTEGUMENTARY SYSTEM

The skin and its associated structures are called the **integumentary system**. It provides the following key functions:

- Protects the body from abrasion and bacterial attack.
- Serves as a control mechanism for internal temperature.
- Provides a reserve of blood vessels that can be used as necessary.
- Produces vitamin D for metabolic purposes.

The top layer of the skin is the epidermis and the layer beneath that is the dermis. The dermis consists of dense connective tissue which protects the body. Skin structure varies widely among animals according to the needs of the particular species. Pigments determine skin color. The process of keratinization results in a new layer of top skin in humans every month or so. This process helps the skin heal itself after minor injuries and forms a barrier against toxic substances and bacterial infections.

> **Review Video: Integumentary System**
> Visit mometrix.com/academy and enter code: 655980

Excretory System

RENAL/URINARY SYSTEM

The renal/urinary system is capable of eliminating excess substances while preserving the substances needed by the body to function. The urinary system consists of the kidneys, urinary ducts, and bladder. The mammalian kidney is a bean-shaped organ attached to the body near the peritoneum. The kidney helps to eliminate water and waste from the body. Within the kidney, there are various tubes and capillaries. Substances exit the bloodstream if they are not needed, and those that are needed are reabsorbed. The unnecessary substances are filtered out into the tubules that

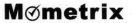

form urine. From theses tubes, urine flows into the bladder and then out of the body through the urethra.

KIDNEYS

The kidneys are bean-shaped structures that are located at the back of the abdominal cavity just under the diaphragm. Each **kidney** consists of three layers: the renal cortex (outer layer), renal medulla (inner layer), and renal pelvis (innermost portion). The **renal cortex** is composed of approximately one million **nephrons**, which are the tiny, individual filters of the kidneys. Each nephron contains a cluster of capillaries called a glomerulus surrounded by the cup-shaped **Bowman's capsule**, which leads to a tubule. The kidneys receive blood from the renal arteries, which branch off the aorta.

In general, the kidneys filter the blood, reabsorb needed materials, and secrete wastes and excess water in the urine. More specifically, blood flows from the **renal arteries** into arterioles into the glomerulus, where it is filtered. The **glomerular filtrate** enters the **proximal convoluted tubule** where water, glucose, ions, and other organic molecules are resorbed back into the bloodstream. Additional substances such as urea and drugs are removed from the blood in the **distal convoluted tubule**. Also, the pH of the blood can be adjusted in the distal convoluted tubule by the secretion of **hydrogen ions**. Finally, the unabsorbed materials flow out from the collecting tubules located in the **renal medulla** to the **renal pelvis** as urine. Urine is drained from the kidneys through the **ureters** to the **urinary bladder**, where it is stored until expulsion from the body through the **urethra**.

Reproductive System

FUNCTION

The **reproductive system** of the human body is responsible solely for the production and utilization of reproductive cells, or **gametes**. The reproductive organs include reproductive organs, the reproductive tract, the perineal structures (external genitalia), and accessory glands and organs responsible for secreting fluids into the reproductive tract.

MALE REPRODUCTIVE SYSTEM

The functions of the male reproductive system are to produce, maintain, and transfer **sperm** and **semen** into the female reproductive tract and to produce and secrete **male hormones**.

The external structure includes the penis, scrotum, and testes. The **penis**, which contains the **urethra**, can fill with blood and become erect, enabling the deposition of semen and sperm into the female reproductive tract during sexual intercourse. The **scrotum** is a sac of skin and smooth muscle that houses the testes and keeps the testes at the proper temperature for **spermatogenesis**. The **testes**, or testicles, are the male gonads, which produce sperm and testosterone.

The internal structure includes the epididymis, vas deferens, ejaculatory ducts, urethra, seminal vesicles, prostate gland, and bulbourethral glands. The **epididymis** stores the sperm as it matures. Mature sperm moves from the epididymis through the **vas deferens** to the **ejaculatory duct**. The **seminal vesicles** secrete alkaline fluids with proteins and mucus into the ejaculatory duct, also. The **prostate gland** secretes a milky white fluid with proteins and enzymes as part of the semen.

The **bulbourethral**, or Cowper's, glands secrete a fluid into the urethra to neutralize the acidity in the urethra.

Additionally, the hormones associated with the male reproductive system include **follicle-stimulating hormone**, which stimulates spermatogenesis; **luteinizing hormone**, which stimulates testosterone production; and **testosterone**, which is responsible for the male sex characteristics.

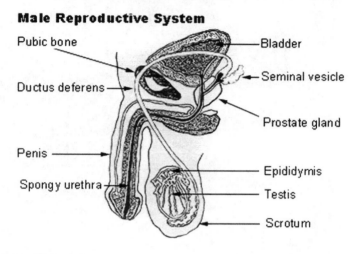

FEMALE REPRODUCTIVE SYSTEM

The functions of the female reproductive system are to produce **ova** (oocytes, or egg cells), transfer the ova to the **fallopian tubes** for fertilization, receive the sperm from the male, and to provide a protective, nourishing environment for the developing **embryo**.

The external portion of the female reproductive system includes the labia majora, labia minora, Bartholin's glands and clitoris. The **labia majora** and the **labia minora** enclose and protect the vagina. The Bartholin's glands secrete a lubricating fluid. The **clitoris** contains erectile tissue and nerve endings for sensual pleasure.

The internal portion of the female reproductive system includes the ovaries, fallopian tubes, uterus, and vagina. The **ovaries**, which are the female gonads, produce the ova and secrete **estrogen** and **progesterone**. The **fallopian tubes** carry the mature egg toward the uterus. Fertilization typically occurs in the fallopian tubes. If fertilized, the egg travels to the **uterus**, where it implants in the uterine wall. The uterus protects and nourishes the developing embryo until birth. The **vagina** is a

167

muscular tube that extends from the **cervix** of the uterus to the outside of the body. The vagina receives the semen and sperm during sexual intercourse and provides a birth canal when needed.

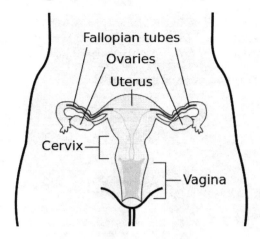

Chemistry

The Atom and The Periodic Table

PROPERTIES OF MATTER

Matter refers to substances that have **mass** and occupy **space** (or volume) the traditional definition of matter describes it as having three states: solid, liquid, and gas These different states are caused by differences in the distances and angles between molecules or atoms, which result in differences in the energy that binds them **Solid** structures are rigid or nearly rigid and have strong bonds Molecules or atoms of **liquids** move around and have weak bonds, although they are not weak enough to readily break Molecules or atoms of **gases** move almost independently of each other, are typically far apart, and do not form bonds the current definition of matter describes it as having four states the fourth is **plasma**, which is an ionized gas that has some electrons that are described as free because they are not bound to an atom or molecule

The following table shows similarities and differences between solids, liquids, and gases:

	Solid	Liquid	Gas
Shape	Fixed shape	No fixed shape (assumes shape of container)	No fixed shape (assumes shape of container)
Volume	Fixed	Fixed	Changes to assume shape of container
Fluidity	Does not flow easily	Flows easily	Flows easily
Compressibility	Hard to compress	Hard to compress	Compresses

Mass: Mass is a measure of the amount of substance in an object

Weight: Weight is a measure of the gravitational pull of Earth on an object

Volume: Volume is a measure of the amount of space occupied There are many formulas to determine volume. For example, the volume of a cube is the length of one side cubed (a^3) and the volume of a rectangular prism is length times width times height ($l \cdot w \cdot h$) the volume of an irregular shape can be determined by how much water it displaces

Density: Density is a measure of the amount of mass per unit volume the formula to find density is mass divided by volume ($D=m/V$) It is expressed in terms of mass per cubic unit, such as grams per cubic centimeter (g/cm^3)

Specific gravity: This is a measure of the ratio of a substance's density compared to the density of water

Both physical changes and chemical reactions are everyday occurrences **Physical changes** do not result in different substances For example, when water becomes ice it has undergone a physical change, but not a chemical change It has changed its form, but not its composition It is still H_2O **Chemical properties** are concerned with the constituent particles that make up the physicality of a substance Chemical properties are apparent when chemical changes occur the chemical properties of a substance are influenced by its electron configuration, which is determined in part by the number of protons in the nucleus (the atomic number) Carbon, for example, has 6 protons and 6

169

electrons It is an element's outermost valence electrons that mainly determine its chemical properties **Chemical reactions** may release or consume energy

STRUCTURE OF ATOMS

All matter consists of **atoms**. Atoms consist of a nucleus and electrons. The **nucleus** consists of protons and neutrons. The properties of these are measurable; they have mass and an electrical charge. The nucleus is positively charged due to the presence of protons. **Electrons** are negatively charged and orbit the nucleus. The nucleus has considerably more mass than the surrounding electrons. Atoms can bond together to make **molecules**. Atoms that have an equal number of protons and electrons are electrically neutral. If the number of protons and electrons in an atom is not equal, the atom has a positive or negative charge and is an **ion**.

Atoms are extremely small. A **hydrogen atom** is about 5×10^{-8} mm in diameter. According to some estimates, five trillion hydrogen atoms could fit on the head of a pin. **Atomic radius** refers to the average distance between the nucleus and the outermost electron. Models of atoms that include the proton, nucleus, and electrons typically show the electrons very close to the nucleus and revolving around it, similar to how the Earth orbits the sun. However, another model relates the Earth as the nucleus and its atmosphere as electrons, which is the basis of the term "**electron cloud**." Another description is that electrons swarm around the nucleus. It should be noted that these atomic models are not to scale. A more accurate representation would be a nucleus with a diameter of about 2 cm in a stadium. The electrons would be in the bleachers.

Atom: The atom is one of the most basic units of matter. An atom consists of a central nucleus surrounded by electrons.

Nucleus: The nucleus of an atom consists of protons and neutrons. It is positively charged, dense, and heavier than the surrounding electrons. The plural form of nucleus is nuclei.

Electrons: These are atomic particles that are negatively charged and orbit the nucleus of an atom.

Protons: Along with neutrons, protons make up the nucleus of an atom. The number of protons in the nucleus determines the atomic number of an element. Carbon atoms, for example, have six protons. The atomic number of carbon is 6. The number of protons also indicates the charge of an atom. The number of protons minus the number of electrons indicates the charge of an atom.

Atomic number (proton number): The atomic number of an element refers to the number of protons in the nucleus of an atom. It is a unique identifier. It can be represented as Z. Atoms with a neutral charge have an atomic number that is equal to the number of electrons.

Neutrons: Neutrons are the uncharged atomic particles contained within the nucleus. The number of neutrons in a nucleus can be represented as "N."

Nucleon: This refers collectively to both neutrons and protons.

Element: An element is matter with one particular type of atom. It can be identified by its atomic number, or the number of protons in its nucleus. There are approximately 117 elements currently known, 94 of which occur naturally on Earth. Elements from the periodic table include hydrogen, carbon, iron, helium, mercury, and oxygen.

Atomic mass: This is also known as the mass number. The atomic mass is the total number of protons and neutrons in the nucleus of an atom. It is referred to as "A." The atomic mass (A) is equal

170

to the number of protons (Z) plus the number of neutrons (N). This can be represented by the equation A = Z + N. The mass of electrons in an atom is basically insignificant because it is so small.

Atomic weight: This may sometimes be referred to as "relative atomic mass," but should not be confused with atomic mass. Atomic weight is the ratio of the average mass per atom of a sample (which can include various isotopes of an element) to 1/12 of the mass of an atom of carbon-12.

> **Review Video: Structure of Atoms**
> Visit mometrix.com/academy and enter code: 905932
>
> **Review Video: Reading Nuclear Equations**
> Visit mometrix.com/academy and enter code: 688890

ISOTOPES

The number of **protons** in an atom determines the element of that atom. for instance, all helium atoms have exactly two protons, and all oxygen atoms have exactly eight protons. If two atoms have the same number of protons, then they are the same element. However, the number of **neutrons** in two atoms can be different without the atoms being different elements. **Isotope** is the term used to distinguish between atoms that have the same number of protons but a different number of neutrons. The names of isotopes have the element name with the mass number. Recall that the **mass number** is the number of protons plus the number of neutrons. for example, carbon-12 refers to an atom that has 6 protons, which makes it carbon, and 6 neutrons. In other words, 6 protons + 6 neutrons = 12. Carbon-13 has six protons and seven neutrons, and carbon-14 has six protons and eight neutrons. Isotopes can also be written with the mass number in superscript before the element symbol. for example, carbon-12 can be written as ^{12}C.

ATOMIC CHARGE

Atomic theory is concerned with the characteristics and properties of atoms that make up matter It deals with matter on a microscopic level as opposed to a macroscopic level Atomic theory, for instance, discusses the kinetic motion of atoms in order to explain the properties of macroscopic quantities of matter **John Dalton** (1766-1844) is credited with making many contributions to the field of atomic theory that are still considered valid This includes the notion that all matter consists of **atoms** and that atoms are indestructible in other words, atoms can be neither created nor destroyed This is also the theory behind the **conservation of matter**, which explains why chemical reactions do not result in any detectable gains or losses in matter This holds true for chemical reactions and smaller scale processes When dealing with large amounts of energy, however, atoms can be destroyed by **nuclear reactions**. This can happen in particle colliders or atom smashers.

Most atoms are **neutral** since the positive charge of the protons in the nucleus is balanced by the negative charge of the surrounding electrons. Electrons are transferred between atoms when they come into contact with each other This creates a molecule or atom in which the number of electrons does not equal the number of protons, which gives it a positive or negative charge. A **negative ion** is created when an atom gains electrons, while a **positive ion** is created when an atom loses electrons An **ionic bond** is formed between ions with opposite charges the resulting compound is neutral. **Ionization** refers to the process by which neutral particles are ionized into charged particles Gases and plasmas can be partially or fully ionized through ionization.

> **Review Video: Nuclear and Chemical Reactions**
> Visit mometrix.com/academy and enter code: 572819

ELECTRONS

Electrons are subatomic particles that orbit the nucleus at various levels commonly referred to as layers, shells, or clouds. The orbiting electron or electrons account for only a fraction of the atom's mass. They are much smaller than the nucleus, are negatively charged, and exhibit wave-like characteristics. Electrons are part of the **lepton** family of elementary particles. Electrons can occupy orbits that are varying distances away from the nucleus, and tend to occupy the lowest energy level they can. If an atom has all its electrons in the lowest available positions, it has a **stable electron arrangement**. The outermost electron shell of an atom in its uncombined state is known as the **valence shell**. The electrons there are called **valence electrons**, and it is their number that determines bonding behavior. Atoms tend to react in a manner that will allow them to fill or empty their valence shells.

PERIODIC TABLE

The periodic table groups elements with similar chemical properties together. The grouping of elements is based on **atomic structure**. It shows periodic trends of physical and chemical properties and identifies families of elements with similar properties. It is a common model for organizing and understanding elements. In the periodic table, each element has its own cell that includes varying amounts of information presented in symbol form about the properties of the element. Cells in the table are arranged in **rows** (periods) and **columns** (groups or families). A cell includes the symbol for the element and its atomic number. The cell for hydrogen, which appears first in the upper left corner, includes an "H" and a "1" above the letter. Elements are ordered by atomic number, left to right, top to bottom.

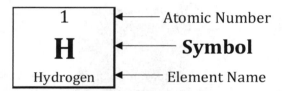

Review Video: **Periodic Table**
Visit mometrix.com/academy and enter code: 154828

In the periodic table, the columns numbered 1 through 18 group elements with similar **outer electron shell configurations**. Since the configuration of the outer electron shell is one of the primary factors affecting an element's chemical properties, elements within the same group have similar chemical properties. Previous naming conventions for groups have included the use of Roman numerals and uppercase letters. Currently, the periodic table groups are: Group 1, alkali metals; Group 2, alkaline earth metals; Groups 3-12, transition metals; Group 13, boron family; Group 14, carbon family; Group 15, pnictogens; Group 16, chalcogens; Group 17, halogens; Group 18, noble gases.

Review Video: **Metals in the Periodic Table**
Visit mometrix.com/academy and enter code: 506502

Review Video: **Noble Gases**
Visit mometrix.com/academy and enter code: 122067

In the periodic table, there are seven **periods** (rows), and within each period there are **blocks** that group elements with the same outer electron subshell. The number of electrons in that outer shell determines which group an element belongs to within a given block. Each row's number (1, 2, 3, etc.) corresponds to the highest number electron shell that is in use. For example, row 2 uses only electron shells 1 and 2, while row 7 uses all shells from 1-7.

Atomic radii will decrease from left to right across a period (row) on the periodic table. In a group (column), there is an increase in the atomic radii of elements from top to bottom. Ionic radii will be smaller than the atomic radii for metals, but the opposite is true for non-metals. From left to right, **electronegativity**, or an atom's likeliness of taking another atom's electrons, increases. In a group, electronegativity decreases from top to bottom. **Ionization energy** or the amount of energy needed to get rid of an atom's outermost electron, increases across a period and decreases down a group. **Electron affinity** will become more negative across a period but will not change much within a group. The **melting point** decreases from top to bottom in the metal groups and increases from top to bottom in the non-metal groups.

Group→	1	2	3	4	5	6	7	8	9	10	11	12	13	14	15	16	17	18
↓Period																		
1	1 H																	2 He
2	3 Li	4 Be											5 B	6 C	7 N	8 O	9 F	10 Ne
3	11 Na	12 Mg											13 Al	14 Si	15 P	16 S	17 Cl	18 Ar
4	19 K	20 Ca	21 Sc	22 Ti	23 V	24 Cr	25 Mn	26 Fe	27 Co	28 Ni	29 Cu	30 Zn	31 Ga	32 Ge	33 As	34 Se	35 Br	36 Kr
5	37 Rb	38 Sr	39 Y	40 Zr	41 Nb	42 Mo	43 Tc	44 Ru	45 Rh	46 Pd	47 Ag	48 Cd	49 In	50 Sn	51 Sb	52 Te	53 I	54 Xe
6	55 Cs	56 Ba	*	72 Hf	73 Ta	74 W	75 Re	76 Os	77 Ir	78 Pt	79 Au	80 Hg	81 Tl	82 Pb	83 Bi	84 Po	85 At	86 Rn
7	87 Fr	88 Ra	**	104 Rf	105 Db	106 Sg	107 Bh	108 Hs	109 Mt	110 Ds	111 Rg	112 Cn	113 Uut	114 Fl	115 Uup	116 Lv	117 Uus	118 Uuo

*	57 La	58 Ce	59 Pr	60 Nd	61 Pm	62 Sm	63 Eu	64 Gd	65 Tb	66 Dy	67 Ho	68 Er	69 Tm	70 Yb	71 Lu
**	89 Ac	90 Th	91 Pa	92 U	93 Np	94 Pu	95 Am	96 Cm	97 Bk	98 Cf	99 Es	100 Fm	101 Md	102 No	103 Lr

ATOMIC MASS UNIT, MOLES, AND AVOGADRO'S NUMBER

Atomic mass unit (**amu**) is the smallest unit of mass, and is equal to 1/12 of the mass of the carbon isotope carbon-12. A **mole (mol)** is a measurement of molecular weight that is equal to the molecule's amu in grams. For example, carbon has an amu of 12, so a mole of carbon weighs 12 grams. One mole is equal to about 6.02×10^{23} elementary entities, which are usually atoms or molecules. This amount is also known as the Avogadro constant or **Avogadro's number (NA)**. Another way to say this is that one mole of a substance is the same as one Avogadro's number of that substance. One mole of chlorine, for example, is 6.02×10^{23} chlorine atoms. The charge on one mole of electrons is referred to as a **Faraday**.

Review Video: Avogadro's Law
Visit mometrix.com/academy and enter code: 360197

Review Video: Mole Concept
Visit mometrix.com/academy and enter code: 593205

Elements, Compounds, and Bonds

ATOMS AND MOLECULES

An **element** is matter with one particular type of atom. Elements from the periodic table such as hydrogen, carbon, iron, helium, mercury, and oxygen are atoms. **Atoms** combine to form **molecules**. For example, two atoms of hydrogen (H) and one atom of oxygen (O) combine to form one molecule of water (H_2O).

THREE STATES OF MATTER

The three states in which matter can exist are solid, liquid, and gas. They differ from each other in the motion of and attraction between individual molecules. In a **solid**, the molecules have little or no motion and are heavily attracted to neighboring molecules, giving them a definite structure. This structure may be ordered/crystalline or random/amorphous. **Liquids** also have considerable attraction between molecules, but the molecules are much more mobile, having no set structure. In a gas, the molecules have little or no attraction to one another and are constantly in motion. They are separated by distances that are very large in comparison to the size of the molecules. **Gases** easily expand to fill whatever space is available. Unlike solids and liquids, gases are easily compressible.

The three states of matter can be traversed by the addition or removal of **heat**. For example, when a solid is heated to its melting point, it can begin to form a liquid. However, in order to transition from solid to liquid, additional heat must be added at the melting point to overcome the latent heat of fusion. Upon further heating to its boiling point, the liquid can begin to form a gas, but again, additional heat must be added at the boiling point to overcome the latent heat of vaporization.

> **Review Video: States of Matter**
> Visit mometrix.com/academy and enter code: 742449
>
> **Review Video: Chemical and Physical Properties of Matter**
> Visit mometrix.com/academy and enter code: 717349

PLASMA

Plasma is an **ionized gas**. However, its properties are different enough from common gas that it is classified as a separate state of matter. It is a gas in which enough energy is provided to free some of the electrons from their atoms. This allows both ions and electrons to coexist. Plasma can be viewed as a cloud of protons, neutrons, and electrons. This enables the plasma to act as a whole rather than as a conglomerate of atoms. This also makes plasma highly **electrically conductive** and easily affected by **electromagnetic fields**. More than 99 percent of the visible universe is made up of plasma, making it the most common state of matter. Plasma is naturally occurring. It is what makes up the sun and the core of stars, and is also found in quasars.

SIX DIFFERENT TYPES OF PHASE CHANGE

A substance that is undergoing a change from a solid to a liquid is said to be **melting**. If this change occurs in the opposite direction, from liquid to solid, this change is called **freezing**. A liquid which is being converted to a gas is undergoing **vaporization**. The reverse of this process is known as **condensation**. Direct transitions from gas to solid and solid to gas are much less common in everyday life, but they can occur given the proper conditions. Solid to gas conversion is known as **sublimation**, while the reverse is called **deposition**.

COMPOUNDS

Compounds are substances containing two or more elements. Compounds are formed by chemical reactions and frequently have different properties than the original elements. Compounds are decomposed by a chemical reaction rather than separated by a physical one.

BINARY COMPOUNDS

Binary compounds refer to compounds that contain only two elements. They can be ionic or covalent. **Binary ionic compounds** are formed by **cations** (metallic positive ions) and **anions** (nonmetal negative ions). Ionic compounds are not molecules. The suffix "ide" is used if there is one anion, as in the case of cuprous oxide, for example. Another example is that fluorine is an element, while fluoride is the negative ion of fluorine. The binary compound barium fluoride would be written as BaF_2. This is because one barium ion has a charge of +2 and one fluoride ion has a charge of -1, so it would take two fluoride ions to balance out the one barium ion. If there is no charge symbol, it is assumed that the charge is 1. The suffixes "ate" or "ite" are used when there is more than one anion, as in the case of mercurous nitrate, for example. A **ternary compound** is one formed of three elements.

INORGANIC COMPOUNDS

The main trait of **inorganic compounds** is that they do not contain **carbon** and **hydrogen**. An example is carbon dioxide. Even though carbon dioxide contains carbon, it is considered inorganic because it does not contain carbon **and** hydrogen. Inorganic compounds also include mineral salts, metals and alloys, non-metallic compounds such as phosphorus, and metal complexes.

Nomenclature refers to the manner in which a compound is named. First, it must be determined whether the compound is **ionic** (formed through electron transfer between cations and anions) or **molecular** (formed through electron sharing between molecules). When dealing with an ionic compound, the name is determined using the standard naming conventions for ionic compounds. This involves indicating the **positive element** first (the charge must be defined when there is more than one option for the valency) followed by the **negative element** plus the appropriate suffix. The rules for naming a molecular compound are as follows: write elements in order of increasing group number and determine the prefix by determining the number of atoms. Exclude mono for the first atom. The name for CO_2, for example, is carbon dioxide. The end of oxygen is dropped and "ide" is added to make oxide, and the prefix "di" is used to indicate there are two atoms of oxygen.

> **Review Video: Ionic Compounds**
> Visit mometrix.com/academy and enter code: 255084

BOND TYPES

Chemical bonds are the attractive forces that bind atoms together into molecules. Atoms form chemical bonds in an attempt to satisfy the octet rule. These bond types include covalent bonds, ionic bonds, and metallic bonds. **Covalent bonds** are formed from the sharing of electron pairs between two atoms in a molecule. **Ionic bonds** are formed from the transferring of electrons between one atom and another, which results in the formations of cations and anions. **Metallic bonding** results from the sharing of delocalized electrons among all of the atoms in a molecule.

IONIC BONDING

Ionic bonding results from the transfer of electrons between atoms. A **cation** or positive ion is formed when an atom loses one or more electrons. An **anion** or negative ion is formed when an atom gains one or more electrons. An **ionic bond** results from the electrostatic attraction between a cation and an anion. One example of a compound formed by ionic bonds is sodium chloride or

NaCl. Sodium (Na) is an alkali metal and tends to form Na⁺ ions. Chlorine is a **halogen** and tends to form Cl⁻ ions. The Na⁺ ion and the Cl⁻ ion are attracted to each other. This **electrostatic attraction** between these oppositely charged ions is what results in the ionic bond between them.

$$Na\cdot + \overset{\times\times}{\underset{\times\times}{Cl}} \times \longrightarrow [Na]^+ [\overset{\times\times}{\underset{\times\times}{Cl}}]^-$$

electron transfer from
sodium to chlorine

COVALENT BONDING

Covalent bonding results from the sharing of electrons between atoms. Atoms seek to fill their **valence shell** and will share electrons with another atom in order to have a full **octet** (except hydrogen and helium, which only hold two electrons in their valence shells). Molecular compounds have covalent bonds. Organic compounds such as proteins, carbohydrates, lipids, and nucleic acids are molecular compounds formed by covalent bonds. Methane (CH_4) is a molecular compound in which one carbon atom is covalently bonded to four hydrogen atoms as shown below.

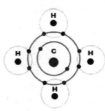

POLAR COVALENT BONDS AND NONPOLAR COVALENT BONDS

Polar covalent bonds result when electrons are shared unequally between atoms. **Nonpolar covalent bonds** result when electrons are shared equally between atoms. The unequal sharing of electrons is due to the differences in the electronegativities of the two atoms sharing the electrons. Partial charges develop due to this unequal sharing of electrons. The greater that the difference is in the electronegativities between the two atoms, the stronger the **dipole** is. For example, the covalent bonds formed between the carbon atom and the two oxygen atoms in carbon dioxide are polar covalent bonds because the electronegativities of carbon and oxygen differ slightly. If the electronegativities are equal, then the covalent bonds are nonpolar. For example, the covalent double bond between two oxygen atoms is nonpolar because the oxygen atoms have the same electronegativities.

RELATIVE BOND LENGTHS OF COVALENT BONDS

The bond length of a covalent bond is the distance between the nuclei of two covalently bonded atoms. The higher the **bond order**, the shorter the bond length. **Single bonds** are between one pair of electrons, and they are the weakest. Because single bonds (bond order 1) are the weakest, they are the longest of the three types of covalent bonds. **Double bonds** are between two pairs of electrons. Because double bonds (bond order 2) are stronger that single bonds, double bonds are shorter than single bonds. **Triple bonds** are between three pairs of electrons. Because triple bonds (bond order 3) are stronger than double bonds and single bonds, triple bonds have the shortest bond length.

RELATIVE BOND STRENGTHS OF COVALENT BONDS

The bond strength determines the amount of energy needed to break a **covalent bond**. Bond strength increases as bond length decreases. The **bond length** is the distance between the nuclei of two covalently bonded atoms. The higher the bond order, the shorter the bond length. **Single**

bonds are between one pair of electrons, and they are the weakest. **Double bonds** are between two pairs of electrons. Double bonds (bond order 2) are stronger that single bonds. **Triple bonds** are between three pairs of electrons. Triple bonds (bond order 3) are stronger than double bonds and single bonds.

METALLIC BONDING

Metallic bonding is a type of bonding between metals. Metallic bonds are similar to covalent bonds in that they are a type of sharing of electrons between atoms. However, in covalent bonding, the electrons are shared with only one other atom. In metallic bonding, the electrons are shared with all the surrounding atoms. These electrons are referred to as **delocalized electrons**. Metallic bonding is responsible for many of the characteristics in metals including conductivity of heat and electricity, malleability, and ductility. An example of metallic bonding is the metallic bond between the copper atoms in a piece of copper wire.

LEWIS STRUCTURE

In order to draw a Lewis structure for a molecule, determine the number of valence electrons for each atom in the molecule and the number of **valence electrons** each atom needs in order to have a full outer shell. All atoms except hydrogen and helium seek to have eight electrons in their outer shells. Hydrogen and helium only have room for two valence electrons. Next, determine the **central atom**. Usually, the central atom is the atom with the largest number of valence openings. Draw the **skeletal structure** with the central atom. Each single bond represents two electrons. Each double bond represents four electrons. Each triple bond represents six electrons. Start with single bonds and change to double or triple bonds as needed to satisfy the **octet rule**. But remember, atoms may only share what they have available. For example, elements in group IIIA have three valence electrons and need an additional five electrons to make eight, but they may only share the three that they have available. Add the remaining valence electrons to all the atoms. Check to make sure that each atom (except hydrogen, helium, and boron) satisfies the octet rule.

MOLECULAR FORMULA

Elements are represented by uppercase letters. If there is no subscript, it indicates there is only one atom of the element. Otherwise, the subscript indicates the number of atoms. In molecular formulas, elements are organized according to the **Hill system**. Carbon is first, hydrogen comes next, and the remaining elements are listed in alphabetical order. If there is no carbon, all elements are listed alphabetically. There are a couple of exceptions to these rules. First, oxygen is usually listed last in oxides. Second, in ionic compounds the positive ion is listed first, followed by the negative ion. In CO_2, for example, C indicates 1 atom of carbon and O_2 indicates 2 atoms of oxygen. The compound is carbon dioxide. The formula for ammonia (an ionic compound) is NH_3, which is one atom of nitrogen and three of hydrogen. H_2O is two atoms of hydrogen and one of oxygen. Sugar is $C_6H_{12}O_6$, which is 6 atoms of carbon, 12 of hydrogen, and 6 of oxygen.

Mixtures and Solutions

IMPORTANT TERMINOLOGY

- A **mixture** is a combination of two or more substances that are not bonded.
- **Suspensions** are mixtures of heterogeneous materials. Particles are usually larger than those found in true solutions. Dirt mixed vigorously with water is an example of a suspension. The dirt is temporarily suspended in water, but the two separate once the mixing is ceased.
- A mixture of large (1 nm to 500 nm) particles is called a **colloidal suspension**.
- The particles are termed **dispersants** and the dispersing medium is similar to the solvent in a solution.
- **Sol** refers to a liquid or a solid that also has solids dispersed through it, such as milk or gelatin. An aerosol spray is a colloid suspension of gas and the solid or liquid being dispersed.
- An **emulsion** refers to a liquid or a solid that has a liquid dispersed through it.
- A **foam** is a liquid that has gas dispersed through it.
- Substances are **immiscible** if they cannot be blended or used to form a single homogeneous substance. They will stay separated or will separate into layers.
- The antonym of immiscible is **miscible**, which refers to substances that can be mixed.

SOLUTIONS

A solution is a homogeneous mixture. A **mixture** is two or more different substances that are mixed together, but not combined chemically. **Homogeneous mixtures** are those that are uniform in their composition. Solutions consist of a **solute** (the substance that is dissolved) and a **solvent** (the substance that does the dissolving). An example is sugar water. The solvent is the water and the solute is the sugar. The intermolecular attraction between the solvent and the solute is called **solvation**. **Hydration** refers to solutions in which water is the solvent. Solutions are formed when the forces between the molecules of the solute and the solvent are as strong as the forces holding the solute together. An example is that salt ($NaCl$) dissolves in water to create a solution. The Na^+ and the Cl^- ions in salt interact with the molecules of water and vice versa to overcome the intramolecular forces of the solute.

> **Review Video: Solutions**
> Visit mometrix.com/academy and enter code: 995937
>
> **Review Video: Stoichiometry**
> Visit mometrix.com/academy and enter code: 801833

PROPERTIES OF SOLUTIONS

Properties of solutions include:

- they have a maximum particle size of one nm
- they do not separate when allowed to stand or when poured through a fiber filter
- they are clear and do not scatter light
- their boiling points increase while their melting points decrease when the amount of solute is increased

SPECIAL SOLUTIONS

A **syrup** is a solution of water and sugar. A **brine** is a solution of table salt, or sodium chloride (NaCl), and water. A **saline solution** is a sterilized solution of sodium chloride in water. A **seltzer** is a solution of carbon dioxide in water.

The term **dilute** is used when there is less solute. Adding more solvent is known as diluting a solution, as is removing a portion of the solute. **Concentrated** is the term used when there is more solute. Adding more solute makes a solution more concentrated, as does removing a portion of the solvent.

CONCENTRATION AND MOLARITY

Concentration can be measured in molarity, molality, or parts per million (ppm). **Molarity** is a measure of the number of moles of solute in a liter of solution. One mole per liter is a 1 M solution. **Molality** is a measure of the number of moles of solute in a kilogram of solution. **Parts per million** is a way of measuring very dilute solutions. One ppm is equal to one gram of solute per one million grams of solution (or, 1 mg/L of water).

> **Review Video: <u>Molarity of a Solution</u>**
> Visit mometrix.com/academy and enter code: 810121

DISTILLATION

Distillation is performed by heating a mixture. Substances differ in their **heat of vaporization**. So when heated, one component of a mixture will generally vaporize before the other. The mixture is put in a flask that's then heated. The component with the lower heat of vaporization is the first to evaporate. A condensing tube circulates water to put the vapor in liquid form. Then the condensate is collected. The flask will contain the left-over component(s) of the mixture.

CHROMATOGRAPHY

Chromatography can be split into the categories of **planar chromatography** and **column chromatography**. It separates compounds by using the differences in the speed of movement of compounds through another medium. In chromatography, a **mobile phase** transports the compound mixture through a **stationary phase**. The stationary phase is responsible for the compound separation.

Chemical Reactions and Catalysts

CHEMICAL REACTIONS

Chemical reactions measured in human time can take place quickly or slowly. They can take fractions of a second or billions of years. The rates of chemical reactions are determined by how frequently reacting atoms and molecules interact. Rates are also influenced by the temperature and various properties (such as shape) of the reacting materials. **Catalysts** accelerate chemical reactions (decrease activation energy), while **inhibitors** decrease reaction rates (increase activation energy). Some types of reactions release energy in the form of heat and light. Some types of reactions involve the transfer of either electrons or hydrogen ions between reacting ions, molecules, or atoms. In other reactions, chemical bonds are broken down by heat or light to form reactive radicals with electrons that will readily form new bonds. Processes such as the formation of ozone and greenhouse gases in the atmosphere and the burning and processing of fossil fuels are controlled by radical reactions.

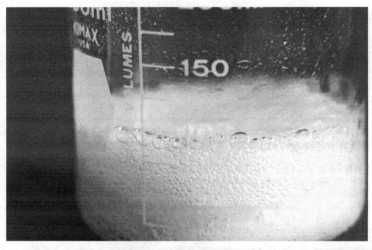

Review Video: Chemical Reactions
Visit mometrix.com/academy and enter code: 579876

Review Video: Catalysts
Visit mometrix.com/academy and enter code: 288189

TYPES OF REACTIONS

One way to organize chemical reactions is to sort them into two categories: **oxidation/reduction reactions** (also called redox reactions) and **metathesis reactions** (which include acid/base reactions). Oxidation/reduction reactions can involve the transfer of one or more electrons, or they can occur as a result of the transfer of oxygen, hydrogen, or halogen atoms. The species that loses electrons is oxidized and is referred to as the reducing agent. The species that gains electrons is reduced and is referred to as the oxidizing agent. The element undergoing oxidation experiences an increase in its oxidation number, while the element undergoing reduction experiences a decrease in its oxidation number. **Single replacement reactions** are types of oxidation/reduction reactions. In a single replacement reaction, electrons are transferred from one chemical species to another. The transfer of electrons results in changes in the nature and charge of the species.

SINGLE SUBSTITUTION, DISPLACEMENT, AND REPLACEMENT REACTIONS

Single substitution, **displacement**, or **replacement reactions** are when one reactant is displaced by another to form the final product (A + BC → AB + C). Single substitution reactions can be cationic or anionic. When a piece of copper (Cu) is placed into a solution of silver nitrate ($AgNO_3$), the solution turns blue. The copper appears to be replaced with a silvery-white material. The equation is $2AgNO_3 + Cu \rightarrow Cu(NO_3)_2 + 2Ag$. When this reaction takes place, the copper dissolves and the silver in the silver nitrate solution precipitates (becomes a solid), resulting in copper nitrate and silver. Copper and silver have switched places in the nitrate.

Double displacement, **double replacement**, **substitution**, **metathesis**, or **ion exchange reactions** are when ions or bonds are exchanged by two compounds to form different compounds (AC + BD → AD + BC). An example of this is that silver nitrate and sodium chloride form two different products (silver chloride and sodium nitrate) when they react. The formula for this reaction is $AgNO_3 + NaCl \rightarrow AgCl + NaNO_3$.

COMBINATION AND DECOMPOSITION REACTIONS

Combination, or **synthesis**, reactions: In a combination reaction, two or more reactants combine to form a single product (A + B → C). These reactions are also called synthesis or **addition reactions**. An example is burning hydrogen in air to produce water. The equation is $2H_2 (g) + O_2 (g) \rightarrow 2H_2O (l)$. Another example is when water and sulfur trioxide react to form sulfuric acid. The equation is $H_2O + SO_3 \rightarrow H_2SO_4$.

Decomposition (or desynthesis, decombination, or deconstruction) reactions: In a decomposition reaction, a reactant is broken down into two or more products (A → B + C). These reactions are also called analysis reactions. **Thermal decomposition** is caused by heat. **Electrolytic decomposition** is due to electricity. An example of this type of reaction is the decomposition of water into hydrogen and oxygen gas. The equation is $2H_2O \rightarrow 2H_2 + O_2$.

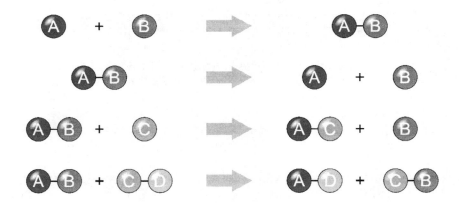

ISOMERIZATION AND NEUTRALIZATION REACTIONS

Isomerization, or **rearrangement**, is the process of forming a compound's isomer. Within a compound, bonds are reformed. The reactant and product have the same molecular formula, but different structural formulas and different properties (A → B or A → A'). For example, butane (C_4H_{10}) is a hydrocarbon consisting of four carbon atoms in a straight chain. Heating it to 100° C or higher in the presence of a catalyst forms isobutane (methylpropane), which has a branched-chain structure. Boiling and freezing points are greatly different for butane and isobutane. A rearrangement reaction occurs within the molecule.

A **neutralization**, **acid-base**, or **proton transfer reaction** is when one compound acquires H^+ from another. These types of reactions are also usually double displacement reactions. The acid has an H^+ that is transferred to the base and neutralized to form a salt.

ACIDS, BASES, AND SALTS

When combined, acids and bases neutralize each other's properties and produce a **salt**. The H^+ cation of the acid combines with the OH^- anion of the base to form water. The cation of the base and the anion of the acid form a salt compound. An example is that hydrochloric acid and sodium hydroxide react to form table salt. The equation for the reaction is $HCl + NaOH \rightarrow H_2O + NaCl$.

The theories related to the classification of acids and bases are the Arrhenius theory, the Brønsted-Lowry theory, and the Lewis theory. The **Arrhenius acid-base theory** states that substances that can ionize to form positive hydrogen ions (H^+) or hydronium ions in an aqueous solution are acids and substances that produce hydroxide ions (OH^-) are bases. The **Brønsted-Lowry theory** states that substances that can act as a proton donor are acids and those that can act as a proton acceptor are bases. The **Lewis theory** states that acids are electron-pair acceptors and bases are electron-pair donors.

PROPERTIES OF ACIDS AND BASES

Some properties of **acids** are that they conduct electricity, change blue litmus paper to red, have a sour taste, react with bases to neutralize them, and react with active metals to free hydrogen. A **weak acid** is one that does not donate all of its protons or disassociate completely. **Strong acids** include hydrochloric, hydriodic, hydrobromic, perchloric, nitric, and sulfuric. They ionize completely. **Superacids** are those that are stronger than 100 percent sulfuric acid. They include fluoroantimonic, magic, and perchloric acids. Acids can be used in pickling, a process used to remove rust and corrosion from metals. They are also used as catalysts in the processing of minerals and the production of salts and fertilizers. Acids may be added to foods as preservatives or to add taste.

Some properties of **bases** are that they conduct electricity, change red litmus paper to blue, feel slippery, and react with acids to neutralize their properties. A **weak base** is one that does not completely ionize in an aqueous solution, and usually has a low pH. **Strong bases** can free protons in very weak acids. Examples of strong bases are hydroxide compounds such as potassium, barium, and lithium hydroxides. Most are in the first and second groups of the periodic table. A **superbase** is extremely strong compared to sodium hydroxide and cannot be kept in an aqueous solution. Superbases are organized into organic, organometallic, and inorganic classes. Bases are used as insoluble catalysts in heterogeneous reactions and as catalysts in hydrogenation.

PH AND PH SCALE

The **potential of hydrogen (pH)** is a measurement of the concentration of hydrogen ions in a substance in terms of the number of moles of H^+ per liter of solution. A lower pH indicates a higher

H^+ concentration, while a higher pH indicates a lower H^+ concentration. Pure water has a neutral pH, which is 7. Anything with a pH lower than water (less than 7) is considered **acidic**. Urine, stomach acid, citric acid, vinegar, hydrochloric acid, and battery acid are acids. Anything with a pH higher than water (greater than 7) is a **base**. Drain cleaner, soap, baking soda, ammonia, egg whites, and sea water are common bases.

PH INDICATORS

A pH indicator is a substance that acts as a detector of hydrogen or hydronium ions. It is halochromic, meaning it changes color to indicate that hydrogen or hydronium ions have been detected. Examples include phenolphthalein, pH paper, and litmus paper.

HYDROLYSIS

Hydrolysis is a chemical reaction between water and another reactant in which both compounds split apart. The water molecules split into hydrogen ions (H+) and hydroxide ions (OH–). The other compound splits into a cation and anion, too. Another way to state this is that hydrolysis is a decomposition reaction of a compound that is combined with water. The general form of a **hydrolysis reaction** is given by $X^-(aq) + H2O(l)(\leftrightarrow)HX(aq) + OH^-(aq)$. A hydrolysis reaction is the reverse process of a neutralization reaction. A neutralization reaction is given by the general form: acid + base → salt + water. In general, a hydrolysis reaction may be thought of as salt + water → acid + base.

ENDOTHERMIC AND EXOTHERMIC REACTIONS

Endothermic reactions are chemical reactions that absorb heat and exothermic reactions are chemical reactions that release heat. The heat difference between endothermic and exothermic reactions is caused by bonds forming and breaking. If more energy is needed to break the reactant bonds than is released when they form, the reaction is **endothermic**. Heat is absorbed and the environmental temperature decreases. If more energy is released when product bonds form than is needed to break the reactant bonds, the reaction is **exothermic**. Heat is released and the environmental temperature increases.

CATALYSTS

Catalysts can increase reaction rates by decreasing the number of steps it takes to form products. The mass of the catalyst should be the same at the beginning of the reaction as it is at the end. The **activation energy** is the minimum amount required to get a reaction started. Activation energy causes particles to collide with sufficient energy to start the reaction. A catalyst enables more particles to react, which lowers the activation energy. Examples of catalysts in reactions are manganese oxide (MnO_2) in the decomposition of hydrogen peroxide, iron in the manufacture of ammonia using the Haber process, and concentrate of sulfuric acid in the nitration of benzene.

> **Review Video: Haber Process for Making Ammonia**
> Visit mometrix.com/academy and enter code: 213059

REACTION RATE

Factors that affect reaction rate include concentration, surface area, and temperature. Increasing the **concentration** of the reactants increases the number of collisions between those reactants and therefore increases the reaction rate. Increasing the **surface area** of contact between the reactants also increases the number of collisions and therefore increases the reaction rate. Finally, increasing the **temperature** of the reactants increases the number of collisions but more significantly also increases the kinetic energy of the reactants, which in turn increases the fraction of molecules

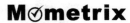

meeting the activation energy requirement. With more molecules at the activation energy, more of the reactants are capable of completing the reaction.

RATE-DETERMINING STEP

Often, when studying specific reactions, only the net reactions are given. Realistically, reactions take place in a series of steps or elementary reactions as shown in the reaction mechanism. Reaction mechanisms show how a reaction proceeds in a series of steps. Some steps are slow, and some are fast. Each step has its own reaction mechanism. The slowest step in the reaction mechanism coincides with the step with the greatest activation energy. This step is known as the **rate-determining step**.

CHEMICAL EQUILIBRIUM

$$N_2 + 3H_2 \leftrightarrow 2NH_3$$

Some chemical reactions are reversible. They can work both ways. Sometimes they can work both ways simultaneously. When a chemical reaction happens in both directions (Forward reaction and Reverse reaction) simultaneously and the rate of reaction is the same on both sides, then a reaction is said to be in a state of **equilibrium**.

Organic Chemistry and Biochemistry

ORGANIC COMPOUNDS

The main trait of organic compounds is that they contain **carbon** *and* **hydrogen**. An example is urea ($CO(NH_2)_2$). Even though urea does not contain carbon-carbon bonds or carbon-hydrogen bonds, it is considered organic because it contains both carbon and hydrogen. Carbon can form long chains, double and triple bonds, and rings. While inorganic compounds tend to have high melting points, organic compounds tend to melt at temperatures below 300° C.

NAMING ALKANES, ALKENES, AND ALKYNES

Hydrocarbons may be classified as alkanes, alkenes, and alkynes based on the type of covalent bonds between the carbon atoms. Molecules with only single bonds between carbon atoms are called **alkanes** with names ending in -*ane*. Molecules with at least one double bond between carbon atoms are called **alkenes** with names ending in -*ene*. Molecules with at least one triple bond between carbon atoms are called **alkynes** with names ending in -*yne*. The prefixes of alkanes, alkenes, alkynes are based on the number of **carbon atoms**. These prefixes are given by the table below. For example, an alkane with one carbon atom would be named methane. An alkane with two carbon atoms would be named ethane. An alkene with two carbon atoms would be named ethene. An alkene with five carbon atoms would be named pentene. An alkyne with four carbon atoms would be named butyne. An alkyne with eight carbon atoms would be named octyne.

Hydrocarbons

#	Prefix	#	Prefix
1	meth-	6	hexa-
2	eth-	7	hepta-
3	prop-	8	octa-
4	but-	9	nona-
5	penta-	10	deca-

NAMING ALCOHOLS, ETHERS, KETONES, ALDEHYDES, AND AMINES

To name an **alcohol**, drop the *-e* from the name of the hydrocarbon and add *-ol*. For example, when the functional group for an alcohol replaces one hydrogen in methane, then the name is changed to methanol. Likewise, ethane becomes ethanol.

Ethers are named for the two hydrocarbons that flank the functional group. The root of the shorter of the two chains is named first. This is followed by *-oxy-*, which is then followed by the name of the longer chain. For example, $CH_3OCH_2CH_3$ is named methoxyethane.

To name a **ketone**, drop *-e* from the name of the hydrocarbon and add *-one*. For example, when the functional group for a ketone is inserted into propane, the name is changed to propanone, which is commonly known as acetone.

To name an **aldehyde**, drop the *-e* from the name of the hydrocarbon and add *-al*. For example, when the functional group for an aldehyde is substituted into methane, the aldehyde name would be methanal.

Amines may be named in more than one way. The two most common ways are either with the prefix *amino-* or the suffix *-amine*. Two simple amines are methylamine (CH_3NH_2) and ethylamine ($CH_3CH_2NH_2$).

CARBOXYLIC ACIDS

Carboxylic acids are organic compounds that contain a **carboxyl functional group** that consists of a carbon atom double-bonded to an oxygen and single-bonded to a hydroxyl (–OH). For example, the simplest carboxylic acid is formic acid, HCO_2H (left). Acetic acid or ethanoic acid, $CH3CO2H$ (right), is commonly known as vinegar. Fatty acids and amino acids are also examples of carboxylic acids.

BENZENE

Benzene is an organic compound that is an aromatic hydrocarbon. **Benzene** has a molecular formula of C_6H_6, where the six carbon atoms are arranged in a "ring" shaped like a hexagon. Each carbon is single-bonded to two other carbons and single-bonded to one hydrogen. The remaining valence electrons from the six carbon atoms are delocalized electrons that are shared among all the carbons in the molecule.

Derivatives of benzene include phenol, which is used in producing carbonates; toluene, which is used as a solvent and an octane booster in gasoline; and aniline, which is used in the production of polyurethane.

BIOMOLECULES

Biomolecules are organic polymers that perform various functions in the human body which are necessary for humans, animals, and plants to function. **Biomolecules** perform various functions including the following:

- Provide a stable structure for the body
- Function as fuel and nutrients for cells
- Serve a role in various reactions as enzymes (biological catalysts)
- Serve to regulate body defense mechanism
- Control genetic functions through heredity

Biomolecules fall within one of the following classes:

- **Carbohydrates** - such as starch (in animals) and cellulose (in plants)
- **Proteins** - such as nucleoprotein, plasma protein, hormones, enzymes and antibodies
- **Nucleic acids** - such as ribonucleic acid (RNA) and deoxyribonucleic acid (DNA)

All biomolecules are **polymers**, which can be hydrolyzed into their base parts, called **monomers**. Polymers are all made up of bound monomers. Carbohydrates are represented by a general formula, (C6H10O5)n, where 40 ≤ n ≤ 3000. Starches produce the monosaccharide glucose (C6H12O6) when hydrolyzed. Glucose remains stored as glycogen in the liver and muscle. Some proteins are structurally synthesized with nucleic acids to form complexes called nucleoproteins.

CLASSIFICATION OF CARBOHYDRATES

Carbohydrates are classified into three categories:

- **Monosaccharide**: Monosaccharides are carbohydrate monomers and are the smallest unit of carbohydrates. They are represented by a general formula (CH2O)n, where n = 3 – 6. Glucose (dextrose), fructose, and galactose are common examples of monosaccharides.
- **Disaccharides**: Disaccharides are made when two monosaccharides are joined together. Disaccharides can also produce two molecules of monosaccharides when hydrolyzed. For example, hydrolyzing sucrose yields one molecule of glucose and one molecule of fructose. Hydrolyzing lactose yields a molecule of glucose and a molecule of galactose. Lastly, hydrolyzing maltose yields two molecules of glucose.
- **Polysaccharides**: Polysaccharides have a high molecular weight for carbohydrates. Polysaccharides can produce many molecules of monosaccharides when hydrolyzed. Examples of polysaccharides are starch, glycogen, and cellulose.

MONOSACCHARIDES

Monosaccharides are named based on the number of **carbon atoms** in the molecule, such as triose (C3), tetrose (C4), pentose (C5), and hexose (C6). Aldoses are the name for a monosaccharide with a group of aldehyde and ketoses are monosaccharides with a ketone group (e.g. fructose).

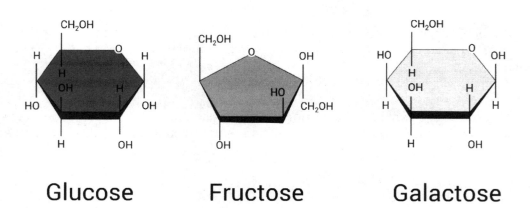

Glucose   Fructose   Galactose

Carbonyl compounds, aldehydes and ketones, can react with –OH group of an alcohol to form hemiacetal and acetal.

Glucose and fructose can form **intramolecular hemiacetal** to produce a cyclic structure because they contain both carbonyl and hydroxyl groups. This hemiacetal formation takes place between the C1 and C5 carbons to form a stable heterocyclic structure. A **pyranose ring**, a six-membered ring consisting of five C atoms and one O atom, forms as a result of the cyclic structure. In a cyclic structure, C1 might have –OH group at the right or left side, and therefore may be termed α-D-glucose and β-D-glucose, respectively.

A **reducing sugar** is a sugar with a free aldehyde or ketone groups which can act as a reducing agent. All monosaccharides are reducing sugars, including glucose, fructose, and galactose. Many disaccharides are also reducing sugars including lactose and maltose (except sucrose). The reducing sugars are able to reduce Fehling's solution and Tollens' reagent.

Fehling's solution is made by mixing a solution of copper sulfate with potassium sodium tartrate in sodium hydroxide (NaOH). When treated with a reducing sugar, the deep blue color of Fehling's solution will fade and subsequently form a red hued precipitate.

Tollen's reagent will cause a silver precipitate when used to head a reducing sugar. The inner surface of the reaction vessel will also form a silver mirror.

LIPIDS

Lipids are a type of biological molecule which is naturally occurring and includes many types of nutrients including fats and vitamins. Lipids are defined as being **hydrophobic**, meaning they will not mix with water well and are unable to bond with the water. Fats, phospholipids, and steroids are the most important types of lipids.

Fats are made of glycerol and fatty acids. A molecule of **glycerol** is a chain of three carbon atoms with a hydroxyl group attached to each atom of carbon. Hydroxyl is one oxygen atom and an atom of hydrogen bonded together. This glycerol atom bonds with **fatty acids** to form fats. Fatty acids are made up of sixteen or eighteen carbon atoms, which are arranged into a backbone structure of long hydrocarbon chains. The carbon atom at the end of a fatty acid makes a double bond with one oxygen atom, using two of its four bonds. This is referred to as a **carboxyl group**. One of the other bonds is used to link to a hydroxyl group. **Fats** are made by joining three molecules of fatty acid and molecule of glycerol.

Glycerol   Fatty Acid

Phospholipids are a type of lipid made when a glycerol molecule is linked to two molecules of fatty acid. One phosphate group is attached to the glycerol molecule's third hydroxyl group. **Phosphate**

groups consist of a single atom of phosphate which is connected to four atoms of oxygen, which results in an overall negative charge. Phospholipids have a peculiar structure resulting from a **hydrophilic phosphate group** head and a **hydrophobic fatty acid** tail. Phospholipids make two layered structures when mixed with water, called **bilayers**, which shield their hydrophobic sections from water. Phospholipids make up **cell membranes** which allow cells to mix with water-based solutions inside and outside. This forms a semi-permeable membrane around a cell, while also making a protective barrier.

Steroids are another type of lipid which is made of four carbon rings that have been fused together. Chemical groups that attach to these rings are what make steroids. Steroids are often found between phospholipid bilayers and help to reinforce the cell membranes while also helping with cell signaling (or communication). Cholesterol is a common example of a steroid found in animal cells.

PROTEINS

Proteins are a type of large biomolecule used for structure, function, and regulation of almost all functions of living beings. Proteins are necessary for a living being to function. The word "protein" traces its etymology to a Greek word for primary or first. Proteins are made from a large set of twenty **amino acids** which are linked together in un-branched polymers. Proteins are diverse because of a wide range of potential combinations. Amino acids form into polymers called **polypeptides**, which derive their name from their peptide bonds. Polypeptides fold up to form coils of molecules used for biological functions. These molecules are called proteins. Proteins have four separate levels of structure:

- **Primary** – The primary structure relates to the sequence of amino acids, which can be arranged in various orders like letters in a word.
- **Secondary** – The secondary structure refers to beta sheets, or alpha helices, which are formed through hydrogen bonding in the polypeptide backbone, between the polar-regions.
- **Tertiary** – The tertiary structure refers to the molecule's overall shape resulting from the interactions between side-chains linked to the polypeptide backbone.
- **Quaternary** – The quaternary structure refers to the structure of the protein when it is made up of two or more polypeptide chains.

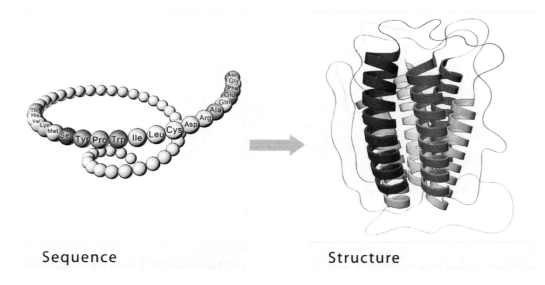

Sequence   Structure

NUCLEIC ACIDS

Nucleic acids are also referred to as **polynucleotides**. This is due to the chains of monomers, called **nucleotides**, which make up nucleic acid. Nucleotides are made up of a nitrogen base, a phosphate group, and a sugar with five carbon atoms. Deoxyribonucleic acid (DNA) and ribonucleic acid (RNA) are the two forms which nucleic acid can take. DNA and RNA are used to store information about and to pass on genetic information to future generations. RNA comes in a single strand of nucleotides which fold onto itself, whereas DNA uses a double-helix structure to hold two strands of nucleotides.

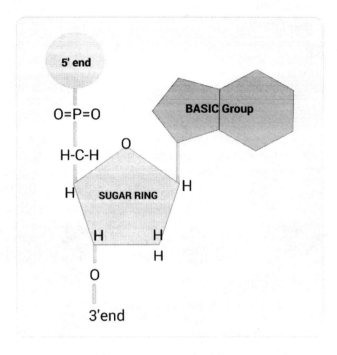

Physics

Classical Mechanics

Mechanics is the study of matter and motion, and the topics related to matter and motion, such as force, energy, and work. Discussions of mechanics will often include the concepts of vectors and scalars. **Vectors** are quantities with both magnitude and direction, while **scalars** have only magnitude. **Scalar quantities** include length, area, volume, mass, density, energy, work, and power. **Vector quantities** include displacement, velocity, acceleration, momentum, and force.

MOTION AND DISPLACEMENT

Motion is a change in the location of an object and is the result of an unbalanced net force acting on the object. Understanding motion requires an understanding of three basic quantities: displacement, velocity, and acceleration.

When something moves from one place to another, it has undergone **displacement**. Displacement along a straight line is a very simple example of a vector quantity. If an object travels from position x = -5 cm to x = 5 cm, it has undergone a displacement of 10 cm. If it traverses the same path in the opposite direction, its displacement is -10 cm. A vector that spans the object's displacement in the direction of travel is known as a **displacement vector**.

> **Review Video: <u>Displacement</u>**
> Visit mometrix.com/academy and enter code: 236197

PROJECTILE, CIRCULAR, AND PERIODIC MOTION

- **Projectile motion**: occurs where an object thrown into the air near the earth's surface moves along an arched path under the effect of gravity alone
- **Circular motion**: movement of an object in a rotating circular path
- **Periodic motion**: motion that is repeated at recurring intervals, such as the swinging of a pendulum

VELOCITY AND ACCELERATIONS

There are two types of velocity to consider: average velocity and instantaneous velocity. Unless an object has a constant velocity or we are explicitly given an equation for the velocity, finding the **instantaneous velocity** of an object requires the use of calculus. If we want to calculate the **average velocity** of an object, we need to know two things: the displacement, or the distance it has covered, and the time it took to cover this distance. The formula for average velocity is simply the distance traveled divided by the time required. In other words, the average velocity is equal to the change in position divided by the change in time. Average velocity is a vector and will always point in the same direction as the displacement vector (since time is a scalar and always positive).

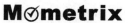

Acceleration is the change in the velocity of an object. Typically, the acceleration will be a constant value. Like position and velocity, acceleration is a vector quantity and will therefore have both magnitude and direction.

Review Video: Speed and Velocity
Visit mometrix.com/academy and enter code: 645590

Review Video: Velocity and Acceleration
Visit mometrix.com/academy and enter code: 671849

ACCELERATION

When an object is thrown upward the acceleration throughout its flight is 9.8 meters per second squared (m/s^2) downward. This is Earth's **gravity** (g) close to its surface. It is the acceleration of all objects when there is no resistance, such as that of air.

If an object is held **stationary**, there is no work performed. This is because the formula for work performed is equal to the force times distance, or **displacement** ($W = F \times d[\cos\theta]$). Displacement is a vector measurement, and there must be displacement for work to be done. If an object is being held up, forces are at work, but are canceling each other out. No work is being done.

NEWTON'S LAWS OF MOTION

FIRST LAW

An object at rest or in motion will remain at rest or in motion unless acted upon by an external force.

This phenomenon is commonly referred to as **inertia**, the tendency of a body to remain in its present state of motion. In order for the body's state of motion to change, it must be acted on by an unbalanced force.

SECOND LAW

An object's **acceleration** is directly proportional to the **net force** acting on the object, and inversely proportional to the object's **mass**.

This law is generally written in equation form F=ma, where F is the net force acting on a body, m is the mass of the body, and a is its acceleration. Note that since the mass is always a positive quantity, the acceleration is always in the same direction as the force.

THIRD LAW

For every force, there is an **equal and opposite** force.

When a hammer strikes a nail, the nail hits the hammer just as hard. If we consider two objects, A and B, then we may express any contact between these two bodies with the equation $F_{AB} = -F_{BA}$, where the order of the subscripts denotes which body is exerting the force. At first glance, this law might seem to forbid any movement at all since every force is being countered with an equal opposite force, but these equal opposite forces are acting on different bodies with different masses, so they will not cancel each other out.

APPLICATIONS OF NEWTON'S LAWS OF MOTION
WEIGHT, MASS, AND ACCELERATION

The **weight** of an object is the force of gravity on the object, and may be defined as the mass times the acceleration of gravity: $w = mg$. **Mass** is the amount of matter an object contains. When an object falls, it will **accelerate** at the same speed regardless of its mass, provided that gravity is the only force working on the object. Where mass can come into play is when there is significant **air resistance**. The force due to air resistance is a function of the object's size, shape, and velocity, but not mass. Thus, the air resistance force on two identically sized and shaped objects of different masses will be the same, but the heavier object will not be as affected, since it requires a greater force to overcome its momentum.

GRAVITATIONAL FORCE AND FRICTION

Gravitational force is a universal force that causes every object to exert a force on every other object. The **gravitational force** between two objects can be described by the formula, $F = Gm_1m_2/r^2$, where m_1 and m_2 are the masses of two objects, r is the distance between them, and G is the gravitational constant, $G = 6.672 \times 10^{-11}$ N-m^2/kg^2. In order for this force to have a noticeable effect, one or both of the objects must be extremely large, so the equation is generally only used in problems involving planetary bodies. For problems involving objects on the earth being affected by earth's gravitational pull, the force of gravity is simply calculated as $F = mg$, where g is 9.8 m/s^2 toward the ground.

Friction is a force that arises as a resistance to motion where two surfaces are in contact. The maximum magnitude of the **frictional force** (f) can be calculated as $f = F_c\mu$, where F_c is the contact force between the two objects and μ is a **coefficient of friction** based on the surfaces' material composition. Two types of friction are static and kinetic. To illustrate these concepts, imagine a book resting on a table. The force of its weight (W) is equal and opposite to the force of the table on the book, or the normal force (N). If we exert a small force (F) on the book, attempting to push it to one side, a frictional force (f) would arise, equal and opposite to our force. At this point, it is a **static frictional force** because the book is not moving. If we increase our force on the book, we will eventually cause it to move. At this point, the frictional force opposing us will be a **kinetic frictional force**. Generally, the kinetic frictional force is lower than static frictional force (because the frictional coefficient for static friction is larger), which means that the amount of force needed to maintain the movement of the book will be less than what was needed to start it moving.

COLLISION AND CONSERVATION OF MOMENTUM

- **Elastic collision**: collision in which the total kinetic energy between two bodies before the collision equals the total kinetic energy after the collision. An example would be a collision between two gas molecules, in which the two molecules only change direction after a collision, but not kinetic energy.
- **Inelastic collision**: collision in which the total kinetic energy between two bodies increases or decreases after a collision. An example would be a collision in which a moving car strikes a parked car, resulting in a single body with a different kinetic energy than either of the original two bodies. In this case, kinetic energy could be lost because of friction between the tires and the road or changes in the car bodies because of the collision.
- **Law of conservation of momentum**: for a collision between two bodies with no external forces, the vector sum of the momentums is not affected by the interaction and remains constant.

DENSITY

A key property determining whether an object will float or sink in water is its **density**. The general rule is that if an object is less dense than water, it floats; if it is denser than water, it sinks. The density of an object is equal to its mass divided by its volume ($d = m/v$). It is important to note the difference between an **object's** density and a **material's** density. Water has a density of one gram per cubic centimeter, while steel has a density approximately eight times that. Despite having a much higher material density, an object made of steel may still float. A hollow steel sphere, for instance, will float easily because the density of the object includes the air contained within the sphere. An object may also float only in certain orientations. An ocean liner that is placed in the water upside down, for instance, may not remain afloat. An object will float only if it can displace a mass of water equal to its own mass.

> **Review Video: Mass, Weight, Volume, Density, and Specific Gravity**
> Visit mometrix.com/academy and enter code: 920570

ENERGY AND WORK

KINETIC AND POTENTIAL ENERGY

The two types of energy most important in mechanics are potential and kinetic energy. **Potential energy** is the amount of energy an object has stored within itself because of its position or orientation. There are many types of potential energy, but the most common is **gravitational potential energy**. It is the energy that an object has because of its height (h) above the ground. It can be calculated as $PE = mgh$, where m is the object's mass and g is the acceleration of gravity. **Kinetic energy** is the energy of an object in motion, and is calculated as $KE = mv^2/2$, where v is the magnitude of its velocity. When an object is dropped, its potential energy is converted into kinetic energy as it falls. These two equations can be used to calculate the velocity of an object at any point in its fall.

> **Review Video: Potential and Kinetic Energy**
> Visit mometrix.com/academy and enter code: 491502

ENERGY TRANSFORMATION

Energy is constantly changing forms and being transferred back and forth. A pendulum swinging is an example of both a kinetic to potential and a potential to kinetic **energy transformation**. When a pendulum is moved from its center point (the point at which it is closest to the ground) to the highest point before it returns, it is an example of a kinetic to potential transformation. When it swings from its highest point toward the center, it is considered a potential to kinetic transformation. The sum of the potential and kinetic energy is known as the **total mechanical energy**. Stretching a rubber band gives it potential energy. That potential energy becomes kinetic energy when the rubber band is released.

Review Video: Energy
Visit mometrix.com/academy and enter code: 677735

TYPES OF ENERGY TRANSFORMATION

Other examples of energy transformations include:

- **Electric to mechanical**: Ceiling fan
- **Chemical to heat**: burning coal
- **Chemical to light**: Phosphorescence and luminescence (which allow objects to glow in the dark) occur because energy is absorbed by a substance (charged) and light is re-emitted comparatively slowly
- **Heat to electricity**: Examples include thermoelectric, geothermal, and ocean thermal.
- **Heat to mechanical**: steam engine
- **Nuclear to heat**: Examples include nuclear reactors and power plants.
- **Mechanical to sound**: Playing a violin or almost any instrument
- **Sound to electric**: Microphone
- **Light to electric**: Solar panels
- **Electric to light**: Light bulbs

WORK

Work can be thought of as the amount of energy expended in accomplishing some goal. The simplest equation for **mechanical work** (W) is $W = Fd$, where F is the force exerted and d is the displacement of the object on which the force is exerted. This equation requires that the force be applied in the same direction as the displacement. If this is not the case, then the work may be calculated as $W = Fd \cos(\theta)$, where θ is the angle between the force and displacement vectors. If force and displacement have the same direction, then work is positive; if they are in opposite directions, then work is negative; and if they are perpendicular, the work done by the force is zero.

If a man pushes a block horizontally across a surface with a constant force of 10 N for a distance of 20 m, the work done by the man is 200 N-m or 200 J. If instead the block is sliding and the man tries to slow its progress by pushing against it, his work done is -200 J, since he is pushing in the direction opposite the motion. If the man pushes vertically downward on the block while it slides, his work done is zero, since his force vector is perpendicular to the displacement vector of the block.

Review Video: Work
Visit mometrix.com/academy and enter code: 681834

SIMPLE MACHINES

Simple machines include the inclined plane, lever, wheel and axle, and pulley. These simple machines have no **internal source of energy**. More complex or compound machines can be formed from them. Simple machines provide a force known as a **mechanical advantage** and make it easier to accomplish a task. The **inclined plane** enables a force less than the object's weight to be used to push an object to a greater height. A **lever** enables a multiplication of force. The **wheel and axle**

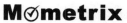

allows for movement with less resistance. Single or double **pulleys** allow for easier direction of force. The wedge and screw are forms of the inclined plane. A **wedge** turns a smaller force working over a greater distance into a larger force. The **screw** is similar to an incline that is wrapped around a shaft.

> **Review Video: <u>Simple Machines</u>**
> Visit mometrix.com/academy and enter code: 950789

MECHANICAL ADVANTAGE

A certain amount of **work** is required to move an object. The amount cannot be reduced, but by changing the way the work is performed a **mechanical advantage** can be gained. A certain amount of work is required to raise an object to a given vertical height. By getting to a given height at an angle, the effort required is reduced, but the distance that must be traveled to reach a given height is increased. An example of this is walking up a hill. One may take a direct, shorter, but steeper route, or one may take a more meandering, longer route that requires less effort. Examples of wedges include doorstops, axes, plows, zippers, and can openers.

> **Review Video: <u>Mechanical Advantage</u>**
> Visit mometrix.com/academy and enter code: 482323

WHEEL AND AXLE

The center of a **wheel and axle** can be likened to a fulcrum on a rotating lever. As it turns, the wheel moves a greater distance than the axle, but with less force. Obvious examples of the wheel and axle are the wheels of a car, but this type of simple machine can also be used to exert a greater force. For instance, a person can turn the handles of a winch to exert a greater force at the turning axle to move an object. Other examples include steering wheels, wrenches, faucets, waterwheels, windmills, gears, and belts. **Gears** work together to change a force. The four basic types of gears are spur, rack and pinion, bevel, and worm gears. The larger gear turns slower than the smaller, but exerts a greater force. Gears at angles can be used to change the direction of forces.

> **Review Video: <u>Simple Machines - Wheel and Axle</u>**
> Visit mometrix.com/academy and enter code: 574045

LEVERS

A lever consists of a bar or plank and a pivot point or fulcrum. Work is performed by the bar, which swings at the pivot point to redirect the force. There are three types of levers: first, second, and third class. Examples of a **first-class lever** include balances, see-saws, nail extractors, and scissors (which also use wedges). In a **second-class lever** the fulcrum is placed at one end of the bar and the work is performed at the other end. The weight or load to be moved is in between. The closer to the fulcrum the weight is, the easier it is to move. Force is increased, but the distance it is moved is decreased. Examples include pry bars, bottle openers, nutcrackers, and wheelbarrows. In a **third-class lever** the fulcrum is at one end and the positions of the weight and the location where the work is performed are reversed. Examples include fishing rods, hammers, and tweezers.

> **Review Video: <u>Levers</u>**
> Visit mometrix.com/academy and enter code: 103910

PULLEYS

A **single pulley** consists of a rope or line that is run around a wheel. This allows force to be directed in a downward motion to lift an object. This does not decrease the force required, just changes its direction. The load is moved the same distance as the rope pulling it. When a **combination pulley** is used, such as a double pulley, the weight is moved half the distance of the rope pulling it. In this way, the work effort is doubled. Pulleys are never 100% efficient because of friction. Examples of pulleys include cranes, chain hoists, block and tackles, and elevators.

> **Review Video: Pulley**
> Visit mometrix.com/academy and enter code: 495865

Thermodynamics

IMPORTANT THERMODYNAMICS TERMINOLOGY

- **Thermodynamics**: This refers to a branch of physics that studies the conversion of energy into work and heat. It is especially concerned with variables such as temperature, volume, and pressure.
- **Thermodynamic equilibrium**: This refers to objects that have the same temperature because heat is transferred between them to reach equilibrium.
- An **open system** is capable of interacting with a surrounding environment and can exchange heat, work (energy), and matter outside their system boundaries.
- A **closed system** can exchange heat and work, but not matter.
- An **isolated system** cannot exchange heat, work, or matter with its surroundings. Its total energy and mass stay the same.
- **Surrounding environment**: In physics, this term refers to everything outside a thermodynamic system (system). The terms "surroundings" and "environment" are also used. The term "boundary" refers to the division between the system and its surroundings.
- **Heat**: Heat is the transfer of energy from a body or system as a result of thermal contact. Heat consists of random motion and the vibration of atoms, molecules, and ions. The higher the temperature is, the greater the atomic or molecular motion will be.
- **Energy**: Energy is the capacity to do work.
- **Work**: Work is the quantity of energy transferred by one system to another due to changes in a system that is the result of external forces, or macroscopic variables. Another way to put this is that work is the amount of energy that must be transferred to overcome a force. Lifting an object in the air is an example of work. The opposing force that must be overcome is gravity. Work is measured in joules (J). The rate at which work is performed is known as power.
- **Thermal energy**: Thermal energy is the energy present in a system due to temperature.
- **Calorie**: This is the amount of energy it takes to raise the temperature of a gram of water by one degree Celsius. A **kilocalorie** refers to the amount of energy it takes to raise the temperature of a kilogram of water by one degree Celsius. A calorie is equal to 4.184 joules.
- **Calorimeter**: This is a measurement device with a thermometer in which chemical or physical processes take place. The resulting change in temperature and the heat capacity can then be determined. Specific heat capacities have already been identified for many materials, and can be viewed in table form.
- **BTU**: This stands for British Thermal Unit. It is a measurement of the amount of energy it takes to raise the temperature of a pound of water by one-degree Fahrenheit. A BTU is equal to 252 calories or 1.054 kilojoules (kJ).
- **Gibbs free energy**: This value is similar to the available energy or maximum work of a closed system.

- **Enthalpy**: This is a measure of heat content in a system. It is usually assumed that the system is closed and the pressure is constant. Enthalpy is represented by the symbol H. The heat of a reaction is the difference between the heat stored in the reactants and in the products. It is represented by ΔH.

> **Review Video: Enthalpy**
> Visit mometrix.com/academy and enter code: 233315

THE LAWS OF THERMODYNAMICS

The laws of thermodynamics are generalized principles dealing with energy and heat.

- The **zeroth law of thermodynamics** states that two objects in thermodynamic equilibrium with a third object are also in equilibrium with each other. Being in thermodynamic equilibrium basically means that different objects are at the same temperature.
- The **first law of thermodynamics** deals with conservation of energy. It states that neither mass nor energy can be destroyed; only converted from one form to another.
- The **second law of thermodynamics** states that the entropy (the amount of energy in a system that is no longer available for work or the amount of disorder in a system) of an isolated system can only increase. The second law also states that heat is not transferred from a lower-temperature system to a higher-temperature one unless additional work is done.
- The **third law of thermodynamics** states that as temperature approaches absolute zero, entropy approaches a constant minimum. It also states that a system cannot be cooled to absolute zero.

The laws of thermodynamics state that **energy** can be exchanged between physical systems as heat or work, and that systems are affected by their **surroundings**. It can be said that the total amount of energy in the universe is constant. The first law is mainly concerned with the conservation of energy and related concepts, which include the statement that energy can only be transferred or converted, not created or destroyed. The formula used to represent the first law is $\Delta U = Q - W$, where ΔU is the change in total internal energy of a system, Q is the heat added to the system, and W is the work done by the system. Energy can be transferred by conduction, convection, radiation, mass transfer, and other processes such as collisions in chemical and nuclear reactions. As transfers occur, the matter involved becomes less ordered and less useful. This tendency towards disorder is also referred to as **entropy**.

GASES

KINETIC THEORY OF GASES

The kinetic theory of gases assumes that gas molecules are small compared to the distances between them and that they are in constant random motion. The attractive and repulsive forces between gas molecules are negligible. Their kinetic energy does not change with time as long as the temperature remains the same. The higher the temperature is, the greater the motion will be. As the temperature of a gas increases, so does the kinetic energy of the molecules. In other words, gas will occupy a greater volume as the temperature is increased and a lesser volume as the temperature is decreased. In addition, the same amount of gas will occupy a greater volume as the temperature increases, but pressure remains constant. At any given temperature, gas molecules have the same **average kinetic energy**.

IDEAL GAS LAW

The ideal gas law is used to explain the properties of a gas under ideal pressure, volume, and temperature conditions. It is best suited for describing monatomic gases (gases in which atoms are not bound together) and gases at high temperatures and low pressures. It is not well-suited for instances in which a gas or its components are close to their condensation point. All collisions are perfectly elastic and there are no intermolecular attractive forces at work. The ideal gas law is a way to explain and measure the macroscopic properties of matter. It can be derived from the kinetic theory of gases, which deals with the microscopic properties of matter. The equation for the ideal gas law is **PV = nRT**, where P is absolute **pressure**, V is absolute **volume**, and T is absolute **temperature**. R refers to the **universal gas constant**, which is 8.3145 J/mol Kelvin, and n is the number of **moles**.

> **Review Video: Ideal Gas Law**
> Visit mometrix.com/academy and enter code: 381353
>
> **Review Video: Ideal Gas vs Real Gas**
> Visit mometrix.com/academy and enter code: 619477

MOLAR MASS, CHARLES'S LAW, AND BOYLE'S LAW

- **Molar mass**: This refers to the mass of one mole of a substance (element or compound), usually measured in grams per mole (g/mol). This differs from molecular mass in that molecular mass is the mass of one molecule of a substance relative to the atomic mass unit (amu).
- **Charles's law**: This states that gases expand when they are heated. It is also known as the law of volumes.
- **Boyle's law**: This states that gases contract when pressure is applied to them. It also states that if temperature remains constant, the relationship between absolute pressure and volume is inversely proportional. When one increases, the other decreases. Considered a specialized case of the ideal gas law, Boyle's law is sometimes known as the Boyle-Mariotte law.

TEMPERATURE, HEAT, AND ENERGY
TEMPERATURE SCALES

There are three main scales for measuring temperature. **Celsius** uses the base reference points of water freezing at 0 degrees and boiling at 100 degrees. **Fahrenheit** uses the base reference points of water freezing at 32 degrees and boiling at 212 degrees. Celsius and Fahrenheit are both relative temperature scales since they use water as their reference point.

The **Kelvin** temperature scale is an absolute temperature scale. Its zero mark corresponds to absolute zero. Water's freezing and boiling points are 273.15 Kelvin and 373.15 Kelvin, respectively. Where Celsius and Fahrenheit are measured is degrees, Kelvin does not use degree terminology.

- Converting Celsius to Fahrenheit: $°F = 9/5°C + 32$
- Converting Fahrenheit to Celsius: $°C = 5/9 (°F − 32)$
- Converting Celsius to Kelvin: $K = °C + 273.15$
- Converting Kelvin to Celsius: $°C = K − 273.15$

HEAT AND TEMPERATURE

Heat is energy transfer (other than direct work) from one body or system to another due to thermal contact. Everything tends to become less organized and less orderly over time (entropy). In all energy transfers, therefore, the overall result is that the energy is spread out uniformly. This transfer of heat energy from hotter to cooler objects is accomplished by conduction, radiation, or convection. **Temperature** is a measurement of an object's stored heat energy. More specifically, temperature is the average kinetic energy of an object's particles. When the temperature of an object increases and its atoms move faster, kinetic energy also increases. Temperature is not energy since it changes and is not conserved. Thermometers are used to measure temperature.

CONDUCTION

Conduction is a form of heat transfer that occurs at the molecular level. It is the result of molecular agitation that occurs within an object, body, or material while the material stays motionless. An example of this is when a frying pan is placed on a hot burner. At first, the handle is not hot. As the pan becomes hotter due to conduction, the handle eventually gets hot too. In this example, energy is being transferred down the handle toward the colder end because the higher speed particles collide with and transfer energy to the slower ones. When this happens, the original material becomes cooler and the second material becomes hotter until equilibrium is reached. **Thermal conduction** can also occur between two substances such as a cup of hot coffee and the colder surface it is placed on. Heat is transferred, but matter is not.

CONVECTION AND RADIATION

- **Convection** refers to heat transfer that occurs through the movement or circulation of fluids (liquids or gases). Some of the fluid becomes or is hotter than the surrounding fluid, and is less dense. Heat is transferred away from the source of the heat to a cooler, denser area. Examples of convection are boiling water and the movement of warm and cold air currents in the atmosphere and the ocean. **Forced convection** occurs in convection ovens, where a fan helps circulate hot air.
- **Radiation** is heat transfer that occurs through the emission of electromagnetic waves, which carry energy away from the emitting object. All objects with temperatures above absolute zero radiate heat.
- **Latent heat** refers to the amount of heat required for a substance to undergo a phase (state) change (from a liquid to a solid, for example).

HEAT CAPACITY AND SPECIFIC HEAT

- **Heat capacity**, also known as thermal mass, refers to the amount of heat energy required to raise the temperature of an object, and is measured in Joules per Kelvin or Joules per degree Celsius. The equation for relating heat energy to heat capacity is $Q = C\Delta T$, where Q is the heat energy transferred, C is the heat capacity of the body, and ΔT is the change in the object's temperature.
- **Specific heat capacity**, also known as specific heat, is the heat capacity per unit mass. Every element and compound has its own specific heat. For example, it takes different amounts of heat energy to raise the temperature of the same amounts of magnesium and lead by one degree. The equation for relating heat energy to specific heat capacity is $Q = mc\Delta T$, where m represents the mass of the object, and c represents its specific heat capacity.

Review Video: Specific Heat Capacity
Visit mometrix.com/academy and enter code: 736791

Waves

WAVE BASICS

TERMINOLOGY

- **Frequency** is a measure of how often particles in a medium vibrate when a wave passes through the medium with respect to a certain point or node. Usually measured in Hertz (Hz), frequency might refer to cycles per second, vibrations per second, or waves per second. One Hz is equal to one cycle per second.
- **Period** is a measure of how long it takes to complete a cycle. It is the inverse of frequency; where frequency is measure in cycles per second, period can be thought of as seconds per cycle, though it is measured in units of time only.
- **Speed** refers to how fast or slow a wave travels. It is measured in terms of distance divided by time. While frequency is measured in terms of cycles per second, speed might be measured in terms of meters per second.
- **Amplitude** is the maximum amount of displacement of a particle in a medium from its rest position, and corresponds to the amount of energy carried by the wave. High-energy waves have greater amplitudes; low energy waves have lesser amplitudes. Amplitude is a measure of a wave's strength.
- **Rest position**, also called equilibrium, is the point at which there is neither positive nor negative displacement.
- **Crest**, also called the peak, is the point at which a wave's positive or upward displacement from the rest position is at its maximum.
- **Trough**, also called a valley, is the point at which a wave's negative or downward displacement from the rest position is at its maximum.
- A **wavelength** is one complete wave cycle. It could be measured from crest to crest, trough to trough, rest position to rest position, or any point of a wave to the corresponding point on the next wave.

TYPES

Waves are divided into types based on the direction of particle motion in a medium and the direction of wave propagation.

- **Longitudinal waves**: These are waves that travel in the same direction as the particle movement. They are sometimes called pressure, compression, or density waves. Longitudinal sound waves are the easiest to produce and have the highest speed. A longitudinal wave consists of compressions and rarefactions, such as those seen by extending and collapsing a Slinky toy.
- **Shear or transverse waves**: These types of waves move perpendicular to the direction of the particle movement. For example, if the particles in a medium move up and down, a transverse wave will move forward. Transverse waves are possible only in solids and are slower than longitudinal waves.
- **Surface (circular) waves**: These waves travel at the surface of a material and move in elliptical orbits. They are a little slower than shear waves.
- **Plate waves**: These waves move in elliptical orbits and only occur in very thin pieces of material.

INTERACTIONS

Waves can be in phase or out of **phase**, which is similar to the concept of being in sync or out of sync. For example, if two separate waves originate from the same point and the peaks (crests) and valleys (troughs) are exactly aligned, they are said to be **in phase**. If the peak of a wave aligns with the valley of another wave, they are **out of phase**. When waves are in phase their displacement is doubled. If they are out of phase, they cancel each other out. If they are somewhere in between being completely in phase and completely out of phase, the wave interaction is a wave that is the sum of the **amplitudes** of all points along the wave. If waves originate from different points, the amplitude of particle displacement is the combined sum of the particle displacement amplitude of each individual wave.

INTERFERENCE

When waves traveling in the same medium interact, it is known as **wave interference**. While a single wave generally remains the same in terms of waveform, frequency, amplitude, and wavelength, several waves traveling through particles in a medium take on a more complicated appearance after they interact. The final properties of a wave are dependent on many factors, such as the points of origin of waves and whether they are in phase, out of phase, or somewhere in between. **Constructive interference** refers to what happens when two crests or two troughs of a wave meet. The resulting amplitude of the crest or trough is doubled. **Destructive interference** is what happens when the crest of one wave and the trough of another that are the same shape meet. When this occurs, the two waves cancel each other out.

DIFFRACTION

Diffraction refers to the bending of waves around small objects and the spreading out of waves past small openings. The narrower the opening, the greater the level of diffraction will be. Larger wavelengths also increase diffraction. A **diffraction grating** can be created by placing a number of slits close together, and is used more frequently than a prism to separate light. Different wavelengths are diffracted at different angles.

> **Review Video: Diffraction of Light Waves**
> Visit mometrix.com/academy and enter code: 785494

WAVEFORMS

Waveforms refer to the shapes and forms of waves as they are depicted on graphs. Forms include sinusoidal, square, triangle, and sawtooth. **Sinusoidal** refers to a waveform in which the amplitude (displacement from the rest position) is proportional to the sine (side opposite of angle/hypotenuse) of a variable such as time. Square, triangle, and sawtooth waveforms are **non-sinusoidal**, and are usually based on formulas. **Square waves** are used to depict digital information. **Pulse waves**, also known as rectangular waves, are a non-sinusoidal form similar to square waves, and are found in synthesizer programming. **Triangle waves**, like square waves, only have odd harmonics. The harmonic of a wave is the integer multiple of a base frequency. **Sawtooth waves** have both even and odd harmonics, and produce a sound particularly suited for synthesizing bowed string instruments.

TRANSFER OF ENERGY IN WAVES

Waves have **energy** and can transfer energy when they interact with matter. Although waves transfer energy, they do not transport **matter**. They are a disturbance of matter that transfers energy from one particle to an adjacent particle. There are many types of waves, including sound, seismic, water, light, micro, and radio waves. The two basic categories of waves are mechanical and electromagnetic. **Mechanical waves** are those that transmit energy through matter. **Electromagnetic waves** can transmit energy through a vacuum. A **transverse wave** provides a good illustration of the features of a wave, which include crests, troughs, amplitude, and wavelength.

PHENOMENON OF SOUND

Sound is a pressure disturbance that moves through a medium in the form of mechanical waves. Sound requires a medium to travel through, such as air, water, or other matter since it is the vibrations that transfer energy to adjacent particles, not the actual movement of particles over a great distance. Sound is transferred through the movement of atomic particles, which can be atoms or molecules. Waves of sound energy move outward in all directions from the source. **Sound waves** consist of **compressions** (particles are forced together) and **rarefactions** (particles move farther apart and their density decreases). A wavelength consists of one compression and one rarefaction. Different sounds have different wavelengths. Sound is a form of kinetic energy.

PITCH, LOUDNESS, TIMBRE, AND OSCILLATION

- **Pitch**: Pitch is the quality of sound determined by frequency. For example, a musical note can be tuned to a specific frequency. Humans can detect frequencies between about 20 Hz to 20,000 Hz.
- **Loudness**: Loudness is a human's perception of sound intensity.
- Sound intensity: Sound intensity is measured as the sound power per unit area, and can be expressed in decibels.
- **Timbre**: This is a human's perception of the type or quality of sound.
- **Oscillation**: This is a measurement, usually of time, against a basic value, equilibrium, or rest point.

DOPPLER EFFECT

The **Doppler effect** refers to the effect the relative motion of the source of the wave and the location of the observer has on waves. The Doppler effect is easily observable in sound waves. What a person hears when a train approaches or a car honking its horn passes by are examples of the Doppler effect. The pitch of the sound is different not because the *emitted frequency* has changed, but because the *received frequency* has changed. The frequency is higher (as is the pitch) as the train approaches, the same as emitted just as it passes, and lower as the train moves away. This is because the wavelength changes. A **redshift** occurs when light or radiation is increased in wavelength. A **blueshift** is a decrease in wavelength.

ELECTROMAGNETIC SPECTRUM

The electromagnetic spectrum is defined by frequency (f) and wavelength (λ). Frequency is typically measured in hertz and wavelength is usually measured in meters. Because light travels at a fairly constant speed, **frequency** is inversely proportional to **wavelength**, a relationship expressed by the formula $f = c/\lambda$, where c is the speed of light (about 300 million meters per second). Frequency multiplied by wavelength equals the speed of the wave; for electromagnetic waves, this is the speed of light, with some variance for the medium in which it is traveling. Electromagnetic waves include (from largest to smallest wavelength) radio waves, microwaves, infrared radiation (radiant heat), visible light, ultraviolet radiation, x-rays, and gamma rays. The energy of electromagnetic waves is carried in packets that have a magnitude inversely proportional to the wavelength. **Radio waves** have a range of wavelengths, from about 10^{-3} to 10^5 meters, while their frequencies range from about 10^3 to 10^{11} Hz.

Review Video: Electromagnetic Radiation Waves
Visit mometrix.com/academy and enter code: 135307

Review Video: Electromagnetic Spectrum
Visit mometrix.com/academy and enter code: 771761

VISIBLE LIGHT

Light is the portion of the electromagnetic spectrum that is visible because of its ability to stimulate the **retina**. It is absorbed and emitted by electrons, atoms, and molecules that move from one energy level to another. **Visible light** interacts with matter through molecular electron excitation (which occurs in the human retina) and through plasma oscillations (which occur in metals). Visible light is between ultraviolet and infrared light on the spectrum. The wavelengths of visible light cover a range from 380 nm (violet) to 760 nm (red). Different wavelengths correspond to different colors. **Dispersion** is the action of distributing radiation according to wavelength, such as light into colors.

> **Review Video: Light**
> Visit mometrix.com/academy and enter code: 900556

PERCEPTION OF COLOR

The human brain interprets or perceives visible light, which is emitted from the sun and other stars, as **color**. For example, when the entire wavelength reaches the retina, the brain perceives the color white. When no part of the wavelength reaches the retina, the brain perceives the color black. The particular color of an object depends upon what is **absorbed** and what is **transmitted** or **reflected**. For example, a leaf consists of chlorophyll molecules, the atoms of which absorb all wavelengths of the visible light spectrum except for green, which is why a leaf appears green. Certain wavelengths of visible light can be absorbed when they interact with matter. Wavelengths that are not absorbed can be transmitted by transparent materials or reflected by opaque materials.

LIGHT AND SOLID OBJECTS

When light waves encounter an object, the light waves are reflected, transmitted, or absorbed. If the light is **reflected** from the surface of the object, the angle at which it contacts the surface will be the same as the angle at which it leaves, on the other side of the perpendicular. If the ray of light is perpendicular to the surface, it will be reflected back in the direction from which it came. When light is **transmitted** through the object, its direction may be altered upon entering the object. This is known as refraction. When light waves are refracted, or bent, an image can appear distorted. The degree to which the light is refracted depends on the speed at which light travels in the object. Light that is neither reflected nor transmitted will be **absorbed** by the surface and stored as heat energy. Nearly all instances of light hitting an object will involve a combination of two or even all three of these.

> **Review Video: Reflection, Transmission, and Absorption of Light**
> Visit mometrix.com/academy and enter code: 109410

LIGHT WAVES AND CHANGING MEDIA

When light waves pass from water to air, the frequency stays the same even though the speed and wavelength increase. This is because frequency is equal to speed (velocity) divided by wavelength ($f = v/\lambda$). In this case, there are two different mediums (water and air), which have different **refractive indexes**. Air has a smaller refractive index. The smaller the refractive index, the faster light moves through the medium. The refractive index of a medium can affect the speed and direction of travel of transmitted light. In air, both the speed and wavelength of the light increase, but the frequency (the number of cycles in a given unit of time) is the same. The **speed** of a wave is equal to its frequency times its wavelength ($v = f \times \lambda$). **Nodes** of a wave are the points at which the amplitude is at its minimum. **Wavelength** is measured as the distance between nodes.

GEOMETRIC OPTICS

Geometric optics uses the concept of rays to determine how light will propagate. **Ray diagrams** can illustrate the path of light through a lens. Different types of lenses refract light, either convergently or divergently, to form images. After passing through a lens, rays converge at a focal point. **Collimated rays** are nearly parallel, and can be thought of as having no focal point. There are many types and combinations of lenses. **Convergent lenses**, also called positive lenses, are thicker in the middle and thinner at the edges. Rays are focused to a point. **Divergent lenses**, also called negative lenses, are thicker at the ends and thinner in the middle. Rays are spread apart, or diverged. A **convex lens** is bowed outward, either at one vertical surface or both. A convex lens with two convex surfaces may also be termed biconvex or double convex. A **concave lens** is bowed inward, while a planar lens is flat.

Electricity, Magnetism, and Beyond

ELECTRICITY AND MAGNETISM

ELECTRIC CHARGE AND ATOMIC STRUCTURE

The attractive force between the electrons and the nucleus is called the **electric force**. A positive (+) charge or a negative (-) charge creates a field of sorts in the empty space around it, which is known as an **electric field**. The direction of a positive charge is away from it and the direction of a negative charge is towards it. An electron within the force of the field is pulled towards a positive charge because an electron has a negative charge. A particle with a positive charge is pushed away, or repelled, by another positive charge. Like charges repel each other and opposite charges attract. **Lines of force** show the paths of charges. The **magnitude** of the force is directly proportional to the magnitude of the charges (q) and inversely proportional to the square of the distance (r) between the two objects: $F = kq_1q_2/r^2$, where $k = 9 \times 10^9$ N-m^2/C^2. This relationship is known as **Coulomb's Law**. **Electric charge** is measured with the unit Coulomb (C). It is the amount of charge moved in one second by a steady current of one ampere (1C = 1A × 1s).

> **Review Video: Electric Charge**
> Visit mometrix.com/academy and enter code: 323587
>
> **Review Video: Electric Force**
> Visit mometrix.com/academy and enter code: 717639

STATIC ELECTRICITY AND CHARGE PRODUCTION

A glass rod and a plastic rod can illustrate the concept of **static electricity** due to friction. Both start with no charge. A glass rod rubbed with silk produces a **positive charge**, while a plastic rod rubbed with fur produces a **negative charge**. The electron affinity of a material is a property that helps determine how easily it can be charged by friction. Materials can be sorted by their affinity for electrons into a triboelectric series. Materials with greater affinities include celluloid, sulfur, and rubber. Materials with lower affinities include glass, rabbit fur, and asbestos. In the example of a glass rod and a plastic one, the glass rod rubbed with silk acquires a positive charge because glass has a lower affinity for electrons than silk. The electrons flow to the silk, leaving the rod with fewer electrons and a positive charge. When a plastic rod is rubbed with fur, electrons flow to the rod and result in a negative charge.

Insulators are materials that prevent the movement of electrical charges, while **conductors** are materials that allow the movement of electrical charges. This is because conductive materials have free electrons that can move through the entire volume of the conductor. This allows an external charge to change the charge distribution in the material. In induction, a neutral conductive material, such as a sphere, can become charged by a positively or negatively charged object, such as a rod. The charged object is placed close to the material without touching it. This produces a force on the **free electrons**, which will either be attracted to or repelled by the rod, polarizing (or separating) the charge. The sphere's electrons will flow into or out of it when touched by a ground. The sphere is now charged. The charge will be opposite that of the charging rod.

Charging by conduction is similar to charging by induction, except that the material transferring the charge actually touches the material receiving the charge. A negatively or positively charged object is touched to an object with a **neutral charge**. Electrons will either flow into or out of the neutral object and it will become charged. Insulators cannot be used to conduct charges. Charging by conduction can also be called charging by contact. The **law of conservation of charge** states that the total number of units before and after a charging process remains the same. No electrons have been created. They have just been moved around. The removal of a charge on an object by conduction is called **grounding**.

MAGNETIC FIELDS AND ATOMIC STRUCTURE

The motions of subatomic structures (nuclei and electrons) produce a **magnetic field**. It is the direction of the spin and orbit that indicates the direction of the field. The strength of a magnetic field is known as the magnetic moment. As electrons spin and orbit a nucleus, they produce a magnetic field.

Pairs of electrons that spin and orbit in opposite directions cancel each other out, creating a **net magnetic field** of zero. Materials that have an unpaired electron are magnetic. Those with a weak attractive force are referred to as **paramagnetic materials**, while **ferromagnetic materials** have a strong attractive force. A **diamagnetic material** has electrons that are paired, and therefore does not typically have a magnetic moment. There are, however, some diamagnetic materials that have a weak magnetic field.

A magnetic field can be formed not only by a magnetic material, but also by electric current flowing through a wire. When a coiled wire is attached to the two ends of a battery, for example, an **electromagnet** can be formed by inserting a ferromagnetic material such as an iron bar within the coil. When electric current flows through the wire, the bar becomes a magnet. If there is no current, the magnetism is lost. A **magnetic domain** occurs when the magnetic fields of atoms are grouped and aligned. These groups form what can be thought of as miniature magnets within a material. This is what happens when an object like an iron nail is temporarily magnetized. Prior to magnetization, the organization of atoms and their various polarities are somewhat random with respect to where the north and south poles are pointing. After magnetization, a significant percentage of the poles are lined up in one direction, which is what causes the magnetic force exerted by the material.

> **Review Video: Magnetic Field Part I**
> Visit mometrix.com/academy and enter code: 953150
>
> **Review Video: Magnetic Field Part II**
> Visit mometrix.com/academy and enter code: 710249

MAGNETS AND MAGNETISM

A magnet is a piece of metal, such as iron, steel, or magnetite (lodestone) that can affect another substance within its field of force that has like characteristics. Magnets can either attract or repel other substances. Magnets have two **poles**: north and south. Like poles repel and opposite poles (pairs of north and south) attract. The magnetic field is a set of invisible lines representing the paths of attraction and repulsion.

Magnetism can occur naturally, or ferromagnetic materials can be magnetized. Certain matter that is magnetized can retain its magnetic properties indefinitely and become a permanent magnet. Other matter can lose its magnetic properties. For example, an iron nail can be temporarily magnetized by stroking it repeatedly in the same direction using one pole of another magnet. Once magnetized, it can attract or repel other magnetically inclined materials, such as paper clips. Dropping the nail repeatedly will cause it to lose its magnetic properties.

VALENCE ELECTRONS AND CONDUCTION

When studying atoms at a microscopic level, it can be seen that some materials such as metals have properties that allow electrons to flow easily. Metals are good **conductors** of electricity because their valence electrons are loosely held in a network of atoms. This is because the valence shells of metal atoms have weak attractions to their nuclei. This results in a "sea of electrons," and electrons can flow between atoms with little resistance. In **insulating** materials such as glass, they hardly flow at all. In between materials can be called **semiconducting materials**, and have intermediate conducting behavior. At low temperatures, some materials become superconductors and offer no resistance to the flow of electrons. **Thermal conductivity** refers to a material's capacity to conduct heat.

> **Review Video: Resistance of Electric Currents**
> Visit mometrix.com/academy and enter code: 668423

ELECTRIC MOTORS

An electric motor converts electric energy into **mechanical energy**. Energy can be provided by an AC or DC source. The power provided has many practical applications. The basic premise of a motor is that the electric current passing through a wire or coil creates a magnetic field that opposes the poles of a permanent magnet. The repelling forces between one pole of the electromagnet and the opposing pole of the fixed magnet cause the coil to move about ½ a turn. As it approaches the pole of like attraction, the coil would normally stop moving. In a motor, however, the current is reversed at this time, which reverses the poles and again forces rotation. In a **DC motor**, a switch or commuter can be used to reverse the charge. In an **AC motor**, the charge alternates on its own. The coil is attached to a shaft that is rotated, which provides the mechanical energy necessary to do work.

ELECTRICAL GENERATORS AND ELECTRIC POTENTIAL

An electrical generator is the opposite of a motor in that it transforms magnetic force into electrical energy. Like a motor, however, it uses an electromagnetic field and a permanent magnet to achieve **electromagnetic induction**. Generators do not create electricity, but rather convert mechanical energy into electric energy. Smaller gas generators are used as backup or primary power sources of electricity for equipment, homes, and other small-scale applications. Larger generators may use mechanical energy from many different sources, including water, steam, wind, compressed air, or even a hand crank.

Electric potential, or electrostatic potential or voltage, is an expression of potential energy per unit of charge. It is measured in volts (V) as a scalar quantity. The formula used is $V = E/Q$, where V is voltage, E is electrical potential energy, and Q is the charge. **Voltage** is typically discussed in the context of electric potential difference between two points in a circuit. Voltage can also be thought of as a measure of the rate at which energy is drawn from a source in order to produce a flow of electric charge.

CIRCUIT BASICS

A circuit is a closed path along which electrons can travel with minimal resistance except at particular locations. **Electric current** is the sustained flow of electrons that are part of an electric charge moving along a path in a circuit. This differs from a **static electric charge**, which is a constant non-moving charge rather than a continuous flow. The rate of flow of electric charge is expressed using the ampere (amp or A) and can be measured using an ammeter. A current of 1 ampere means that 1 coulomb of charge passes through a given area every second. Electric charges typically only move from areas of high electric potential to areas of low electric potential.

DIRECT AND ALTERNATING CURRENT

Direct current (DC) is the flow of an electric charge in one direction. Batteries and solar cells typically use direct current.

Alternating current (AC) is current that periodically reverses direction. AC is typically used in houses and other buildings.

OHM'S LAW

Electric currents experience **resistance** as they travel through a circuit. Resistance is the hindrance to the flow of an electric charge. Different objects have different levels of resistance. The **ohm** (Ω) is the measurement unit of electric resistance. The symbol is the Greek letter omega. **Ohm's Law**, which is expressed as $I = V/R$, states that current flow (I, measured in amps) through an object is equal to the potential difference from one side to the other (V, measured in volts) divided by resistance (R, measured in ohms). An object with a higher resistance will have a lower current flow through it given the same potential difference.

SIMPLE CIRCUITS

Movement of electric charge along a path between areas of high electric potential and low electric potential, with a resistor or load device between them, is the definition of a **simple circuit**. It is a closed conducting path between the high and low potential points, such as the positive and negative terminals on a battery. One example of a circuit is the flow from one terminal of a car battery to the other. The electrolyte solution of water and sulfuric acid provides work in chemical form to start the flow. A frequently used classroom example of circuits involves using a D cell (1.5 V) battery, a small light bulb, and a piece of copper wire to create a circuit to light the bulb.

SERIES CIRCUITS

Series circuits are circuits in which there is only one path through which electrons can flow. An example of a **series circuit** is a string of old-fashioned Christmas tree lights. If a load in this type of circuit is removed, disabled, or switched off, the circuit is open and electricity does not flow. In the series circuit below, three resistors are in series, and their equivalent **resistance** is:

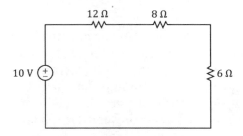

$$R_{eq} = R_1 + R_2 + \cdots + R_n = 12 + 8 + 6 = 26\Omega$$

PARALLEL CIRCUIT

A parallel circuit is one in which there is more than one path through which electrons can travel. In a parallel circuit, the same voltage exists across all parallel paths, though the current may be vastly different among them. For the **parallel circuit** below, the equivalent **resistance** is:

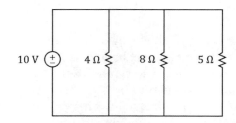

$$R_{eq} = \frac{1}{\dfrac{1}{R_1} + \dfrac{1}{R_2} + \cdots + \dfrac{1}{R_n}} = \frac{1}{\dfrac{1}{4} + \dfrac{1}{8} + \dfrac{1}{5}}$$

POWER, WATT, AND TRANSFORMER

- **Power**: Measured in watts, electric power refers to the rate at which electrical energy is transferred by an electric circuit. It can be calculated using **Joule's law**: P = VI, where *P* is power, *V* is the potential difference (in volts) and *I* is current (in amps). Power can be generated, transmitted, and converted into various forms of light.
- **Watt**: A watt is the unit used to measure power. One watt is equal to one joule of energy per second.
- **Transformer**: A transformer is a device that uses induction to transfer current from one circuit to another. Two wound coils act as a pair of **inductors**. Voltage can be modified to be transferred to another circuit (as in transmission lines) or to a load, such as an electrical device plugged into a socket.

NUCLEAR PHYSICS

NUCLEAR BINDING ENERGY

The nuclear binding energy of an atom is the energy that would be required to disassemble the nucleus into its **constituent nucleons**. They are held together by a strong nuclear force in the nucleus. Nuclear binding energy may be calculated by determining the difference in mass between the nucleus and the sum of the masses of its constituent particles. This mass, m, is converted to energy by the equation E = mc², where c is the speed of light in a vacuum.

Nuclei may be **transformed** by a rearrangement of nucleons. These nuclear transformations may occur by many different means, including radioactive decay, nuclear fusion, and nuclear fission. In nuclear fusion, two light nuclei merge into a single nucleus that is heavier. In nuclear fission, a single large nucleus divides into two or more smaller nuclei. In either case, if the mass of the nuclei before transformation is greater than the mass after transformation, then it is an exothermic process. Conversely, if the mass is greater after transformation, the process is endothermic. Nickel and iron have the most stable nuclei of any elements, having the largest binding energies.

NUCLEAR REACTIONS

The particles of an atom's nucleus (the protons and neutrons) are bound together by **nuclear force**, also known as **residual strong force**. Unlike chemical reactions, which involve electrons, nuclear reactions occur when two nuclei or nuclear particles collide. This results in the release or absorption of energy and products that are different from the initial particles. The energy released in a nuclear reaction can take various forms, including the release of kinetic energy of the product particles and the emission of very high energy photons known as **gamma rays**. Some energy may also remain in the nucleus. **Radioactivity** refers to the particles emitted from nuclei as a result of nuclear instability. There are many nuclear isotopes that are unstable and can spontaneously emit some kind of radiation. The most common types of radiation are alpha, beta, and gamma radiation, but there are several other varieties of radioactive decay.

RADIOACTIVITY

Radioactive decay: This occurs when an unstable atomic nucleus spontaneously loses energy by emitting ionizing particles and radiation. Decay is a form of energy transfer, as energy is lost. It also results in different products. Before decay there is one type of atom, called the **parent nuclide**. After decay there are one or more different products, called the **daughter nuclide(s)**.

Radioactivity: This refers to particles that are emitted from nuclei as a result of nuclear instability.

> **Review Video: Radioactivity**
> Visit mometrix.com/academy and enter code: 537142

Radioactive half-life is the time it takes for half of the radioactive nuclei in a sample to undergo radioactive decay. Radioactive decay rates are usually expressed in terms of half-lives. The different types of radioactivity lead to different decay paths, which transmute the nuclei into other chemical elements. **Decay products** (or daughter nuclides) make radioactive dating possible. **Decay chains** are a series of decays that result in different products. for example, uranium-238 is often found in granite. Its decay chain includes 14 daughter products. It eventually becomes a stable isotope of lead, which is why lead is often found with deposits of uranium ore. Its first half-life is equivalent to the approximate age of the earth, about 4.5 billion years. One of its products is radon, a radioactive gas. **Radiation** is when energy is emitted by one body and absorbed by another. Nuclear weapons, nuclear reactors, and radioactive substances are all examples of things that involve ionizing radiation. Acoustic and electromagnetic radiation are other types of radiation.

Stable isotopes: Isotopes that have not been observed to decay are stable, or non-radioactive, isotopes. It is not known whether some stable isotopes may have such long decay times that observing decay is not possible. Currently, 80 elements have one or more stable isotopes. There are 256 known stable isotopes in total. Carbon, for example, has three isotopes. Two (carbon-12 and carbon-13) are stable and one (carbon-14) is radioactive.

Radioactive isotopes: These have unstable nuclei and can undergo spontaneous nuclear reactions, which results in particles or radiation being emitted. It cannot be predicted when a specific nucleus will decay, but large groups of identical nuclei decay at predictable rates. Knowledge about rates of decay can be used to estimate the age of materials that contain radioactive isotopes.

Ionizing radiation is that which can cause an electron to detach from an atom. It occurs in radioactive reactions and comes in three types: alpha (α), beta (β), and gamma (γ). Alpha rays are positive, beta rays are negative, and gamma rays are neutral. **Alpha particles** are larger than beta particles and can cause severe damage if ingested. Because of their large mass, however, they can be stopped easily. Even paper can protect against this type of radiation. **Beta particles** can be beta-minus or beta-plus. Beta-minus particles contain an energetic electron, while beta-plus particles are emitted by positrons and can result in gamma photons. Beta particles can be stopped with thin metal. **Gamma rays** are a type of high energy electromagnetic radiation consisting of photons. Gamma radiation rids the decaying nucleus of excess energy after it has emitted either alpha or beta radiation. Gamma rays can cause serious damage when absorbed by living tissue, and it takes thick lead to stop them. Alpha, beta, and gamma radiation can also have positive applications.

Nuclear fission and nuclear fusion are similar in that they occur in the nucleus of an atom, can release great amounts of energy, and result in the formation of different elements (known as nuclear transmutation). They are different in that one breaks apart a nucleus and the other joins nuclei. **Nuclear fission** is the splitting of a large nucleus into smaller pieces. **Nuclear fusion** is the joining of two nuclei, which occurs under extreme temperatures and pressures. Fusion occurs naturally in stars, and is the process responsible for the release of great amounts of energy. When fusion occurs, many atomic nuclei with like charges are joined together, forming a heavier nucleus. When this occurs, energy can be absorbed and/or released.

Review Video: Nuclear Fusion
Visit mometrix.com/academy and enter code: 381782

Radioactive waste is a waste product that is considered dangerous because of either low levels or high levels of radioactivity. Radioactive waste could include discarded clothing that was used as protection against radiation or decay products of substances used to create electricity through nuclear fission. Small amounts of radioactive material can be ingested as a method of tracing how the body distributes certain elements. Other radioactive materials are used as light sources because they glow when heated. Uncontrolled radiation or even small amounts of radioactive material can cause sickness and cancer in humans. **Gamma wave radiation** is fast moving radiation that can cause cancer and damage genetic information by crashing into DNA molecules or other cells. Low-level radiation also occurs naturally. When related to everyday occurrences, radiation is measured in millirems per hour (mrem/hr). Humans can be exposed to radiation from stone used to build houses, cosmic rays from space, x-rays and other medical devices, and nuclear energy products.

ALPHA DECAY OF RADON

The alpha decay of radon (Rn) to polonium (Po), which is part of the uranium-238 decay chain, is a good example of **conservation of mass number**. Two protons and two neutrons are lost when a nucleus emits an alpha particle, meaning the mass number will be four less and the atomic number (Z), protons, will be 2 less. When the atomic number (Z) and mass number (A) are diagrammed in a formula, the mass number is in superscript in front of the symbol for the element and the atomic number is in subscript. When Rn, with a mass number of 222 and an atomic number of 86, emits an alpha particle, it loses four from its mass number. It becomes polonium, which has a mass number of 218 and an atomic number of 84. Since an alpha particle with two protons and two neutrons is also a result of the reaction, the mass number is **conserved**.

THEORY OF RELATIVITY

Albert Einstein proposed two theories of relativity: the general theory of relativity (1916) and the special theory of relativity (1905). **Special relativity** is based on two basic premises. The first is that the laws of physics are the same for all observers in uniform motion relative to one another. This is also known as the principle of relativity. The second is that the speed of light in a vacuum is also the same for all observers and their relative motion or the motion of the source of the light does not affect this. **General relativity** is the generally accepted explanation of gravity as a property of space and time, or spacetime. Einstein was born in Germany in 1879 and received the Nobel Prize in Physics in 1921. He died in April of 1955.

Health

Human Growth and Development

EARLY CHILDHOOD PHYSICAL GROWTH AND DEVELOPMENT

From birth to 3 years, children typically grow to twice their height and gain four times their weight. Whereas infants' heads are nearly one-fourth of their full body length, toddlers develop more balanced proportions similar to those of adults. They overcome the disequilibrium of changing so rapidly: generally, children usually start walking around 1 year, climb stairs holding banisters around 18 months, and master running around 2 years. Three-year-olds have normally mastered sitting, walking, toilet training, eating with spoons, scribbling, and demonstrating enough eye-hand coordination to throw and catch a ball. Most children develop sufficient gross motor skills for balancing on one foot and skipping; fine motor skills for controlling scissors, crayons, and pencils; and further refinement of their body proportions between 5 and 8 years old. Implications of the period from birth to 8 years include its being a critical time for developing many **fundamental skills**; hence it is also a critical time for **developmental delays** to be identified and to receive early intervention, which has proven more effective than later intervention.

PHYSICAL GROWTH AND DEVELOPMENT DURING MIDDLE CHILDHOOD

When contrasted with the rapid, obvious, and dramatic changes of early childhood, **middle childhood** is a period of slower physical growth and development. Children continue to grow, but at a slower and steadier rate than when they were younger. In middle childhood, muscle mass develops and children grow stronger. Their **strength** and **coordination in motor skills** advance, evidenced by gradually improving skills for tasks like accurately throwing baseballs; walking on tiptoes; broad-jumping; skipping; lacing and tying shoes; cutting and pasting paper; and drawing people including heads, bodies, arms, and legs. Children can typically dress themselves unassisted, skip using both feet, ride bicycles, skate, and bounce a ball four to six times by the time they are 6. By the time they are around 9, children usually can learn to sew and build models; by age 10, children are capable of catching fly balls. Their hair darkens slightly, and their skin appearance and texture more closely approximate those of adults. Girls and boys in middle childhood are usually similar in height until **puberty**, which frequently begins near the end of middle childhood, averaging around 10 years in girls and 11 years in boys.

PHYSICAL GROWTH AND DEVELOPMENT IN ADOLESCENCE

The most salient physical growth and development aspects of adolescence undoubtedly involve **puberty**. Girls today develop the first signs of puberty, breast buds, before adolescence in late middle childhood, at an average of 10 years within a range between 8 and 13 years; peak growth in height, weight, muscle mass, etc. is around a year after puberty's onset and menarche about two years after, averaging before age 13. Boys begin puberty around a year later than girls, averaging around 11 years within a range of 9-14 years, with peak growth around two years after onset. The first signs are testicular enlargement and scrotal reddening and thinning. Both girls and boys go through a series of **stages** that make up puberty. These stages incorporate changes to almost all of their body systems, including most notably the **skeletal, muscular, and reproductive systems**. Voices deepen, and body hair and other secondary sex characteristics develop. Acne often plagues adolescents. Whereas girls and boys are about the same heights in middle childhood, girls frequently become taller in their early teens. However, boys catch up within one or two years, typically growing taller than girls. Puberty accounts for around 25 percent of individual growth in height.

Personal Hygiene

Good personal hygiene promotes good health by preventing and limiting exposure to bacterial and viral **microorganisms**. In addition to **physical benefits**, good bodily hygiene also supports good **mental health** by promoting psychological well-being and feeling good about oneself. When people neglect their personal hygiene, they develop body odors, bad breath, damaged and lost teeth, and unkempt hair and clothing. Other people then view them as unhealthy; as a result, they can encounter social and employment discrimination. Some components of good personal hygiene include bathing, nail care, and foot care. Not everybody needs to bathe or shower daily; for some people, this can remove too many body oils, exacerbating dry skin. However, individuals should wash their bodies and hair regularly as often as they find necessary. The skin is continually shedding dead cells, which must be removed. If it accumulates, it can cause health problems. Trimming the fingernails and toenails regularly averts problems like hangnails and infected nailbeds. Keeping the feet clean and dry, and wearing clean flip-flops at public facilities, gyms, health clubs, spas, and around swimming pools prevents contracting athlete's foot and other fungal infections.

ORAL HYGIENE, HAND WASHING, AND SLEEP

Ideally, we should brush our teeth after every time we eat. Health professionals recommend brushing and flossing the teeth twice a day at a minimum. **Brushing teeth** removes plaque and reduces mouth bacteria, inhibiting tooth decay. This prevents not only tooth cavities, but also gum disease. **Flossing and gum massage** keep gums healthy and strong. If oral bacteria build up, it can cause gum disease. Gum disease not only causes irreversible bone loss in the jaw; the bacteria can travel from the gums directly to the heart, causing serious heart valve disorders. Unhealthy gums can loosen teeth, causing difficulty chewing, eating, and tooth loss. Most people need dental cleanings and checkups twice yearly, some more often. **Hand washing** prevents bacteria and viruses from spreading. We should wash our hands after using the bathroom; before preparing food and eating; after sneezing or coughing; and after handling garbage. Having alcohol-based hand sanitizing gels on hand is recommended when water is inaccessible. **Sleeping** enough and well must not be overlooked as a component of personal hygiene: insufficient or inadequate sleep impairs the immune system, inviting illness.

Chronic and Communicable Diseases

HIV/AIDS

The **human immunodeficiency virus** (HIV) impairs or destroys an infected individual's immune system, raising infection risk and ruining infection defenses. As HIV advances, its final stage is **AIDS**, acquired immune deficiency syndrome. The World Health Organization (WHO) estimated that by the end of 2013, 35 million humans were living with HIV. Of these, 23.4-26.2 million lived in sub-Saharan Africa. Global health community efforts include research and development of new medications to address symptoms for people already infected, as well as preventing new infections; outreach and education to stop HIV spread; and supporting children and families who have lost parents to AIDS deaths. **Anti-retroviral therapy (ART) drugs** have enabled many HIV patients to survive 15+ years before developing AIDS symptoms. WHO estimated 12.9 million people were receiving these by the end of 2013, 11.7 million of them in low-income and middle-income nations. The most successful global health effort, this program has been significantly helped by the **President's Emergency Plan for AIDS Relief (PEPFAR)**. Additionally, the US Department of Health and Human Services (HHS), National Institutes of Health (NIH) offices, Gates Foundation, and Centers for Disease Control and Prevention (CDC) are all actively involved in global HIV/AIDS research, researcher training, coordination, and vaccine development.

CYSTIC FIBROSIS

In cystic fibrosis (**CF**), a defective gene produces a protein causing the body to secrete **mucus** that is much thicker and stickier than normal. This mucus clogs up the lungs, resulting in infections that can cause or threaten death. It also blocks the **pancreas** from delivering enzymes that help break down and absorb necessary nutrients from foods. Over 75 percent of CF patients are diagnosed by age 2. Today, almost half of CF patients are aged 18 or more. Around 1,000 new CF cases are diagnosed annually. Symptoms include shortness of breath; wheezing; chronic persistent coughing, including phlegm-productive coughs; slow weight gain and inadequate growth despite good appetite; frequently developing lung infections; difficult, bulky, greasy, and/or frequent bowel movements; and skin with an extremely salty taste. Most children with CF died before entering elementary school during the 1950s. Today, significant progress in the understanding and treatment of CF has dramatically improved longevity and life quality in CF patients. Many now live into middle adulthood or older; life expectancy has doubled in the past three decades. The **Cystic Fibrosis Foundation**, whose support has enabled almost all available CF treatment medications, views research for a cure as "promising."

SICKLE CELL ANEMIA

Anemia means the blood has fewer **red blood cells (RBC)** than normal. RBCs, which transport oxygen in **hemoglobin** (an iron-rich protein) through the bloodstream and remove the waste product carbon dioxide, are produced in the bone marrow, normally living about four months. **Sickle cell** is one genetic type of anemia, inherited when both parents have the gene. When one parent has this gene but the other's is normal, children inherit sickle cell trait; they do not have the disease, but pass the sickle hemoglobin gene to their children. In America, sickle cell anemia is commonest in African-Americans (around one in 500). It also affects Hispanic-Americans (around one in 36,000); and people of Caribbean, Mediterranean, Indian, and Saudi Arabian descent. Normal RBCs are disc-shaped and travel easily through blood vessels. Sickle cells are crescent-shaped, sticky, and stiff, impeding blood flow. This causes organ damage, pain, and increased risk of infections. Some patients have chronic fatigue and/or pain. A few patients may receive future cures through stem cell transplants, but no widespread cure currently exists. Symptoms and complications are managed through treatments. Improved care and treatments enable some patients to live into their 40s, 50s, or older.

TAY-SACHS DISEASE

Tay-Sachs disease is a rare genetic disorder, inherited through an **autosomal recessive pattern**; i.e., both parents carry copies of a mutated gene and are usually asymptomatic, but pass these to their children. **Tay-Sachs** is rare overall, and more common among Eastern/Central European Jewish, certain Quebec French-Canadian, Old-Order Pennsylvania Dutch/Amish, and Louisiana Cajun populations. The genetic defect prevents an enzyme from breaking down a toxic substance, which builds up in the brain and spinal cord, progressively destroying **neurons**. The commonest form appears in infancy, typically around 3-6 months. A typical sign is a "cherry-red spot" eye abnormality, detectable through eye examination. Babies' motor muscles weaken; development slows; they lose motor skills like turning over, sitting up, and crawling; and develop exaggerated startle reactions to loud sounds. As it progresses, this disease causes seizures, loss of vision and hearing, intellectual impairment, and paralysis. Most children with the commoner infantile form of Tay-Sachs disease typically only survive until early childhood. Later-onset forms of the disease are extremely rare, typically with milder, highly variable symptoms including muscular weakness, poor coordination, other motor symptoms, speech difficulties, and mental illness.

TYPE 2 DIABETES

Historically, **type 1 diabetes**, which has a greater genetic component, was called "juvenile diabetes" because symptoms appeared during childhood, contrasting with type 2 "adult-onset diabetes." However, these terms were abandoned as more cases of **type 2 diabetes** are occurring in childhood and adolescence—evidence of the contributions of **lifestyle factors** including obesity, poor nutrition, and physical inactivity. When people consume large amounts of refined carbohydrates (simple sugars and starches processed to remove all fibers) with no fiber slowing digestion, these enter the bloodstream rapidly, causing a sudden spike in blood sugar, experienced by some as an energy rush. However, with quick metabolism and the pancreas' secretion of extra insulin to neutralize excessive blood sugar, sugars exit as fast as they entered, causing a precipitous blood-sugar drop, or "crash," with fatigue, sleepiness, irritability, depression and cycle-perpetuating cravings for more sugar or starch. Moreover, **metabolic syndrome** eventually develops—insulin resistance to the pancreas' attempts to neutralize repeated artificial blood sugar elevation. In type 1 diabetes, the pancreas fails to produce insulin; in type 2, the body becomes immune to insulin, causing chronically high, unstable blood sugar. Blindness, limb loss, shock, coma, and death are a few of many sequelae from uncontrolled diabetes.

CHRONIC, NONCOMMUNICABLE DISEASES

According to the World Health Organization (WHO, 2013), over 36 million people die annually from **noncommunicable diseases (NCDs)**, with almost 80 percent (29 million) in low-income and middle-income nations. Of these, over 9 million are before age 60. Of these premature deaths, 90 percent are in low-income and middle-income nations. Roughly 80 percent of all NCD deaths are due to four disease types: **cardiovascular diseases**, e.g., strokes and heart attacks, which cause the majority (17.3 million yearly); **cancers** (7.6 million yearly); **respiratory diseases** like asthma and chronic obstructive pulmonary disease (COPD) (4.2 million yearly); and **diabetes** (1.3 million yearly). These four disease groups have four **risk factors** in common: tobacco use, physical inactivity, harmful alcohol use, and poor nutrition. WHO projects the greatest increases in NCD mortality by 2020 will be in African countries, where NCDs are also predicted to surpass maternal and infant mortality from childbirth and nutritional and communicable diseases combined as the most common killers by 2030. Behavioral risk factors for NCDs that can be modified are tobacco use, physical inactivity, unhealthy diets, and harmful alcohol consumption.

MEASURES TAKEN BY WHO TO PREVENT NCDS

WHO's *Action Plan of the global strategy for the prevention and control of noncommunicable diseases* gives member states and international partners steps for preventing and addressing NCDs in world nations. WHO is also working to reduce **NCD risk factors**, including: implementing anti-tobacco measures identified in the WHO Framework Convention on Tobacco Control in world nations to decrease public tobacco exposure; helping world communities lower rates of death and disease from physical inactivity and unhealthy diets through the WHO *Global strategy on diet, physical activity and health aims to promote and protect health;* identifying action areas with priority and recommending measures of protection against the harmful consumption of alcohol through the WHO *Global strategy to reduce the harmful use of alcohol;* responding to the United Nations Political Declaration on NCDs by developing a comprehensive framework for global NCD prevention, monitoring, and control, which includes a group of global voluntary targets and a list of indicators; and responding to the World Health Assembly's resolution (WHA 64.11) by developing a 2013-2020 **Global NCD Action Plan** with comprehensive guidance for implementing the United Nations High-Level Meeting's political commitments. WHA endorsed this plan, urging member state, Director-General and Secretariat implementation and future WHA progress reports.

DISEASE ETIOLOGY

Etiology is defined in medicine as the study of origins or causes of diseases or pathological conditions. Early writings attributed diseases to various unproven "causes" including spells, curses, and imbalances in bodily humors. Ancient Greek physicians Galen and Hippocrates often associated disease with unidentified components in the air, influencing miasmatic perspectives on disease etiology of Medieval European physicians. Ancient Roman scholar Marcus Terentius Varro suggested **microorganisms** caused diseases in his book *On Agriculture* in the 1st century BCE. German physician Robert Koch (1843-1910), modern bacteriology founder, discovered scientific evidence of microorganisms causing the infectious diseases anthrax, cholera, and tuberculosis. As in all experimental science, in **epidemiology**, statistical correlation between/among variables does not prove causation. Sir Austin Bradford-Hill, the epidemiologist who proved causal relationship between tobacco smoking and lung cancer, defined criteria for showing causation. American epidemiologist Alfred Evans proposed the **Unified Concept of Causation**, synthesizing previous thinking. **Etiology** can contribute to causal chains including independent co-factors and promoters. For example, stress, once believed to cause peptic ulcer disease, was belatedly identified as a promoter, with excess stomach acid a prerequisite and *Helicobacter pylori* infection the primary etiology.

INFLUENZA

Influenza (**flu**) is an infectious viral respiratory illness. Its symptoms can range from mild to fatal. Young children, seniors, and people with some health conditions have greatest risk for serious complications. Annual **vaccination** is the best way to prevent it. The US Department of Health and Human Services' (HHS) Office of Global Affairs, International Influenza Unit (IIU) is an international partnership to enhance global flu identification and response, coordinated by HHS personnel and Operation Divisions including National Institutes of Health (NIH); Centers for Disease Control and Infection (CDC); Food and Drug Administration (FDA); Office of the Assistant Secretary for Preparedness and Response, Biomedical Advanced Research and Development Authority (ASPR/BARDA); the US Departments of State (DOS), Defense (DOD), Agriculture (USDA), Commerce, and Treasury; the US Agency for International Development (USAID); foreign governments; the international World Health Organization (WHO), World Bank, International Partnership on Avian and Pandemic Influenza (IPAPI), Global Health Security Action Group (GHSAG), UN System Influenza Coordination (UNSIC), Pan-American Health Organization (PAHO); and nonprofits like PATH and the Gates Foundation. **Influenza pandemics**—world outbreaks—occur when a new virus with little or no human immunity emerges. There were three in the 20th century and one so far in the 21st.

First Aid, Safety, and Nutrition

BASIC FIRST-AID PROCEDURES IN VARIOUS SITUATIONS

The following are first-aid procedures in various situations:

- **Anaphylaxis (allergic shock)** - Immediately call 9-1-1. Administer epinephrine (EpiPen) per autoinjector if the person has one. Begin cardiopulmonary resuscitation (CPR) if in respiratory arrest.
- **Animal bites**
  - *Minor* (if no concern about rabies): Wash with soap and water and apply antibiotic cream/ointment and bandage.
  - *Major*: Apply pressure to stop the bleeding with a dry clean bandage, and transport to the emergency department, or call 9-1-1 if severe.

- **Black eye** - Apply cold compress, avoiding pressure on eye. If blood is noted in the eye itself or if vision is impaired, transport to the emergency department.
- **Chemical burns/eye splashes** - Remove contaminated belongings and flush the burn area with a copious amount of tap water for at least 10 minutes. Transport to the emergency department or call 9-1-1 if burns are severe, the patient feels faint, or the burn is more than three inches in diameter. Flush the eyes for at least 20 minutes, and then transport to the emergency department.
- **Cut/Scrapes** - Apply pressure with a clean bandage to stop the bleeding. Rinse with clear water and wash around the wound with soap and water. Apply antibiotic ointment and dressing. If the wound is deep and requires suturing; transport to the emergency department.
- **Heat cramps, heat exhaustion, heat stroke**
    - *Heat cramps and exhaustion*: Remove the person to the shade, lay flat, and elevate legs; cool by spraying with cold water, and have the person drink cool water.
    - *Heat stroke*: Call 9-1-1. Spray or immerse in cool water and fan; administer CPR if necessary.
- **Hypothermia** - Call 9-1-1. Remove wet clothing, warm gradually with warm compresses to the trunk; give warm drinks. Do not warm too quickly, and do not massage limbs.
- **Insect bites/stings** - Remove stingers, wash with soap and water, and apply a cool compress. Apply cortisone cream to reduce itching. If a severe reaction or bite with a known dangerous insect (such as a scorpion), call 9-1-1. Administer an EpiPen if the person has one for allergies to insects.
- **Bleeding**
    - *Minor*: Apply pressure with a clean bandage to stop the bleeding and apply dry dressing.
    - *Severe*: Call 9-1-1. Remove any large debris from the wound. Apply pressure with a clean bandage to stop the bleeding but not if debris is imbedded in the wound, and don't apply pressure to an eye. In these cases, simply cover with a clean dressing. Lie the person flat and elevate the feet. Apply a tourniquet for bleeding that is life-threatening only if trained to do so.
- **Snakebites (venomous)** - Call 9-1-1. Position the injury below the level of the heart if possible. Cover the wound with a dry dressing. DO NOT apply ice, cut the skin, or apply a tourniquet. Report a description of the snake to first responders.
- **Spider bite** - Cleanse the bite with soap and water, and apply antibiotic ointment and cool compress. Transport to the emergency department if a poisonous spider, such as a black widow or brown recluse, is suspected.
- **Sprains/Fractures/Dislocations**
    - *Sprains*: RICE (rest, ice, compress, elevate). Transport to the emergency department if unable to bear weight or use the joint.
    - *Fractures*: Call 9-1-1 or transport to the emergency department. Apply pressure to stop any bleeding, cover with a dry dressing, immobilize the injured limb, and apply an ice pack.
    - *Dislocation*: Transport to the emergency department. Do not attempt to move the joint. Apply an ice compress to the joint.

- **Shock (any cause)** - Call 9-1-1. Lay the person flat, elevate the legs and feet, and keep still. Loosen clothing. Begin CPR if cardiac or respiratory arrest exist.
- **Stroke** - Call 9-1-1. Keep the head elevated.
- **Nosebleeds** - Sit the person upright and pinch nostrils for 5 to 10 minutes. Transport to the emergency department if bleeding follows an accident or if it persists for more than 20 minutes.

CPR

Hands-only **cardiopulmonary resuscitation** (CPR) is recommended for nonmedical rescuers for unconscious teens or adults who have no pulse or respirations. The rescuer should call 9-1-1 and place the victim supine on a hard surface. To find the correct hand position, run two fingers along the ribs to the center chest, place two fingers over the xiphoid process, and place the palm of the other hand on the sternum directly above the fingers. Then place the other hand on top of the first, fingers linked and elbows locked, to begin **compressions**, which should be done in a rocking movement, using the body to apply pressure. (Note: Use two fingers for infants.) The rate of compressions is at least 100 per minute and at least two inches deep (one-third chest depth for infants and small children). This rate corresponds roughly to the beat of the Bee Gees' song "Staying Alive" (dum, dum, dum, dum, stayin' alive, stayin' alive….). With two trained rescuers, **rescue breathing** may be added at a compression to breathing rate of 30:2.

HEIMLICH MANEUVER

The universal sign of choking is when a person clutches his or her throat and appears to be choking or gasping for breath. If the person can speak ("Can you speak?") or cough, the **Heimlich maneuver** is not usually necessary. The Heimlich maneuver can be done with the victim sitting, standing, or supine. The Heimlich procedure for children (≥1 year) and adults is as follows:

- Wrap arms around the victim's waist from the back if sitting or standing. Make a fist and place the thumb side against the victim's abdomen slightly above the umbilicus. Grasp this hand with the other and thrust sharply upward to force air out of the lungs.
- Repeat as needed and call 9-1-1 if there is no response.
- If the victim loses consciousness, ease him or her into a supine position on the floor, place hands similarly to CPR but over the abdomen while sitting astride the victim's legs. Repeat upward compressions five times. If no ventilation occurs, attempt to sweep the mouth and ventilate the lungs mouth to mouth. Repeat compressions and ventilations until recovery or emergency personnel arrive.

Indications of **choking** in infants younger than one year include lack of breathing, gasping, cyanosis, and inability to cry. Procedures for the **Heimlich chest thrusts** include the following:

- Position the infant in the prone (face-down) position along the forearm with the infant's head lower than the trunk, being sure to support the head so the airway is not blocked.
- Using the heel of the hand, deliver five forceful upward blows between the shoulder blades.
- Sandwich the child between your two arms, turn the infant into the supine position, and drape him or her over your thigh with the head lower than the trunk and the head supported.
- Using two fingers (as in CPR compressions), give up to five thrusts (about 1.5 inches deep) to the lower third of the sternum.

- Only do a finger sweep and remove any foreign object if the object is visible. Repeat five back blows, five chest thrusts, repeating until the foreign body is ejected or until emergency personnel take over.
- If the infant loses consciousness, begin CPR. If a pulse is noted but spontaneous respirations are absent, continue with ventilation only.

HEALTH AND SAFETY OF INDIVIDUALS RESPONDING TO MEDICAL EMERGENCIES

When responding to a medical emergency, it's important to take measures to **prevent self-injury or infection**. Precautions include the following:

- Assess the **safety risks** of the situation before rendering aid (gunshots, gang activity, fire, fallen electrical wires, severe storm conditions), and do not give aid unless the situation is safe.
- Avoid contact with **body fluids** (blood, urine, feces, semen), and use gloves if available; otherwise, attempt to find some type of barrier (plastic bag, towel) to use to prevent direct contact.
- Use a **face mask** if possible if in danger of airborne pathogens, such as when a person has a severe cough.
- **Standard precautions**: Hand hygiene with soap and water or alcohol scrub should be carried out if possible before touching a person, but this is not always possible in an emergent situation. Hands and any contaminated body parts should be washed with soap and water as soon as possible after contact, especially if contaminated by body fluids.

FOOD PRODUCT LABELS

The FDA, under the Federal Food, Drug, and Cosmetic Act, regulates **product labeling**. Labels on food products contain information specific to the product, but the same type of information is contained for all food products:

- **Serving size, servings per container, and calories**: The calories are based on the serving size, so if there are three servings and the calorie count is 150, then the entire product has 450 calories. The calorie count also indicates the number of calories derived from fat.
- **Nutrients**: This includes the amount of fat, carbohydrates, and protein per serving as well as cholesterol, sodium, sugar, and fiber. The amounts are indicated in grams or milligrams but also as a percentage of the daily recommended value. Grams of dietary fiber can be subtracted from the total carbohydrate grams because fiber is carbohydrate that is not digested.
- **Vitamins and minerals**: These are listed as a percentage of daily recommended value per serving.
- **Footnote**: This explains how the percentages displayed are based on a 2,000-calorie diet.

INTERPRETATION OF SIGNS AND SYMBOLS

Sign/Symbol	Interpretation

Flame: Includes flammable materials and gases and those that are self-heating or self-reactive.

Corrosion: Includes substances that can cause skin burns, metal corrosion, and eye damage.

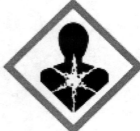

Health hazard: Includes carcinogens, toxic substances, and respiratory irritants.

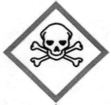

Poison: Includes materials, gases, or substances that are extremely toxic and may result in death or severe illness.

Irritant: Includes material, gases, or substances that are irritants to skin, eyes, and/or respiratory tract, acutely toxic, or have a narcotic effect.

Biohazard: Includes biological substances, such as body fluids, that pose a threat to humans. Appears on sharps containers that hold contaminated needles.

Science Chapter Quiz

1. What is the name for any substance that stimulates the production of antibodies?

    a. collagen
    b. hemoglobin
    c. lymph
    d. antigen

2. Which of the answer choices provided best defines the following statement?

    For a given mass and constant temperature, an inverse relationship exists between the volume and pressure of a gas?

    a. Ideal Gas Law
    b. Boyle's Law
    c. Charles' Law
    d. Stefan-Boltzmann Law

3. Which of the following structures has the lowest blood pressure?

    a. arteries
    b. arteriole
    c. venule
    d. vein

4. What kind of bond connects sugar and phosphate in DNA?

    a. hydrogen
    b. ionic
    c. covalent
    d. overt

5. Which law of classical thermodynamics states that energy can neither be created nor destroyed?

    a. Zeroth
    b. First
    c. Second
    d. Third

6. A cyclist is riding over a hill. At what point is his potential energy greatest?

    a. at the base of the hill
    b. halfway up the hill
    c. at the very top of the hill
    d. on the way down the hill

7. Which kind of radiation has no charge?

    a. beta
    b. alpha
    c. delta
    d. gamma

8. Which type of cholesterol is considered to be the best for health?

    a. LDL
    b. HDL
    c. VLDL
    d. VHDL

9. The atomic number of an element is defined by:

    a. The total number of protons and electrons it contains.
    b. The total number of electrons it contains.
    c. The total number of protons it contains.
    d. The total number of neutrons it contains.

10. Which of the following devices changes chemical energy into electrical energy?

    a. battery
    b. closed electric circuit
    c. generator
    d. transformer

Science Chapter Quiz Answers

1. D: The name for a substance that stimulates the production of antibodies is an *antigen*. An antigen is any substance perceived by the immune system as dangerous. When the body senses an antigen, it produces an antibody. *Collagen* is one of the components of bone, tendon, and cartilage. It is a spongy protein that can be turned into gelatin by boiling. *Hemoglobin* is the part of red blood cells that carries oxygen. In order for the blood to carry enough oxygen to the cells of the body, there has to be a sufficient amount of hemoglobin. *Lymph* is a near-transparent fluid that performs a number of functions in the body: It removes bacteria from tissues, replaces lymphocytes in the blood, and moves fat away from the small intestine. Lymph contains white blood cells.

2. B: Boyle's law states that for a constant mass and temperature, pressure and volume are related inversely to one another: $PV = c$, where c = constant.

3. D: Of the given structures, veins have the lowest blood pressure. *Veins* carry oxygen-poor blood from the outlying parts of the body to the heart. An *artery* carries oxygen-rich blood from the heart to the peripheral parts of the body. An *arteriole* extends from an artery to a capillary. A *venule* is a tiny vein that extends from a capillary to a larger vein.

4. C: The sugar and phosphate in DNA are connected by covalent bonds. A *covalent bond* is formed when atoms share electrons. It is very common for atoms to share pairs of electrons. Hydrogen bonds are used in DNA to bind complementary bases together, such as adenine with thymine or guanine with cytosine. An *ionic bond* is created when one or more electrons are transferred between atoms. *Ionic bonds*, also known as *electrovalent bonds*, are formed between ions with opposite charges. There is no such thing as an *overt bond* in chemistry.

5. B: The first law of classical thermodynamics states that energy can neither be created nor destroyed. The zeroth law is concerned with thermodynamic equilibrium, and the second and third laws discuss entropy.

6. C: Potential energy is stored energy. At the top of the hill, the cyclist has the greatest amount of potential energy (and the least amount of kinetic energy) because his motion is decreased and he has the potential of motion in any direction.

7. D: Gamma radiation has no charge. This form of electromagnetic radiation can travel a long distance and can penetrate the human body. Sunlight and radio waves are both examples of gamma radiation. Alpha radiation has a 2+ charge. It only travels short distances and cannot penetrate clothing or skin. Radium and uranium both emit alpha radiation. Beta radiation has a 1– charge. It can travel several feet through the air and is capable of penetrating the skin. This kind of radiation can be damaging to health over a long period of exposure. There is no such thing as delta radiation.

8. B: High-density lipoproteins (*HDL*) are considered to be the healthiest form of cholesterol. This type of cholesterol actually reduces the risk of heart disease. A lipoprotein is composed of both lipid and protein. These substances cannot move through the bloodstream by themselves; they must be carried along by some other substance. Although most people think of cholesterol as an unhealthy substance, it helps to maintain cell walls and produce hormones. Cholesterol is also important in the production of vitamin D and the bile acids that aid digestion. The other answer choices are low-density lipoproteins (*LDL*), very-low-density lipoproteins (*VLDL*), and very-high-density lipoproteins (*VHDL*).

9. C: The atomic number of an element is defined by the total number of protons it contains, and elements are arranged on the periodic table by atomic number. The atomic mass of an element is the sum total of its protons and neutrons.

10. A: In a Zn-Cu battery, the zinc terminal has a higher concentration of electrons than the copper terminal, so there is a potential difference between the locations of the two terminals. This is a form of electrical energy brought about by the chemical interactions between the metals and the electrolyte the battery uses. Creating a circuit and causing a current to flow will transform the electrical energy into heat energy, mechanical energy, or another form of electrical energy, depending on the devices in the circuit. A generator transforms mechanical energy into electrical energy and a transformer changes the electrical properties of a form of electrical energy.

PAX Practice Test

Verbal Review

READING COMPREHENSION

The next six questions are based on the following passage.

The Bermuda Triangle

The area known as the Bermuda Triangle has become such a part of popular culture that it can be difficult to separate fact from fiction. The interest first began when five Navy planes vanished in 1945, officially resulting from "causes or reasons unknown." The explanations about other accidents in the Triangle range from the scientific to the supernatural. Researchers have never been able to find anything truly mysterious about what happens in the Bermuda Triangle, if there even is a Bermuda Triangle. What is more, one of the biggest challenges in considering the phenomenon is deciding how much area actually represents the Bermuda Triangle. Most consider the Triangle to stretch from Miami out to Puerto Rico and to include the island of Bermuda. Others expand the area to include all of the Caribbean islands and to extend eastward as far as the Azores, which are closer to Europe than they are to North America.

The problem with having a larger Bermuda Triangle is that it increases the odds of accidents. There is near-constant travel, by ship and by plane, across the Atlantic, and accidents are expected to occur. In fact, the Bermuda Triangle happens to fall within one of the busiest navigational regions in the world, and the reality of greater activity creates the possibility for more to go wrong. Shipping records suggest that there is not a greater than average loss of vessels within the Bermuda Triangle, and many researchers have argued that the reputation of the Triangle makes any accident seem out of the ordinary. In fact, most accidents fall within the expected margin of error. The increase in ships from East Asia no doubt contributes to an increase in accidents. And as for the story of the Navy planes that disappeared within the Triangle, many researchers now conclude that it was the result of mistakes on the part of the pilots who flew into storm clouds, likely became discomposed, and then simply got lost.

1. **Which of the following describes this type of writing?**
   a. Narrative
   b. Persuasive
   c. Expository
   d. Technical

2. Which of the following sentences is most representative of a summary sentence for this passage?

    a.   The problem with having a larger Bermuda Triangle is that it increases the odds of accidents.

    b.   The area that is called the Bermuda Triangle happens to fall within one of the busiest navigational regions in the world, and the reality of greater activity creates the possibility for more to go wrong.

    c.   One of the biggest challenges in considering the phenomenon is deciding how much area actually represents the Bermuda Triangle.

    d.   Researchers have never been able to find anything truly mysterious about what happens in the Bermuda Triangle, if there even is a Bermuda Triangle.

3. With which of the following statements would the author most likely agree?

    a.   There is no real mystery about the Bermuda Triangle because most events have reasonable explanations.

    b.   Researchers are wrong to expand the focus of the Triangle to the Azores, because this increases the likelihood of accidents.

    c.   The official statement of "causes or reasons unknown" in the loss of the Navy planes was a deliberate concealment from the Navy.

    d.   Reducing the legends about the mysteries of the Bermuda Triangle will help to reduce the number of reported accidents or shipping losses in that region.

4. Which of the following represents an opinion statement on the part of the author?

    a.   The problem with having a larger Bermuda Triangle is that it increases the odds of accidents.

    b.   The area known as the Bermuda Triangle has become such a part of popular culture that it can be difficult to sort through the myth and locate the truth.

    c.   The increase in ships from East Asia no doubt contributes to an increase in accidents.

    d.   Most consider the Triangle to stretch from Miami to Puerto Rico and include the island of Bermuda.

5. Which of the following is a common argument that researchers make about the validity of the Bermuda Triangle's reputation?

    a.   It cannot be scientifically verified, since accidents happen for "causes or reasons unknown."

    b.   The boundaries of the area must be established and agreed upon before any test of the reputation would be possible

    c.   The supernatural nature of the Bermuda Triangle is well established in popular culture.

    d.   Since the number of accidents attributed to the area is within a normal margin of error, there is nothing extraordinary about the Bermuda Triangle

6. As it is used in the context of the passage, 'discomposed' most nearly means:

    a.   inverted

    b.   forgetful

    c.   broken down

    d.   disoriented

The next six questions are based on the following passage.

In the United States, the foreign language requirement for high school graduation is decided at the state level. This means the requirement varies, with some states deciding to forego a foreign language requirement altogether (www.ncssfl.org). It is necessary that these states reconsider their position and amend their requirements to reflect compulsory completion of a course of one or more foreign languages. Studying a foreign language has become increasingly important for the global economy. As technology continues to make international business relations increasingly easy, people need to keep up by increasing their communication capabilities. High school graduates with foreign language credits have been shown to have an increased college acceptance rate. In addition, students who have mastered more than one language typically find themselves in greater demand when they reach the job market. Students who did not study a foreign language often find themselves unable to obtain a job at all.

7. What is the main idea of this passage?
   a. Studying a foreign language will help graduating students find jobs after high school.
   b. Studying a foreign language should be a mandatory requirement for high school graduation.
   c. Studying a foreign language helps students gain an understanding of other cultures.
   d. Studying a foreign language is essential if a student hopes to get into college.

8. Which of the following statements represents the best summary of the claims made in this passage?
   a. Studying a foreign language is important if you want to graduate from high school and get a job.
   b. Studying a foreign language is important for the global economy because of the technological advances that have been made in international communications.
   c. Studying a foreign language is important for the global economy, college acceptance rates, and becoming a sought-after candidate in the job market.
   d. Studying a foreign language is important for college acceptance rates and obtaining a job after college.

9. Which of the following statements represents an EXAGGERATED claim in support of the argument presented in this passage?
   a. In the United States, the foreign language requirement for high school graduation is decided at the state level.
   b. Studying a foreign language has become increasingly important for the global economy.
   c. High school graduates with foreign language credits have been shown to have an increased college acceptance rate.
   d. Students who did not study a foreign language often find themselves unable to obtain a job at all.

10. Which of the following would be a useful source of information to determine the validity of the argument presented in this passage?

  a. A survey of high school students' preferences with regard to foreign language requirements.
  b. A comparison of the correlation between a second language introduced at home and subsequent college acceptance rates.
  c. A survey that asks parents to select the foreign language they would like their children to study in high school.
  d. A comparison of the correlation between high school students' study of a foreign language and subsequent college acceptance rates.

11. Which of the following would be the best concluding statement for this passage?

  a. States should consider how important foreign languages are for the global economy when making their policies regarding foreign language requirements for graduation from high school.
  b. Policies regarding a foreign language requirement for graduation from high school should take into account the importance of foreign languages for the global economy and the correlation between foreign languages and increased college acceptance rates and employment opportunities.
  c. High school graduation requirements should include a foreign language class because of the influence knowledge of a second language has on college acceptance rates.
  d. Policies regarding a foreign language requirement for graduation from high school should take into account how difficult it is to obtain a job in today's economy for those who do not have knowledge of more than one language.

12. Based on this passage, the author would most likely agree with which of the following?

  a. Learning a foreign language is only for fun and it should be up to the individual to decide whether or not they wish to learn one.
  b. Learning a foreign language should be a basic requirement for all students, because studies have shown that it improves the local economy.
  c. Learning a foreign language is an unreasonable expectation for the government to place upon students, since most people find no need to speak more than one language.
  d. Learning a foreign language needs to be compulsory for all students in the United States.

The next six questions are based on the following passage.

In 1603, Queen Elizabeth I of England died. She had never married and had no heir, so the throne passed to a distant relative: James Stuart, the son of Elizabeth's cousin and one-time rival for the throne, Mary, Queen of Scots. James was crowned King James I of England. At the time, he was also King James VI of Scotland, and the combination of roles would create a spirit of conflict that haunted the two nations for generations to come.

The conflict developed as a result of rising tensions among the people within the nations, as well as between them. Scholars in the 21st century are far too hasty in dismissing the role of religion in political disputes, but religion undoubtedly played a role in the problems that faced England and Scotland. By the time of James Stuart's succession to the English throne, the English people had firmly embraced the teachings of Protestant theology. Similarly, the Scottish Lowlands was decisively Protestant. In the Scottish Highlands, however, the clans retained their Catholic faith. James acknowledged the Church of England and still sanctioned the largely Protestant translation of the Bible that still bears his name.

James's son King Charles I proved himself to be less committed to the Protestant Church of England. Charles married the Catholic Princess Henrietta Maria of France, and there were suspicions among the English and the Lowland Scots that Charles was quietly a Catholic. Charles's own political troubles extended beyond religion in this case, and he was beheaded in 1649. Eventually, his son King Charles II would be crowned, and this Charles is believed to have converted secretly to the Catholic Church. Charles II died without a legitimate heir, and his brother James ascended to the throne as King James II.

James was recognized to be a practicing Catholic, and his commitment to Catholicism would prove to be his downfall. James's wife Mary Beatrice lost a number of children during their infancy, and when she became pregnant again in 1687 the public became concerned. If James had a son, that son would undoubtedly be raised a Catholic, and the English people would not stand for this. Mary gave birth to a son, but the story quickly circulated that the royal child had died and the child named James's heir was a foundling smuggled in. James, his wife, and his infant son were forced to flee; and James's Protestant daughter Mary was crowned the queen.

In spite of a strong resemblance to the king, the young James was generally rejected among the English and the Lowland Scots, who referred to him as "the Pretender." But in the Highlands the Catholic princeling was welcomed. He inspired a group known as *Jacobites*, to reflect the Latin version of his name. His own son Charles, known affectionately as Bonnie Prince Charlie, would eventually raise an army and attempt to recapture what he believed to be his throne. The movement was soundly defeated at the Battle of Culloden in 1746, and England and Scotland have remained ostensibly Protestant ever since.

13. Which of the following sentences contains an opinion on the part of the author?
a. James was recognized to be a practicing Catholic, and his commitment to Catholicism would prove to be his downfall.
b. James' son King Charles I proved himself to be less committed to the Protestant Church of England.
c. The movement was soundly defeated at the Battle of Culloden in 1746, and England and Scotland have remained ostensibly Protestant ever since.
d. Scholars in the 21st century are far too hasty in dismissing the role of religion in political disputes, but religion undoubtedly played a role in the problems that faced England and Scotland.

14. Which of the following is a logical conclusion based on the information that is provided within the passage?
a. Like Elizabeth I, Charles II never married and thus never had children.
b. The English people were relieved each time that James II's wife Mary lost another child, as this prevented the chance of a Catholic monarch.
c. Charles I's beheading had less to do with religion than with other political problems that England was facing.
d. Unlike his son and grandsons, King James I had no Catholic leanings and was a faithful follower of the Protestant Church of England.

15. Based on the information that is provided within the passage, which of the following can be inferred about King James II's son?

    a. Considering his resemblance to King James II, the young James was very likely the legitimate child of the king and the queen.

    b. Given the queen's previous inability to produce a healthy child, the English and the Lowland Scots were right in suspecting the legitimacy of the prince.

    c. James "the Pretender" was not as popular among the Highland clans as his son Bonnie Prince Charlie.

    d. James was unable to acquire the resources needed to build the army and plan the invasion that his son succeeded in doing.

16. Which of the following best describes the organization of the information in the passage?

    a. Cause-effect

    b. Chronological sequence

    c. Problem-solution

    d. Comparison-contrast

17. Which of the following best describes the author's intent in the passage?

    a. To persuade

    b. To entertain

    c. To express feeling

    d. To inform

18. Who does the passage say ascended the throne because someone else did not have a legitimate heir?

    a. King James Stuart

    b. Queen Elizabeth I

    c. King Charles II

    d. King James II

The next six questions are based on the following passage.

Global warming and the depletion of natural resources are constant threats to the future of our planet. All people have a responsibility to be proactive participants in the fight to save Earth by working now to conserve resources for later. Participation begins with our everyday choices. From what you buy to what you do to how much you use, your decisions affect the planet and everyone around you. Now is the time to take action.

When choosing what to buy, look for sustainable products made from renewable or recycled resources. The packaging of the products you buy is just as important as the products themselves. Is the item minimally packaged in a recycled container? How did the product reach the store? Locally grown food and other products manufactured within your community are the best choices. The fewer miles a product traveled to reach you, the fewer resources it required.

You can continue to make a difference for the planet in how you use what you bought and the resources you have available. Remember the locally grown food you purchased? Don't pile it on your plate at dinner. Food that remains on your plate is a wasted resource, and you can always go back for seconds. You should try to be aware of your consumption of water and energy. Turn off the water when you brush your teeth, and limit your showers to five minutes. Turn off the lights, and don't leave appliances or chargers plugged in when not in use.

Together, we can use less, waste less, recycle more, and make the right choices. It may be the only chance we have.

19. What is the author's tone?

a.   The author's tone is optimistic.
b.   The author's tone is pessimistic.
c.   The author's tone is matter-of-fact.
d.   The author's tone is angry.

20. Why does the author say it is important to buy locally grown food?

a.   Buying locally grown food supports people in your community.
b.   Locally grown food travels the least distance to reach you, and therefore uses fewer resources.
c.   Locally grown food uses less packaging.
d.   Locally grown food is healthier for you because it has been exposed to fewer pesticides.

21. What does the author imply will happen if people do not follow his suggestions?

a.   The author implies we will run out of resources in the next 10 years.
b.   The author implies water and energy prices will rise sharply in the near future.
c.   The author implies global warming and the depletion of natural resources will continue.
d.   The author implies local farmers will lose their farms.

22. "You should try to be aware of your consumption of water and energy."
What does the word "consumption" mean in the context of this selection?

a.   Using the greatest amount
b.   Illness of the lungs
c.   Using the least amount
d.   Depletion of goods

23. The author makes a general suggestion to the reader: "You should try to be aware of your consumption of water and energy." Which of the following is one way the author specifies that this suggestion be carried out?

a. Food that remains on your plate is a wasted resource, and you can always go back for a second helping.
b. Locally grown food and other products manufactured within your community are the best choices.
c. Turn off the lights, and don't leave appliances or chargers plugged in when not in use.
d. Participation begins with our everyday choices.

24. How does the author make a connection between the second and third paragraphs?

a. The author indicates he will make suggestions for how to tell other people what to buy.
b. The author indicates he will continue to give more examples of what you should buy.
c. The author indicates he will make suggestions for how to keep from buying more items.
d. The author indicates he will now make suggestions for how to use what you bought.

The next six questions are based on this passage.

In the United States, where we have more land than people, it is not at all difficult for persons in good health to make money. In this comparatively new field there are so many avenues of success open, so many vocations which are not crowded, that any person of either sex who is willing, at least for the time being, to engage in any respectable occupation that offers, may find lucrative employment.

Those who really desire to attain an independence, have only to set their minds upon it, and adopt the proper means, as they do in regard to any other object which they wish to accomplish, and the thing is easily done. But however easy it may be found to make money, I have no doubt many of my hearers will agree it is the most difficult thing in the world to keep it. The road to wealth is, as Dr. Franklin truly says, "as plain as the road to the mill." It consists simply in expending less than we earn; that seems to be a very simple problem. Mr. Micawber, one of those happy creations of the genial Dickens, puts the case in a strong light when he says that to have annual income of twenty pounds per annum, and spend twenty pounds and sixpence, is to be the most miserable of men; whereas, to have an income of only twenty pounds, and spend but nineteen pounds and sixpence is to be the happiest of mortals.

Many of my readers may say, "we understand this: this is economy, and we know economy is wealth; we know we can't eat our cake and keep it also." Yet I beg to say that perhaps more cases of failure arise from mistakes on this point than almost any other. The fact is, many people think they understand economy when they really do not.

25. Which of the following statements best expresses the main idea of the passage?

a. Getting a job is easier now than it ever has been before.
b. Earning money is much less difficult than managing it properly.
c. Dr. Franklin advocated getting a job in a mill.
d. Spending money is the greatest temptation in the world.

26. What would this author's attitude likely be to a person unable to find employment?

    a. descriptive
    b. conciliatory
    c. ingenuous
    d. incredulous

27. According to the author, what is more difficult than making money?

    a. managing money
    b. traveling to a mill
    c. reading Dickens
    d. understanding the economy

28. Who is the most likely audience for this passage?

    a. economists
    b. general readers
    c. teachers
    d. philanthropists

29. Which word best describes the author's attitude towards those who believe they understand money?

    a. supportive
    b. incriminating
    c. excessive
    d. patronizing

30. This passage is most likely taken from a(n) ____.

    a. self-help manual
    b. autobiography
    c. epistle
    d. novel

WORD KNOWLEDGE

1. The data in the graph exhibited an *aberration*.

  ***Aberration* means:**

   a. deviation from course
   b. linear appearance
   c. inverted appearance
   d. circular theme

2. The prince *abjured* the ambassador.

  ***Abjured* means:**

   a. congratulated
   b. renounced
   c. relieved
   d. fired

3. The chemist attempted to practice *alchemy*.

  ***Alchemy* means:**

   a. turning metal into gold
   b. separating ions
   c. fusion
   d. isolating chemical components

4. The man at the bar was *belligerent*.

  ***Belligerent* means:**

   a. friendly
   b. courteous
   c. angry
   d. talkative

5. The ships formed a *blockade* near the mouth of the Mississippi River.

  ***Blockade* means:**

   a. prevent passage
   b. fishing convoy
   c. whaling expedition
   d. zigzag formation

6. The men erected a *bulwark* near the opening.

  ***Bulwark* means:**

   a. trap
   b. obstacle
   c. barn
   d. runway

7. The group embarked on a *clandestine* operation.

Clandestine means:

a. environmental expedition
b. shipping adventure
c. scary
d. secretive

8. The agent of the government was *choleric*.

Choleric means:

a. easily provoked
b. undercover
c. cooperative
d. late

9. Some members of the organization broke away and created a grass roots *caucus*.

Caucus means:

a. group with political aims
b. environmental group
c. management organization
d. religious movement

10. The circumstances were open to *conjecture*.

Conjecture means:

a. discussion
b. guessing
c. argument
d. public

11. The news anchor attempted to *disseminate* the story.

Disseminate means:

a. to convey
b. to deny
c. to rebuke
d. to review

12. The stockpiles for the occupation began to *dwindle*.

Dwindle means:

a. to increase
b. to decrease
c. to rot
d. to be self-limiting

13. The chemicals began to *effervesce*.

Effervesce means:

a. to combine
b. to catalyze
c. to break down
d. to bubble up

14. The witness began to *evince* critical details.

Evince means:

a. to hide
b. to cover secretly
c. exaggerate
d. to make manifest

15. The front line troops began to *extricate* from the enemy.

Extricate means:

a. confront
b. surrender
c. disentangle
d. deploy

16. The congressman from Ohio started a *filibuster*.

Filibuster means:

a. bill
b. congressional investigation
c. an attempt to disrupt legislation
d. program related to welfare

17. The soldier showed *fortitude* during the engagement with the enemy.

Fortitude means:

a. patient courage
b. willingness for action
c. endurance
d. professionalism

18. The southern lady was *genteel* when hosting northern businessmen.

Genteel means:

a. rude
b. refined
c. reserved
d. resentful

19. The lawyer launched into a *harangue* when speaking to the witness.

Harangue means:

a. discussion
b. monologue
c. dialogue
d. tirade

20. Some believe our destinies are *immutable*.

Immutable means:

a. professional
b. conversational
c. unchangeable
d. unerring

21. The baby was diagnosed with *jaundice*.

    ***Jaundice* means:**

    a. yellowing condition
    b. condition of glucose intolerance
    c. condition of nutritional deficiency
    d. condition of dermatitis

22. The criminal was known for his *knavery*.

    ***Knavery* means:**

    a. quickness
    b. light-footedness
    c. burglary ability
    d. deceitfulness

23. The patient exhibited signs of *languor*.

    ***Languor* means:**

    a. confusion
    b. anxiety
    c. depression
    d. deceitfulness

24. The Romans were able to *macadamize* a large portion of the Italian peninsula.

    ***Macadamize* means:**

    a. to pave
    b. to supply
    c. to connect
    d. to protect

25. The patient's lower extremity began to show signs of *necrosis*.

    ***Necrosis* means:**

    a. maceration
    b. tissue death
    c. induration
    d. redness

26. The traffic official began to *obviate* the construction.

    ***Obviate* means:**

    a. clear away
    b. identify
    c. reproduce
    d. delegate

27. The general *presaged* the battle plan to his subordinate officers.

    ***Presaged* means:**

    a. delegated
    b. clarified
    c. foretold
    d. introduced

28. **The orange grove was under** *quarantine*, **because of a local virus.**

    ***Quarantine* means:**

    a. pressure
    b. demolition
    c. reconstruction
    d. isolation

29. **The defendant was asked to** *remunerate* **the damage he caused during the robbery.**

    ***Remunerate* means:**

    a. reconstruct
    b. renounce
    c. pay for
    d. repeat

30. **The welding machine** *scintillated* **into the dark shop.**

    ***Scintillated* means:**

    a. emitted gases
    b. emitted light
    c. emitted fumes
    d. emitted noise

Mathematics Review

(no calculator)

1. **897.54 – 48.39 =**
   a. 849.15
   b. 813.15
   c. 859.15
   d. 814.15

2. **1053.33 – 545.69 =**
   a. 519.64
   b. 517.54
   c. 508.64
   d. 507.64

3. **893.42 + 82.77 =**
   a. 976.09
   b. 976.29
   c. 986.19
   d. 976.19

4. **94.31 + 973.37 =**
   a. 1067.68
   b. 1167.68
   c. 1067.78
   d. 1167.78

5. **A senior paid $3.47, $9.50 and $2.50 for lunch during a basketball tournament. What was the average amount he paid over three days?**
   a. $5.18
   b. $5.25
   c. $5.16
   d. $5.37

6. **89.35 x 32.75 =**
   a. 2826.23
   b. 2925.31
   c. 2926.21
   d. 2837.41

7. **Using the following equation, solve for (x). 3x – 4y = 25 and (y)=2**
   a. x =10
   b. x = 11
   c. x = 12
   d. x = 13

8. Using the following equation, solve for (y). 5y – 3x = 24 and (x) = 7

    a. y = 8
    b. y = 9
    c. y = 10
    d. y = 11

9. An armoire was purchased for $340.32 at an auction, subject to a 5% tax rate. What was the additional tax charged on the armoire?

    a. $15.82
    b. $16.02
    c. $16.39
    d. $17.02

10. 894 + ((3)(12)) =

    a. 730
    b. 932
    c. 930
    d. 945

11. Round to the nearest 2 decimal places, 892/15 =

    a. 60.47
    b. 59.47
    c. 62.57
    d. 59.57

12. Round to the nearest 2 decimal places, 999.52/13 =

    a. 76.89
    b. 76.97
    c. 86.87
    d. 86.97

13. Round to the nearest 2 decimal places, 9.42/3.47 =

    a. 2.63
    b. 2.71
    c. 2.81
    d. 2.94

14. Jonathan Edwards ate 8.32 lbs. of food over 3 days. What was his average intake?

    a. 2.66 lbs.
    b. 2.77 lbs.
    c. 2.87 lbs.
    d. 2.97 lbs.

15. Which of the following decimals equals 9.47%?

    a. .000947
    b. .00947
    c. .0947
    d. .9470

16. .10 equals which of the following fractions?
   a. 1/100
   b. 1/10
   c. 1/50
   d. 1/5

17. What is the area of a rectangle with sides 34 meters and 12 meters?
   a. 408 m^2
   b. 2.83 m^2
   c. 22 m^2
   d. 40.8 m^2

18. The standard ratio of (number of treatments) and (total mL dose) is 3.5 to 2 mL. If only 2 treatments are given, how many total mL doses are given?
   a. 1.58 mL
   b. 2.34 mL
   c. 1.14 mL
   d. 2.58 mL

19. If one side of a triangle equals 4 inches and the second side equals 5 inches, what does the third side equal?
   a. 9 inches
   b. 1 inches
   c. 6.4 inches
   d. 4.6 inches

20. If x=75 + 0, and y= (75)(0), then
   a. x>y
   b. x=y
   c. x<y
   d. x+y = 0

21. If x=3, the x^2+x=
   a. 9
   b. 15
   c. 12
   d. 10

22. If a=4 and b=5, then a (a^2+b)=
   a. 52
   b. 84
   c. 62
   d. 64

23. If x= ¼, y=1/2, and z= 2/3, then $x + y - z$ =
   a. 1/8
   b. 2/9
   c. 1/12
   d. 2/5

24. If $x = \frac{1}{2}$, $y = 1/3$, $z = 3/8$, then $x(y-z) =$

    a. 1/48
    b. -1/48
    c. 1/64
    d. -1/64

25. 2/3 cup of oil is needed for a cake recipe, and you have 1/4 cup. How much more oil do you need?

    a. 1/2
    b. 2/7
    c. 3/8
    d. 5/12

26. 8 ¾ + 6 ½ =

    a. 32
    b. 15 ¼
    c. 14 ½
    d. 17 ¾

27. A senior citizen was billed $ 3.85 for a long-distance phone call. The first 10 minutes cost $3.50, and 35 cents was charged for each additional minute. How long was the telephone call?

    a. 17 minutes
    b. 20 minutes
    c. 15 minutes
    d. 11 minutes

28. A ½ cup of skim milk is 45 calories. Approximately how many calories would ¾ cup of skim milk provide?

    a. 67 ½
    b. 68
    c. 76 ½
    d. 60

29. $10b = 5a - 15$. If $a = 3$, then $b =$

    a. 7
    b. 5
    c. 1
    d. 0

30. (5 x 4) ÷ (2 x 2) =

    a. 6
    b. 7.2
    c. 5
    d. 4

31. Which of these numbers is a prime number?

  a. 12
  b. 4
  c. 15
  d. 11

32. 12 members of a weight loss club are female; there are 23 members altogether. Approximately what percentage of members are males?

  a. 59%
  b. 48%
  c. 36%
  d. 44%

33. A person travels an average of 57 miles daily, and this morning he traveled 14 miles. What percentage of his daily average of mile traveled did he travel this morning?

  a. 25%
  b. 22%
  c. 27%
  d. 32%

34. 75 is 60% of what number?

  a. 130
  b. 125
  c. 45
  d. 145

35. A student invests $3000 of his student loan and receives 400 dollars in interest over a 4-year period. What is his average yearly interest rate?

  a. 3.3%
  b. 2.1%
  c. 5%
  d. 4.2%

The next question refers to the following graph.

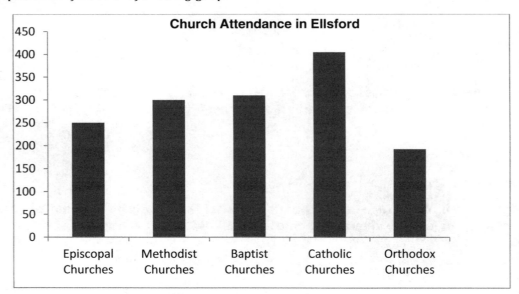

36. The graph above shows the weekly church attendance among residents in the town of Ellsford, with the town having five different denominations: Episcopal, Methodist, Baptist, Catholic, and Orthodox. Approximately what percentage of church-goers in Ellsford attends Catholic churches?

a. 23%
b. 28%
c. 36%
d. 42%

37. Solve for *x*:

$$2x + 4 = x - 6$$

a. $x = -12$
b. $x = 10$
c. $x = -16$
d. $x = -10$

38. A can has a radius of 1.5 inches and a height of 3 inches. Which of the following best represents the volume of the can?

a. 17.2 in^3
b. 19.4 in^3
c. 21.2 in^3
d. 23.4 in^3

39. Four more than a number, x, is 2 less than $\frac{1}{3}$ of another number, y. Which of the following algebraic equations correctly represents this sentence?

    a. $x + 4 = \frac{1}{3}y - 2$

    b. $4x = 2 - \frac{1}{3}y$

    c. $4 - x = 2 + \frac{1}{3}y$

    d. $x + 4 = 2 - \frac{1}{3}y$

40. The table below shows the cost of renting a bicycle for 1, 2, or 3 hours. Which answer choice shows the equation that best represents the data? Let C represent the cost of the rental and h stand for the number of hours of rental time.

Hours	1	2	3
Cost	$3.60	$7.20	$10.80

    a. $C = 3.60h$

    b. $C = h + 3.60$

    c. $C = 3.60h + 10.80$

    d. $C = \frac{10.80}{h}$

Science Review

1. The heart is divided into __ chambers.

   a. 2
   b. 3
   c. 4
   d. 5

2. Blood leaves the right ventricle and goes to the ____.

   a. lungs
   b. kidneys
   c. right atrium
   d. arterial circulation to the body

3. Which of the following does not help determine heart rate?

   a. body temperature
   b. physical activity
   c. concentration of ions
   d. anaerobic cellular metabolism

4. Which of the following is not considered a layer of the heart?

   a. epicardium
   b. endocarcium
   c. myocardium
   d. vasocardium

5. The hormone _____ can promote increased blood volume, and increased blood pressure.

   a. estrogen
   b. testosterone
   c. aldosterone
   d. dopamine

6. Which of the following terms matches the definition: an abnormally slow heartbeat.

   a. tachycardia
   b. bradycardia
   c. fibrillation
   d. myocardial infarct

7. Blood is made of approximately __% hematocrit and ____% plasma.

   a. 45, 55
   b. 55, 45
   c. 75, 25
   d. 25, 75

8. The right lung has ___ lobes and the left lung has ___ lobes.

   a. 2, 3
   b. 3, 2
   c. 4, 2
   d. 2, 4

9. Aerobic respiration in cells occurs in the _____.

a. cytoplasm
b. nucleus
c. mitochondria
d. cell membrane

10. Which of the following terms matches the definition: collapse of a lung.

a. anoxia
b. atelectasis
c. dyspnea
d. hypercapnia

11. The central nervous system is composed of the _____ and the _____.

a. brain, spinal cord
b. brain, peripheral nerves
c. spinal cord, peripheral nerves
d. spinal cord, musculature system

12. The brain is made of _____ lobes.

a. 2
b. 3
c. 4
d. 5

13. _____ is a state of equilibrium within tissues.

a. peristalsis
b. stomatitis
c. homeostasis
d. synergy

14. _____ is a state of inflammation of the mouth.

a. diverticulitis
b. hepatitis
c. enteritis
d. stomatitis

15. _____ is the most important male hormone

a. estrogen
b. aldosterone
c. progesterone
d. testosterone

16. Which of the following functions are not related to the kidneys?

a. filtration
b. bile production
c. secretion
d. re-absorption

17. Which of the following terms matches the definition: uncontrolled urination.

a. enuresis
b. dieuretic
c. pyuria
d. ureteritis

18. Auditory impulses are interpreted in the _____ lobes.

a. frontal
b. parietal
c. temporal
d. occipital

19. The outer layer of the eye is the ____.

a. cornea
b. sclera
c. retina
d. rods

20. The inner layer of the eye is the ____.

a. cornea
b. sclera
c. retina
d. rods

21. Which of the following elements are not halogens?

a. Chlorine
b. Bromide
c. Iodine
d. Cesium

22. The horizontal rows of the periodic table are called ____.

a. periods
b. columns
c. rows
d. families

23. A/an ____ is the simplest unit of an element.

a. atom
b. molecule
c. electron
d. neutron

24. Compounds with various structures, but the same shape are called ____.

a. polar compounds
b. isomers
c. variables
d. transient compounds

25. Converting gas into a liquid is known as _____.

    a. evaporation
    b. transitioning
    c. condensation
    d. sublimation

26. Which of the following terms matches the definition: the volume of a gas varies indirectly with temperature with pressure constant.

    a. Boyle's law
    b. Charles law
    c. Johnson's law
    d. Avogadro's law

27. Which of the following terms matches the definition: energy is conserved with every process.

    a. 1st Law of Thermodynamics
    b. 2nd Law of Thermodynamics
    c. 3rd Law of Thermodynamics
    d. 4th Law of Thermodynamics

28. An acid is a substance that increases the _____ count in water.

    a. chloride ion
    b. hydroxide ion
    c. hydrogen ion
    d. oxygen

29. Which of the following is not true of a reaction catalyst's potential?

    a. it can speed up a reaction
    b. it can cause a reaction
    c. it is never destroyed
    d. it is always found on the right side of an equation

30. Using the 2nd Law of Newton identify the formula that is applicable.

    a. $F = ma$
    b. $Speed = \frac{Distance}{Time}$
    c. $Power = \frac{F \times D}{T}$
    d. $Watts = Voltage \times Amperes$

31. Which of the following is NOT consistent with the scientific method?

    a. Observe the data, noting potential outliers, and then analyze the results.
    b. Develop a new hypothesis based on a conclusion from a previous experiment.
    c. Conduct an experiment and then make a hypothesis that fits the results.
    d. Communicate the results of an experiment that did not confirm the hypothesis.

32. What are the two types of measurement important in science?

    a. quantitative and numerical
    b. qualitative and descriptive
    c. numerical and scientific
    d. quantitative and qualitative

The next question refers to the following graphic.

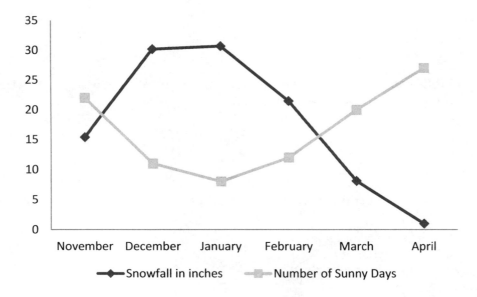

33. The chart above shows the average snowfall in inches for a town on Michigan's Upper Peninsula, during the months November through April. Which of the following can be concluded based on the information that is provided in the chart?

    a. April is not a good month to go skiing in the Upper Peninsula.

    b. Snowfall blocks the sunshine and reduces the number of sunny days.

    c. The fewest sunny days occur in the months with the heaviest snowfall.

    d. There is no connection between the amount of snowfall and the number of sunny days.

34. What is the name of the structure that prevents food from entering the airway?

    a. trachea

    b. esophagus

    c. diaphragm

    d. epiglottis

35. Which substance makes up the pads that provide support between the vertebrae?

    a. bone

    b. cartilage

    c. tendon

    d. fat

36. The two criteria for classifying epithelial tissue are *cell layers* and _____.
Which of the following completes the sentence above?

    a. Cell composition

    b. Cell absorption

    c. Cell shape

    d. Cell stratification

37. Organized from high to low, the hierarchy of the human body's structure is as follows: organism, organ systems, organs, tissues. Which of the following comes next?

- a. Molecules
- b. Atoms
- c. Cells
- d. Muscle

The next two questions are based on the periodic table.

1 IA																	18 VIIIA
1 **H** 1.01	2 IIA											13 IIIA	14 IVA	15 VA	16 VIA	17 VIIA	2 **He** 4.00
3 **Li** 6.94	4 **Be** 9.01											5 **B** 10.81	6 **C** 12.01	7 **N** 14.01	8 **O** 16.00	9 **F** 19.00	10 **Ne** 20.18
11 **Na** 22.99	12 **Mg** 24.31	3 IIIB	4 IVB	5 VB	6 VIB	7 VIIB	8	9 VIIIB	10	11 IB	12 IIB	13 **Al** 26.98	14 **Si** 28.09	15 **P** 30.97	16 **S** 32.07	17 **Cl** 35.45	18 **Ar** 39.95
19 **K** 39.1	20 **Ca** 40.08	21 **Sc** 44.96	22 **Ti** 47.88	23 **V** 50.94	24 **Cr** 52.00	25 **Mn** 54.94	26 **Fe** 55.85	27 **Co** 58.93	28 **Ni** 58.69	29 **Cu** 63.55	30 **Zn** 65.39	31 **Ga** 69.72	32 **Ge** 72.61	33 **As** 74.92	34 **Se** 78.96	35 **Br** 79.90	36 **Kr** 83.80
37 **Rb** 85.47	38 **Sr** 87.62	39 **Y** 88.91	40 **Zr** 91.22	41 **Nb** 92.91	42 **Mo** 95.94	43 **Tc** (98)	44 **Ru** 101.07	45 **Rh** 102.91	46 **Pd** 106.42	47 **Ag** 107.87	48 **Cd** 112.41	49 **In** 114.82	50 **Sn** 118.71	51 **Sb** 121.76	52 **Te** 127.6	53 **I** 126.9	54 **Xe** 131.29
55 **Cs** 132.9	56 **Ba** 137.3	57 **La*** 138.9	72 **Hf** 178.5	73 **Ta** 180.9	74 **W** 183.9	75 **Re** 186.2	76 **Os** 190.2	77 **Ir** 192.2	78 **Pt** 195.1	79 **Au** 197.0	80 **Hg** 200.6	81 **Tl** 204.4	82 **Pb** 207.2	83 **Bi** 209	84 **Po** (209)	85 **At** (210)	86 **Rn** (222)
87 **Fr** (223)	88 **Ra** (226)	89 **Ac^** (227)	104 **Rf** (261)	105 **Db** (262)	106 **Sg** (263)	107 **Bh** (264)	108 **Hs** (265)	109 **Mt** (268)	110 **Ds** (271)	111 **Rg** (272)							

	58 **Ce** 140.1	59 **Pr** 140.9	60 **Nd** 144.2	61 **Pm** (145)	62 **Sm** 150.4	63 **Eu** 152.0	64 **Gd** 157.3	65 **Tb** 158.9	66 **Dy** 162.5	67 **Ho** 164.9	68 **Er** 167.3	69 **Tm** 168.9	70 **Yb** 173.0	71 **Lu** 175.0
^	90 **Th** 232.0	91 **Pa** (231)	92 **U** 238.0	93 **Np** (237)	94 **Pu** (244)	95 **Am** (243)	96 **Cm** (247)	97 **Bk** (247)	98 **Cf** (251)	99 **Es** (252)	100 **Fm** (257)	101 **Md** (258)	102 **No** (259)	103 **Lr** (260)

Note: The row labeled with * is the <u>Lanthanide Series</u>, *and the row labeled with ^ is the* <u>Actinide Series</u>.

38. On average, how many neutrons does one atom of bromine (Br) have?

- a. 35
- b. 44.90
- c. 45
- d. 79.90

39. On average, how many protons does one atom of zinc (Zn) have?

- a. 30
- b. 35
- c. 35.39
- d. 65.39

40. In your garden, you noticed that the tomato plants did better on the north side of your house than the west side and you decided to figure out why. They are both planted with the same soil that provides adequate nutrients to the plant, and they are watered at the same time during the week. Over the course of a week, you begin to measure the amount of sunlight that hits each side of the house and determine that the north side gets more light because the sunlight is blocked by the house's shadow on the west side. What is the name of the factor in your observations that affected the tomato plants growth?

    a.   The control
    b.   The independent variable
    c.   The dependent variable
    d.   The conclusion

41. Which of the following cannot exist in RNA?

    a.   Uracil
    b.   Thymine
    c.   Cytosine
    d.   Guanine

42. In the development of genetic traits, one gene must match to one _____ for the traits to develop correctly.

    a.   Codon
    b.   Protein
    c.   Amino acid
    d.   Chromosome

43. Which of the following best describes the careful ordering of molecules within solids that have a fixed shape?

    a.   Physical bonding
    b.   Polar molecules
    c.   Metalloid structure
    d.   Crystalline order

44. Which of the following describes the transport network that is responsible for the transference of proteins throughout a cell?

    a.   Golgi apparatus
    b.   Endoplasmic reticulum
    c.   Mitochondria
    d.   Nucleolus

45. During the *anaphase* of mitosis, the _____, originally in pairs, separate from their daughters and move to the opposite ends (or poles) of the cell.

    a.   Chromosomes
    b.   Spindle fibers
    c.   Centrioles
    d.   Nuclear membranes

46. A(n) _____ is the physical and visible expression of a genetic trait.

    a.   Phenotype
    b.   Allele
    c.   Gamete
    d.   Genotype

47. A substance is considered *acidic* if it has a pH of less than which of the following?

    a.   12
    b.   9
    c.   7
    d.   4

48. A triple beam balance would show the units of measurement in which form?

    a.   Liters
    b.   Grams
    c.   Meters
    d.   Gallons

49. Which of the following best describes a section that divides the body into equal upper and lower portions?

    a.   Coronal
    b.   Transverse
    c.   Oblique
    d.   Median

50. Which of the following best describes one of the roles of RNA?

    a.   Manufacturing the proteins needed for DNA
    b.   Creating the bonds between the elements that compose DNA
    c.   Sending messages about the correct sequence of proteins in DNA
    d.   Forming the identifiable "*double helix*" shape of DNA

51. Which of the following do *catalysts* alter to control the rate of a chemical reaction?

    a.   Substrate energy
    b.   Activation energy
    c.   Inhibitor energy
    d.   Promoter energy

52. The Punnett square shown here indicates a cross between two parents, one with alleles BB and the other with alleles Bb. Select the correct entry for the upper right box in the Punnett square, which is indicated with the letter, *x*:

	B	B
B		*x*
b		

    a.   Bb
    b.   bB
    c.   BB
    d.   bb

53. Which part of the cell is often called the cell "power house" because it provides energy for cellular functions?

 a. Nucleus
 b. Cell membrane
 c. Mitochondria
 d. Cytoplasm

54. What function do ribosomes serve within the cell?

 a. Ribosomes are responsible for cell movement.
 b. Ribosomes aid in protein synthesis.
 c. Ribosomes help protect the cell from its environment.
 d. Ribosomes have enzymes that help with digestion.

55. What is the most likely reason that cells differentiate?

 a. Cells differentiate to avoid looking like all the cells around them.
 b. Cells differentiate so that simple, non-specialized cells can become highly specialized cells.
 c. Cells differentiate so that multicellular organisms will remain the same size.
 d. Cells differentiate for no apparent reason.

56. How is meiosis similar to mitosis?

 a. Both produce daughter cells that are genetically identical.
 b. Both produce daughter cells that are genetically different.
 c. Both occur in humans, other animals, and plants.
 d. Both occur asexually.

57. In the suburban neighborhood of Northwoods, there have been large populations of deer, and residents have complained about them eating flowers and garden plants. What would be a logical explanation, based on observations, for the large increase in the deer population over the last two seasons?

 a. Increased quantity of food sources
 b. Decreased population of a natural predator
 c. Deer migration from surrounding areas
 d. Increase in hunting licenses sold

58. What type of chemical bond connects the oxygen and hydrogen atoms in a molecule of water?

 a. Static bond
 b. Aquatic bond
 c. Ionic bond
 d. Covalent bond

59. Two cars driving in opposite directions collide. If you ignore friction and any other outside interactions, which of the following statements is always true?

 a. The total momentum is conserved.
 b. The sum of the potential and kinetic energy are conserved.
 c. The total velocity of the cars is conserved.
 d. The total impulse is conserved.

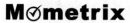

60. What is the speed of a wave with a frequency of 12 Hz and a wavelength of 3 meters?

    a.   12 meters per second

    b.   36 meters per second

    c.   4 meters per second

    d.   0.25 meters per second

Answer Key and Explanations

Verbal Review

Reading Comprehension

Number	Answer
1	C
2	D
3	A
4	C
5	D
6	B
7	B
8	C
9	D
10	D
11	B
12	D
13	D
14	C
15	A
16	B
17	D
18	D
19	C
20	B
21	C
22	D
23	C
24	D
25	B
26	D
27	A
28	B
29	D
30	A

Word Knowledge

Number	Answer
1	A
2	B
3	A
4	C
5	A
6	B
7	D
8	A
9	A
10	B
11	A
12	B
13	D
14	D
15	C
16	C
17	A
18	B
19	D
20	C
21	A
22	D
23	C
24	A
25	B
26	A
27	C
28	D
29	C
30	B

Mathematics Review

Number	Answer
1	A
2	D
3	D
4	A
5	C
6	C
7	B
8	B
9	D
10	C
11	B
12	A
13	B
14	B
15	C
16	B
17	A
18	C
19	C
20	A
21	C
22	B
23	C
24	B
25	D
26	B
27	D
28	A
29	D
30	C
31	D
32	B
33	A
34	B
35	A
36	B
37	D
38	C
39	A
40	A

Science Review

Number	Answer	Number	Answer
1	C	31	B
2	A	32	D
3	D	33	C
4	D	34	D
5	C	35	B
6	B	36	C
7	A	37	C
8	B	38	B
9	C	39	A
10	B	40	B
11	A	41	B
12	C	42	B
13	C	43	D
14	D	44	B
15	D	45	A
16	B	46	A
17	A	47	C
18	C	48	B
19	B	49	B
20	C	50	C
21	D	51	B
22	A	52	C
23	A	53	C
24	B	54	B
25	C	55	B
26	B	56	C
27	A	57	B
28	C	58	D
29	D	59	A
30	A	60	B

Verbal Review

READING COMPREHENSION

1. C: The passage is expository in the sense that it looks more closely into the mysteries of the Bermuda Triangle and exposes information about what researchers have studied and now believe.

2. D: This sentence is the best summary statement for the entire passage, because it wraps up clearly what the author is saying about the results of studies on the Bermuda Triangle.

3. A: Of all the sentences provided, this is the one with which the author would most likely agree. The passage suggests that most of the "mysteries" of the Bermuda Triangle can be explained in a reasonable way. The passage mentions that some expand the Triangle to the Azores, but this is a point of fact, and the author makes no mention of whether or not this is in error. The author quotes the Navy's response to the disappearance of the planes, but there is no reason to believe the author questions this response. The author raises questions about the many myths surrounding the Triangle, but at no point does the author connect these myths with what are described as accidents that fall "within the expected margin of error."

4. C: The inclusion of the statement about the ships from East Asia is an opinion statement, as the author provides no support or explanation. The other statements within the answer choices offer supporting evidence and explanatory material, making them acceptable for an expository composition.

5. D: The most compelling argument from researchers stated in the passage is about the fact that the number of accidents in the Bermuda Triangle is within expected margins.

6. B: The best substitute for discomposed in the passage would be disoriented. There is no evidence given that the planes became inverted or that the pilots were forgetful. There is no way to know if the planes or pilots broke down prior to becoming lost.

7. B: The passage does not say that studying a foreign language will help students find jobs after high school (choice A) or gain an understanding of other cultures (choice C). The passage does say that studying a foreign language is important for college acceptance (choice D), but this point alone is not the main idea of the passage.

8. C: The passage does not claim that studying a foreign language is essential to high school graduation (choice A). Choices B and D represent claims made in the passage, but do not include all of the claims made.

9. D: Although students may find knowledge of a foreign language helpful in obtaining a job, it is an obvious exaggeration to claim that students who did not study a foreign language would be unemployable.

10. D: Choices A and C represent options that would provide information regarding the opinions of students and parents, but not actual evidence regarding the influence of studying a foreign language on future success. Choice B specifies a second language taught at home, whereas the passage focuses specifically on a foreign language taught in high school.

11. B: Choices A, C, and D do not offer a complete summary of the claims made in this passage.

12. D: The author makes their position clear that they believe learning a foreign language should be required of all students in the country, not just for those in the states that choose to have that requirement.

13. D: All other sentences in the passage offer some support or explanation. Only the sentence in answer choice D indicates an unsupported opinion on the part of the author.

14. C: The author actually says, "Charles's own political troubles extended beyond religion in this case, and he was beheaded in 1649." This would indicate that religion was less involved in this situation than in other situations. There is not enough information to infer that Charles II never married; the passage only notes that he had no legitimate children. (In fact, he had more than ten illegitimate children by his mistresses.) And while the chance of a Catholic king frightened many in England, it is reaching beyond logical inference to assume that people were relieved when the royal children died. Finally, the author does not provide enough detail for the reader to assume that James I had no Catholic leanings. The author only says that James recognized the importance of committing to the Church of England.

15. A: The author notes, "In spite of a strong resemblance to the king, the young James was generally rejected among the English and the Lowland Scots, who referred to him as "the Pretender." This indicates that there was a resemblance, and this increases the likelihood that the child was, in fact, that of James and Mary Beatrice. Answer choice B is too much of an opinion statement that does not have enough support in the passage. The passage essentially refutes answer choice C by pointing out that James "the Pretender" was welcomed in the Highlands. And there is little in the passage to suggest that James was unable to raise an army and mount an attack.

16. B: The passage is composed in a chronological sequence with each king introduced in order of reign.

17. D: The passage is largely informative in focus, and the author provides extensive detail about this period in English and Scottish history. There is little in the passage to suggest persuasion, and the tone of the passage has no indication of a desire to entertain. Additionally, the passage is historical, so the author avoids expressing feelings and instead focuses on factual information (with the exception of the one opinion statement).

18. D: Paragraph three states that "Charles II died without a legitimate heir, and his brother James ascended to the throne as King James II."

19. C: The author does not make predictions of a radically rejuvenated planet (choice A) or the complete annihilation of life as we know it (choice B). The author is also not accusatory in his descriptions (choice D). Instead, the author states what he believes to be the current state of the planet's environment, and makes practical suggestions for making better use of its resources in the future.

20. B: As the passage states: "Locally grown food and other products manufactured within your community are the best choices. The fewer miles a product traveled to reach you, the fewer resources it required."

21. C: The author does not mention running out of resources in a specific time period (choice A), the cost of water and energy (choice B), or the possibility of hardship for local farmers (choice D).

22. D: As the passage states: "You should try to be aware of your consumption of water and energy. Turn off the water when you brush your teeth, and limit your showers to five minutes. Turn off the lights, and don't leave appliances or chargers plugged in when not in use." The contexts of these sentences indicate that consumption means the depletion of goods (e.g., water and energy).

23. C: Of the choices available, this is the only sentence that offers specific ideas for carrying out the author's suggestion to the reader of limiting consumption of energy.

24. D: The author begins the third paragraph with, "You can continue to make a difference for the planet in how you use what you bought and the resources you have available." This sentence makes the connection between the second paragraph which deals with what people should buy and the third paragraph which makes suggestions for how to use what they have.

25. B: The author asserts both that earning money is increasingly easy and that managing money is difficult.

26. D: The author seems to believe that there are plenty of lucrative jobs for everyone.

27. A: The author insists that many people who have no trouble earning money waste it through lavish spending.

28. B: This passage is clearly intended for a non-expert adult readership.

29. D: The author suggests that many people who believe they understand economy in fact do not.

30. A: It seems clear that the author is about to describe the correct means of personal economy for a self-help manual.

WORD KNOWLEDGE

1. A: Aberration means a deviation from what is normal or typical. Its Latin roots are ab-, meaning away from, and errare, meaning to err or stray. Combined, these make up the Latin verb aberrare, to go astray (from). There are no other meanings.

2. B: To abjure means "to renounce." The original Latin roots are ab-, meaning away from, and jurare, meaning to swear, which is also the root of the English word jury. Hence "swearing away from" is renouncing, rejecting, or repudiating someone or something, abstaining from or avoiding something, or taking something back.

3. A: Alchemy refers to the hypothetical process of turning base metals into gold. While this process does not exist in reality, it was a famously popular pursuit during the Middle Ages. Today this word is also used figuratively to mean turning something common into something precious, or any mysterious transformation. The Medieval Latin alchymia derived from the Arabic al-kimiya, originating from the Late Greek word chemeia.

4. C: Belligerent means angry or hostile. Its original sense had to do with waging war. Belligerare in Latin means "to wage war," from bellum, which means war (as in the English word "antebellum," meaning prewar), and gerare, which means to wage. "Hostilities" in English can refer to warfare and to anger. An English synonym of belligerent from the same root is "bellicose." Both mean warlike, aggressive, combative, etc.

5. A: Blockade refers to preventing passage or blocking it. Its similarity to the word "block" makes it easier to define. One difference between "block" and "blockade" is that "blockade" was originally, and is still often, used to refer specifically to military maneuvers intended to block physically the transportation, trade, and communications of enemy nations. It also refers to obstruction of physiological processes and, generally, to any obstruction. It can be used as a transitive verb or a noun.

6. B: The choice closest to the meaning of bulwark is obstacle. A bulwark is a protective, defensive, or supportive structure that is like a wall. Synonyms include rampart, breakwater, and seawall. The (usually) plural term "bulwarks" can also refer to a ship's sides above the upper deck. It is also used abstractly, as in "Democratic ideals provide a bulwark against despotism."

7. D: The adjective clandestine means secretive or in secret. The Latin source word clandestinus derived from clam, meaning secretly. Secret, and synonyms like covert, furtive, undercover, stealthy, surreptitious, etc., represent the only meaning of this word.

8. A: Choleric means easily provoked. Synonyms include hot-tempered, irate, irritable, angry, etc. In ancient Greek civilization, Hippocrates and other physicians subscribed to the theory that the body contained four essential substances they called humors: blood, phlegm (mucus), yellow bile, and black bile, which should be balanced. The physician Galen named four temperaments resulting from unbalanced dominance of one humor: sanguine with blood, phlegmatic with mucus, melancholic with yellow bile, and choleric with black bile. This is the origin of the word and its meaning.

9. A: A caucus is a group with political aims. For example, the National Women's Political Caucus, the National Black Caucus, the National Caucus of Environmental Legislators, the Tea Party Caucus, etc. The origin of this word is unknown. It can mean a closed group meeting of members of a political party or faction to make policy decisions or choose candidates, or a group promoting a cause. There are no other meanings.

10. B: Conjecture means guessing or speculation. Synonyms include supposition, inference, and surmise. The Latin conjectura is the past participle of the verb conicere, meaning literally to throw together. The English word is a noun. It has no alternate meanings.

11. A: The closest choice is "to convey." Disseminate means to spread or distribute, or to disperse throughout, as is done when sowing seeds. Indeed, the Latin root of this word is semen, which means "seed" in English and is the English biological term for male spermatic fluid, i.e., human or animal "seed."

12. B: To dwindle means "to decrease," usually steadily. It can be a transitive or intransitive verb, e.g., to make less or to become less. It is thought to originate from the Old English verb dwinan, to waste away, probably derived from the Old Norse words dvina, to pine away, and/or deyja, to die. This word has no alternate definitions.

13. D: To bubble up is a synonym for "to effervesce." The related adjective is effervescent, meaning bubbly—literally as in bubbly liquids, or figuratively, as in bubbly personalities. The origin is the Latin verb fervere, meaning "to boil." The formatives ex- meaning out, and fervescere, meaning to begin to boil, combined to produce effervescere, meaning to effervesce or boil out, as when steam escapes.

14. D: Evince means "to make manifest or demonstrate." Other synonyms include: to show, display, or reveal. The Latin verb vincere means to conquer (e.g., Julius Caesar's "Veni, vidi, vici" meaning "I came, I saw, I conquered"). Derived from this is evincere, to vanquish or win a point.

15. C: Disentangle is the best choice as a synonym for extricate. It means to remove from entanglement, or to differentiate from something related. Its roots are the Latin ex-, meaning out, and tricae, meaning trifles or perplexities. These combine to form the verb extricare, whose past participle is extricatus.

16. C: A filibuster is an attempt to disrupt legislation. In United States government, it commonly takes the form of engaging in a lengthy speech on the floor of the Senate, House of Representatives, state legislature, and so on, to delay or prevent voting to pass a law or similar actions. This word's origin, the Spanish filibustero, meaning freebooter, is also the source of its other meaning: an irregular military adventurer, specifically an American inciting rebellion in 1850s Latin America. These are the only two definitions.

17. A: Fortitude refers to strength of mind or of character that enables someone to have courage in the face of adversity. Its root is the same as the words "fort" and "fortify." Fort means strong in French. All these come from the Latin fortis, also meaning strong. (In Shakespeare's play Hamlet, the name of the supporting character Fortinbras transliterates to "strong in arm" in English.) If you chose "endurance" as the answer, this is understandable, as one can "endure" hardship; however, endurance refers more to lasting a long time, wearing well, etc., related to durable and duration, from Latin durare, to harden or last, from durus, or hard, rather than referring to strength. The original meaning of fortitude was simply strength, now considered obsolete, superseded by the current definition of non-physical strength.

18. B: Genteel means refined and comes from the French gentil, meaning gentle, as in gentilhomme, for gentleman. It can mean aristocratic, polite, elegant, or related to the gentry or upper class. Other meanings are connected with appearing or trying to appear socially superior or respectable; being falsely delicate, prudish, or affected; or being conventionally and/or ineffectually pretty, as in artistic style.

19. D: A tirade is the nearest synonym to a harangue. A harangue can simply mean a speech addressing a public assembly. It can also mean a lecture. A third meaning, most commonly used in contemporary English, is a spoken or written rant. While a monologue is also delivered by one person, it does not include the ranting connotations of harangue and tirade. Diatribe and philippic are other synonyms.

20. C: Immutable means unchangeable. The Latin verb mutare means to change. Its past participle is mutates, the root of the English verb "mutate" and noun "mutation," as used in biology when genes or viruses mutate, or change in form or characteristics.

21. A: Jaundice is a yellowing condition. The French adjective jaune means yellow. The Latin root for the French and English words is galbinus, or greenish-yellow. When people or animals develop jaundice, their skin and the whites of their eyes turn yellowish. Jaundice is usually due to liver damage or dysfunction; the yellow color comes from a buildup of bile. This word is also used figuratively to mean a feeling of distaste, hostility, or being fed up, as in "a jaundiced attitude" or "a jaundiced view" of something or someone.

22. D: Deceitfulness is closest to knavery in meaning. In the Middle Ages, a roguish, rascally, mischievous, or tricky, deceitful fellow was called a knave. The Jack in a deck of playing cards was also formerly called the Knave. This Middle English word derived from the Old English cnafa.

23. C: The closest choice to languor is depression. Languor means listlessness, apathy, inertia, slowness, sluggishness, or weakness/weariness of the body or mind. The related adjective is "languid." The root is Latin.

24. A: Macadamize means "to pave." The related word "macadam" refers to paving material. It originates from the name of John L. McAdam, a nineteenth-century Scottish engineer who turned road construction into a science and invented the process of macadamization. Over time, macadamize and macadam have evolved to refer to a variety of processes and materials for building roads.

25. B: Necrosis refers to tissue death. It shares roots with words like necropsy, necrophilia, and so on. The original root is the Greek nekros, meaning dead body. The "necro-" root is used in medical terminology and refers to death.

26. A: Preclude is the only synonym for obviate among these choices. To obviate means to prevent, avert, or forestall; or to render unnecessary. Both meanings incorporate the element of anticipating something in advance. The root is the Latin verb obviare, which meant to meet or withstand; the past participle is obviatus.

27. C: Presaged means foretold. You may recognize the Latin prefix pre-, meaning before. The Latin root word sagus means prophetic, which is also the root of the English word "seek." Presage can be a verb or a noun.

28. D: Quarantine means isolation. Quadraginta is the original Latin root. Quarantine developed from the Latinate languages French, whose quarante means forty, and Italian, with its cognate quaranta. It was a custom in the seventeenth century to isolate ships for 40 days to prevent diseases and pests from spreading. In fact, another definition of quarantine is a 40-day period.

29. C: To remunerate means to pay for something, as in remunerating someone's services or paying someone. Synonyms include to pay, to compensate, or to recompense. In Latin, munus means gift. The verb for this noun is munerare, to give. Combined with re- for back, remunerare is to give back, and its past participle is remuneratus, the root of remunerate.

30. B: To scintillate is to emit light—literally, to sparkle. The Latin noun scintilla means spark. This word is also in the English vocabulary. The Latin verb "to sparkle" is scintillare; its past participle is scintillatus, the English word's root. The adjective "scintillating" is commonly used figuratively to describe a sparkling personality, conversation, or witticism.

Mathematics Review

1. A: The correct remainder is 849.15. When subtracting numbers with a decimal point, you borrow the same way as you do when there is no decimal. Thus, the first digits to the left of the decimal are 7 – 8; you borrow 1 from the 9 to the left of the 7, making the 7 into 17. 17 – 8 = 9. The borrowed-from 9 becomes an 8; 8 – 4 = 4.

2. D: The correct remainder is 507.64. When subtracting larger digits from smaller ones, you must borrow from the next digit to the left, adding a 1 to the smaller digit. In the decimal system, the borrowed 1 adds a unit of 10 to the digit to make it >10—big enough to subtract any digit from 1 to 9 in the subtrahend from it. Hence the rightmost 3 in the minuend borrows 1 from the 3 to its left, making it 13. 13 – 9 = 4. The borrowed-from 3 becomes 2. You borrow 1 from the 3 to the left; 12 – 6 = 6; etc. Borrowing continues across the decimal point in numbers with decimals.

3. D: The correct sum is 976.19. When adding numbers with decimal points, you add them the same way as numbers with no decimal. Thus, adding the 7 + 4 to the right of the decimal point, the sum is 11; you write 1 and then carry the other 1 to the left of the decimal point. So, 3 + 2 + carried 1 = 6. Two places left of the decimal, 8 + 9 = 17; write 7 and carry the 1; so, 8 + carried 1 = 9.

4. A: The correct sum is 1076.68. When adding numbers with a decimal point in any place in which the sum is >10, you write down the right-hand digit and carry the left-hand digit over to the next place to the left. Thus, when adding the 7 two places to the left of the decimal in 973.37 with the 9 in 94.31, 7 + 9 = 16, so you write down a 6 and carry the 1 to the next place, where 9 + 1 = 10.

5. C: This word problem requires an average. You add $3.47 + $9.50 + $2.50. This equals $15.47. Since there were three amounts, you then divide $15.47 by 3, and the result is $5.1567. When working with amounts of money, you round off anything beyond two digits to the right of the decimal to get a usable number of cents. If the third digit to the right is 1 through 4, you ignore it and leave the second digit as is. If the third digit is 5 or more, you round the second digit up, as in this case; so, $5.1567 becomes $5.16.

6. C: The correct product is 2926.21. When multiplying numbers with multiple digits, you first multiply every digit in the multiplicand respectively by the rightmost digit in the multiplier; then by the multiplier's second digit to the left, then by the third, and so on. You write each product below and one place to the left of the previous product, and add all products together. First, multiply 89.35 by the 5 in 32.75, getting 446.75. Then multiply 89.35 by the 7 in 32.75, getting 625.45, which you write below and one place to the left of 446.75. 89.35 x 2 = 178.70, written below and one place to the left of 625.45. 89.35 x 3 = 268.05, written below and one place to the left of 178.70.

Temporarily removing the decimal points may make it easier to add the staggered columns, replacing the point in the final summed product:

$$
\begin{array}{r}
8935 \\
\times \quad 3275 \\
\hline
44675 \\
62545 \\
17870 \\
28605 \\
\hline
29262125
\end{array}
$$

After multiplying two numbers with two decimal places each, 2 x 2 = 4, so place the decimal point 4 places from the end, = 2926.2125. Discard the final 25 = 2926.21.

7. B: In this equation, the unknown quantity is (x). (y) = 2. In the equation, substitute 2 for y: 3x – 4*2 = 25. 4y, or 4*2 = 8. So 3x – 8 = 25. If 25 is the remainder of 3x – 8, add 8 back to 25: 25 + 8 = 33. This means that 3x = 33. 33 ÷ 3 = 11. Therefore, x = 11.

8. B: In this equation, (x) = 7 and (y) is unknown. 3x = 3*7 = 21. Therefore, 5y – 21 = 24. It follows that if 5y – 21 = 24, then 24 + 21 = 5y. 24 + 21 = 45, so 45 = 5y. 45 / 5 = 9, so (y) = 9.

9. D: To determine the tax, you must calculate 5% of $340.32. 5% = .05. So, you multiply $340.32 by .05, getting $17.0160. When multiplying two numbers, each with two decimal places, you also multiply the decimal places, so the product has four places right of the point. Since you want cents here, you eliminate the final (rightmost) zero; the digit 6 rounds up the 1 left of it to a 2, and is then discarded, yielding a final product of $17.02.

10. C: First, multiply the two multiples, (3)(12). 3*12 = 36. Then add 894 + 36. The sum is 930. Whenever two or more figures are in parentheses as they are here, this means the operation (in this case, multiplication) with these figures is performed first. The operation outside of the parentheses (in this case, addition) is performed afterward on the result of the first operation.

11. B: With 892 ÷ 15, you get 59.4666, and so on (you will get an endless recurrence of 6 in the last place if you continue to divide). The convention with digits > 5 is to round up to the next higher number. Since this problem specifies to the nearest two decimal places, you round .46 up to .47.

12. A: 999.52 ÷ 13 yields 76.886 (with many more digits continuing to the right before getting to an even quotient with nothing left over to be divided further). The convention is to round up digits > 5. So rounding to the nearest two decimal places, 76.88 is rounded up to 76.89 because the third digit was a 6.

13. B: 9.42 ÷ 3.47 gives a quotient of 2.714697 followed by many more digits before reaching an even division. Since the third decimal place has a 4, you do not round the second decimal place up because only half of 10 or more, i.e., > 5, will round up the next decimal place. Since 4 < 5, the 1 is left as is, yielding 2.71.

14. B: To get the average, divide the 8.32 pounds of food by the 3 days. 8.32/3 = 2.773333..... Since you will keep getting a 3 by continuing to divide, and 3 < 5, you do not round up the previous decimal places. Rounding off to two decimal places, the average = 2.77 pounds.

15. C: The correct version is .0947. An even 9% = .09 because percentages are per 100; the first decimal place equals tenths, the second equals hundreds, and so on. When we use the % sign, we eliminate the decimal point and any leading zeros as redundant. We write either .09 or 9%. So, since 9% already equals 9/100 or .09, in the figure 9.47, the .47 represents 47 hundredths of a percent. 9% does not equal the whole number 9; it equals 9/100. Decimal points are not repeated within one number. Instead, each successive decimal place equals another tenth (tens, hundreds, thousands, ten-thousands, hundred-thousands, millions, et cetera) Therefore, 9-and-47-hundredths percent = .0947.

16. B: .10 equals 1/10. In the decimal system, whole numbers are left of the decimal point. One decimal place (to the right of the point) = tenths; two places = hundredths; three places = thousandths, and so on. 1/100 would be .010; 1/50 would be .02; and 1/5 would be .20.

17. A: To obtain the area of a rectangle, multiply the two lengths of the sides:
$$34 \text{ m} \times 12 \text{ m} = 408 \text{ m}^2$$

18. C: The standard ratio given is 3.5 treatments : 2 milliliters. To find out how many milliliters are in one dose, 2 ÷ 3.5 = 0.57 of a milliliter. If only two doses are given, multiply 0.57 ml * 2 = 1.14 total milliliters given.

19. C: An obtuse triangle has one angle >90°. An acute triangle has all angles <90°. With a 4" side and a 5" side, the third side must be either >5" or <4" for it to be an obtuse triangle. 1" is too short: the sides could not meet unless they were parallel, that is, a 180° angle. 9" is too long to connect with 4" and 5" sides; at the widest possible angle, the 4" side would still be too short to meet the others. 4.6" is in between 4" and 5", so this makes an acute angle; therefore, the triangle would be acute, not obtuse. 6.4" is longer than the 5" side (the longer of the two sides given), so the angle is >90° and is therefore obtuse.

20. A: This problem illustrates the property of zero and the identity property. Any number + 0 = the same number, so 75 + 0 = 75. Any number multiplied by zero = 0, so (75)(0) = 0. Therefore x = 75 and y = 0; 75 > 0, so x > y.

21. C: If x = 3, then x2 = 9. To square a number, multiply it by itself. If x = 3 and x2 = 9, then x2 + x = 9 + 3 = 12.

22. B: If a = 4, then a2 = 16. The square of a number is that number multiplied by itself. You always perform the operation in parentheses first. So a2 + b = 16 + 5 = 21. Multiply 21 by 4 (the value of a). 21 * 4 = 84.

23. C: When adding and subtracting fractions, first you must find a common denominator. In this problem, there are fourths, halves, and thirds. Three does not divide evenly into 8, and 4 does not divide evenly into 6. But 4 * 3 = 12, and 12 is evenly divisible by 2, so use 12ths. Divide each denominator into 12, then multiply that quotient by each numerator: 1/4 = 3/12; 1/2 = 6/12; and 2/3 = 8/12. To solve this problem, respectively add and subtract the numerators: 3/12 + 6/12 = 9/12; 9/12 – 8/12 = 1/12, so the answer is 1/12.

24. B: To get a common denominator for /2, /3, and /8, multiply /8 * /3 = /24. Then 1/2 = 12/24; 1/3 = 8/24, and 3/8 = 9/24. The first operation is the one in parentheses. If y = 8/24 and z = 9/24, y – z = 8/24 – 9/24. 8 – 9 yields a negative number, -1, or -1/24. If x = 12/24, then x * -1/24 = 12 * -1 in the numerator, or -12, and 24 * 24 in the denominator, or 576, giving -12/576. To reduce this fraction to the lowest possible numerator and denominator, divide each by 12. So, -12/576 = -1/48.

25. D: To compare these two quantities, you need a common denominator. Multiply the first denominator, the 3 in 2/3, times the second denominator, the 4 in 1/4. 3 * 4 = 12. Divide the first original denominator into the common denominator, i.e., 12 ÷ 3 = 4, and multiply 4 * 2, the first numerator. 4 * 2 = 8. So, 2/3 = 8/12. Do the same with the second fraction: 1/4 = 3/12. So, if you have 3/12 cup of oil and you need a total of 8/12 cup, you need 5/12 cup more.

26. B: The common denominator for /4 and /2 = 4 * 2, or 8. Divide each fraction's denominator into the common denominator and multiply that quotient by each fraction's numerator. So, 3/4 = 6/8, and 1/2 = 4/8. 6/8 + 4/8 = 10/8. 8 divides into 10 once, so 8/8 = 1 with 2/8 left over, making 1 and 2/8 or, reduced, 1¼. Add the whole numbers: 8 + 6 = 14. Then 14 + 1¼ = 15¼.

27. D: If the first 10 minutes of the call cost $3.50 and the total charge was $3.85, just subtract $3.50 from $3.85 and you get $.35. Each additional minute cost $.35. So, the call was 10 minutes plus 1 additional minute, for a total of 11 minutes.

28. A: If ½ cup of skim milk has 45 calories, then 1 cup has 90 calories (45 * 2 = 90, or 45 + 45 = 90). So ¼ cup is 90 calories ÷ 4 = 22.5 calories. For ¾, multiply 22.5 calories times 3 = 67.5 calories, that is, 67½. Another way to solve this is: ¼ = 25% or .25, so ¾ = 75% or .75. Multiply 90 * .75 = 67.5.

29. D: If a = 3, then 5a = 5 * 3 = 15. If 5a = 15, then 5a – 15 = 15 – 15 = 0. Because any number multiplied by 0 = 0, if 10b = 0, then b must also = 0.

30. C: Always perform the operations within the parentheses first before performing the operation between the parenthetical values. In this problem, 5 * 4 = 20 and 2 * 2 = 4. So, 20 ÷ 4 = 5.

31. D: A prime number is any natural number that can only be divided evenly by 1 or by itself and not by any other numbers. For example, 2, 3, 5, 7, 11, 13, 17, and 19 are the first eight prime numbers in ascending order. Therefore, out of the choices given, 11 is the only prime number. 12 can be evenly divided by 2, 3, 4, and 6; 4 is evenly divisible by 2; and 15 is evenly divisible by 3 and 5. Furthermore, they are all evenly divisible by 1 and by themselves, so they are not prime numbers.

32. B: From the total of 23 club members, subtract the 12 females. 23 – 12 = 11, so there are 11 male members. To get the percentage of males, 11 ÷ 23 =0.478, which rounds up to 0.48, or 48%. You can always get a percentage by dividing the smaller number by the larger number.

Copyright © Mometrix Media. You have been licensed one copy of this document for personal use only. Any other reproduction or redistribution is strictly prohibited. All rights reserved.

33. A: To obtain the percentage, divide the smaller number by the larger number. So, 14 ÷ 57 = 0.245, which rounds up to 0.25, or 25%. (Always round up when the next decimal place > 5.)

34. B: One simple way to figure this out is: 60% = 6/10. So, if 75 = 6/10, find out how much 1/10 is: 75 ÷ 6 = 12.5. So, 12.5 = 1/10 of the unknown number. To get that number, just multiply the 1/10 by 10: 12.5 * 10 = 125. With decimal numbers, you simply move the decimal point one place to the right instead, which is the same as multiplying by 10.

35. A: If the student receives $400.00 over 4 years, the average amount is $100.00 per year. ($400 ÷ 4 = $100.) Percentages can be calculated by dividing the smaller number by the bigger number. So, to find out what percent $100.00 is of $3,000.00: 100 ÷ 3,000 = 0.033, or 3.3%, which is the average annual interest rate.

36. B: Adding up the number of church-goers in Ellsford results in about 1450 residents who attend a church in the town each week. There are approximately 400 people in Ellsford who attend a Catholic church each week. This number represents about 28% of the 1450 church-goers in the town.

37. D: Begin by subtracting 4 from both sides:

$$2x + 4 - 4 = x - 6 - 4$$
$$2x = x - 10$$

Then, subtract x from both sides:

$$2x - x = x - 10 - x$$

You are left with:

$$x = -10$$

38. C: The volume of a cylinder may be calculated using the formula $V=\pi r^2 h$, where r represents the radius and h represents the height. Substituting 1.5 for r and 3 for h gives $V=\pi(1.5)^2 (3)$, which simplifies to $V \approx 21.2$.

39. A: The expression "Four more than a number, x" can be interpreted as x+4. This is equal to "2 less than 1/3 of another number, y," or 1/3 y-2. Thus, the equation is x+4=1/3 y-2.

40. A: This equation is a linear relationship that has a slope of 3.60 and passes through the origin. The table shows that for each hour of rental, the cost increases by $3.60. This matches with the slope of the equation. Of course, if the bicycle is not rented at all (0 hours), there will be no charge ($0). If plotted on the Cartesian plane, the line would have a y intercept of 0. Choice A is the only one that follows these requirements.

Science Review

1. C: The heart's four chambers are the left and right atria, and the left and right ventricles. The left atrium and right atrium each hold blood returning to the heart via blood vessels, and each empties into the corresponding left or right ventricle at the right time. The ventricles are muscular and pump blood out of the heart. The right ventricle pumps blood to the lungs, and the left ventricle pumps blood to all the other organs.

2. A: Blood leaves the heart's right ventricle and goes to the lungs. The kidneys and the rest of the body receive blood from the left ventricle. The right atrium, as well as the left atrium, holds blood coming to the heart via the blood vessels; each atrium empties into the corresponding ventricle.

3. D: Anaerobic cellular metabolism refers to processes of breaking things down and converting them to other substances (metabolites) in the body's cells. Anaerobic means these processes do not use or require oxygen. Metabolic processes not involving oxygen do not affect heart rate. Increases in body temperature and physical activity increase the heart rate as the heart works harder to pump blood-supplying oxygen to the body. The concentrations of calcium, sodium, and potassium ions do affect heart rate. These ions, known as electrolytes, must stay in balance to regulate heart rate. If they are balanced, heart function is not affected, but with imbalance, cardiac function will be elevated (excess calcium) or depressed (excess potassium or sodium). Sodium deficiency causes cardiac fibrillation.

4. D: The three layers of the heart are the epicardium (outermost), myocardium (middle), and endocardium (innermost). "Vasocardium" is not a layer of the heart or even a legitimate term. The adjectives "vasocardial" or "vasocardiac" are used to refer to anything related to both blood vessels (vaso-) and heart (cardiac), as with the "vasocardial system." A related term with the order of parts reversed is "cardiovascular system."

5. C: The hormone aldosterone is secreted by the adrenal glands and regulates the levels of sodium and potassium ions (electrolytes). Aldosterone stimulates excretion of potassium and reabsorption of sodium into the bloodstream. It maintains blood pressure and body fluids. Too much aldosterone can increase the blood volume and hence the blood pressure. Estrogen is a hormone of the female reproductive system and testosterone is a hormone of the male reproductive system. Dopamine is a neurotransmitter associated with the brain's pleasure and reward circuits, and also with the regulation of motor control.

6. B: Bradycardia means a slower heartbeat than normal. The combining form brady- is from the Greek bradys meaning slow. Tachycardia means a faster heartbeat than normal. (Tachy- from Greek tachos means speed, as also in "tachometer.") Fibrillation means uncoordinated, ineffectual heart movements. A myocardial infarct is a type of heart attack.

7. A: Hematocrit is the red blood cell portion of the blood. Plasma is mainly water, plus some plasma proteins, blood glucose, and so on. Normal levels of hematocrit are around 36% to 45% for women, and about 40% to 50% for men. Thus, an approximate normal level is around 45%. A hematocrit >50% can cause blood clots and heart attacks with exertion. If a hematocrit is 45%, it follows that the remaining plasma portion of the blood would be 55%.

8. B: The slightly bigger right lung has three lobes: the superior lobe, middle lobe, and inferior lobe. The left lung has two lobes: the superior lobe and the inferior lobe. So, 3, 2 is the correct answer.

9. C: The aerobic respiration process has four steps. The first step, glycolysis, occurs in the cytoplasm. The second through fourth steps (the formation of acetyl coenzyme A, the citric acid cycle, and the electric transport chain and chemosmosis) occur in the mitochondria. Mitochondria are the cells' power producers. They create energy for cellular functions and processes, such as aerobic respiration, which involves the oxidation of glucose molecules.

10. B: Atelectasis is the medical term for collapse of a lung. Its Greek roots are ateles, incomplete or defective, and ektasis, extension or stretching out, as a collapsed lung cannot inflate and expand properly. Anoxia literally means no oxygen. It commonly refers to a lack of oxygen to the brain, especially in a fetus before or during childbirth. Dyspnea means difficulty breathing. Hypercapnia means too much carbon dioxide (a waste product of aerobic respiration) in the blood.

11. A: The central nervous system is another term for the brain and the spinal cord. It does not include the peripheral nerves (peripheral is the opposite of central) or the muscular system. Choices omitting the brain are necessarily incorrect.

12. C: The brain is composed of four lobes: the frontal lobe, the parietal lobe in the midbrain, the temporal lobe at the bottom, and the occipital lobe at the back. Some people also refer specifically to the left and right of each lobe. This is because the brain has two hemispheres (left and right), so each lobe also has two hemispheres. Each lobe has different functions.

13. C: Homeostasis is a state of equilibrium, or balance, within the body. The natural tendency is to maintain or restore homeostasis. Peristalsis is the wavelike muscular contractions of the digestive system to process food. Stomatitis is an inflammation of the mouth's mucosa.

14. D: Stomatitis is a state of oral inflammation, usually caused by viral or bacterial infection. Diverticulitis is inflammation of a diverticulum, or an abnormal pouch, in the wall of the large intestine. Hepatitis is inflammation of the liver. Enteritis is inflammation of the small intestine.

15. D: The most important male hormone is testosterone. Estrogen is the most important female hormone. Aldosterone is a hormone that regulates blood volume and pressure in both sexes. Progesterone is the second most important female hormone.

16. B: Bile production is a function of the liver, not of the kidneys. The kidneys filter the blood to clean it, removing waste products like urea and ammonium, excreting them in urine. They secrete hormones such as renin, calcitriol, and erythropoietin. The kidneys also reabsorb water, glucose, and amino acids.

17. A: Enuresis is the medical term for uncontrolled urination. A diuretic is an agent (a drug or substance) that stimulates urination. (Diuretics are not the same as enuresis but can cause it.) Pyuria means pus in the urine. Ureteritis means an inflammation of the ureter(s), muscular tubes that send urine from the kidneys into the bladder.

18. C: Auditory impulses, meaning sounds received through the ears, are interpreted in the brain's temporal lobes. Acoustic impulses travel through the external ear canal, are amplified and transmitted by the middle ear mechanism, converted into electrical energy in the inner ear's cochlea, and sent via the auditory nerve to the primary auditory cortex in the temporal lobe for analysis.

19. B: The eye's outer layer is the sclera, or the white of the eye. The cornea is the clear, protuberant, main refractive surface at the eye's front. The retina is a layered sensory tissue lining the eye's inner surface that is sensitive to light that creates images of what the eye sees. The retina contains two kinds of photoreceptors: rods and cones. Cones are responsible for color vision and high visual acuity. Rods are responsible for peripheral vision, night vision/low-light vision, and detecting motion.

20. C: The inner layer of the eye is the retina. The cornea is the main refractive surface on the front of the eye. The sclera is the outermost layer, or white of the eye. The rods are one of two kinds of photoreceptors found within the retina. (The other photoreceptors are cones.)

21. D: Halogens are nonmetallic chemical elements. There are five halogens: fluorine, chlorine, bromine, iodine, and astatine. At room temperature, iodine and astatine are solids, bromine is a liquid, and fluorine and chlorine are gases. Cesium is not a halogen; it is a metal element.

22. A: In the periodic table of the chemical elements, the numbers of the periods 1, 2, 3, and so forth, are listed vertically in a column on the left, and each period runs horizontally across the table. The groups 1, 2, 3, et cetera, are listed horizontally, and each group runs vertically down the table.

23. A: The simplest unit of an element is an atom, i.e. the smallest particle to which it can be broken down. A molecule contains at least two atoms bonded together chemically (covalent bonding). Electrons, along with protons and neutrons, are particles found within the nucleus of an atom.

24. B: Isomers are compounds with the same shapes even if their structures vary. Polar compounds are molecules with polar covalent bonds; electromagnetically, their electrons are not equally shared in chemical bonds. Variables in the sciences are any entities or factors that can change. Experimenters manipulate variables to determine their effects on other variables. In research, a variable can be a logical set of attributes. A transient compound is one that disappears rapidly in the body.

25. C: Condensation is the process whereby gas is converted to liquid. For example, when water vapor (a gas) in the air is cooled, it becomes liquid. This is how condensation forms on the outside of a glass containing cold liquid. Evaporation is the opposite: the process of a liquid becoming a gas, as when water evaporates into the air. Sublimation is the process of a solid becoming a gas, as with dry ice.

26. B: Charles' Law is also known as the law of volumes. It describes how gases expand when heated. Boyle's law states that for a given mass at a constant temperature, the product of pressure times volume is a constant. Johnson's Law, attributed to California Senator Hiram Johnson (1918), states that "the first casualty when war comes is truth." Dr. Samuel Johnson (1730) had stated the same principle in much wordier terms. Avogadro's Law states that when a gas is at a constant temperature and pressure, its volume is in direct proportion to the number of moles of gas. These are all gas laws except Johnson's.

27. A: The First Law of Thermodynamics states that neither matter nor energy can be created or destroyed. They can only be converted from one form to the other. Therefore, matter and energy are always conserved. The Second Law of Thermodynamics is the law of entropy: Energy moves away from its source, which means energy, or heat, cannot flow from a colder to a hotter body. The Third Law of Thermodynamics states that all energy processes cease as temperature approaches absolute zero. There is a "Zeroth" Law of Thermodynamics (if each of two systems is in equilibrium with a third system, the first two are in equilibrium with each other), but there is no "Fourth Law of Thermodynamics."

28. C: Acids increase the number of hydrogen ions in water. The pH scale measures how acidic or basic a liquid is. Hydrogen ions and hydroxide ions are the focus of pH. The strongest acids have low pH values: 0–4. High pH values (10–14) are found in the strongest bases or alkali, the opposites of acids. Sodium hydroxide is a base or alkaline compound. When dissolved in water, acids break down to hydrogen (H+) ions and another compound, while bases break down to hydroxide (OH-) ions and another compound.

29. D: A catalyst is a substance that increases the rate of a reaction. A reaction will not occur without the minimum activation energy it needs. A catalyst can provide an alternative means for the reaction to occur that requires a lower level of activation energy, so in this sense, a catalyst can also initiate a reaction. Another property of catalysts is that they do not change chemically after a reaction has completed, so they are never destroyed. Catalysts are not always on the right of the equation. For example, a car's catalytic converter takes harmful carbon monoxide and nitrogen oxide molecules and converts them, using platinum, palladium, and rhodium, to more harmless carbon dioxide and nitrogen molecules:

$2CO + 2NO$ Pt/Pd/Rh $\rightarrow 2CO_2 + N_2$

The catalysts platinum (Pt), palladium (Pd), and rhodium (Rh) are in the middle of the equation.

30. A: Newton's Second Law of Motion states that when all existing forces are not balanced, the acceleration of an object depends on the net force acting on the object and the object's mass. When net force is represented as Fnet and mass as m, and acceleration as a, net force is the product of mass times acceleration, or F net = ma (or m * a). Speed = Distance/Time is the equation of the basic formula for calculating velocity. Power = F * D/T is the basic equation for work done, that is, force times distance divided by time. The formula of voltage times amperes is for calculating watts, or units of power, in the measurement of electrical energy.

31. C: According to the principles of the scientific method, it is imperative that the hypothesis be established prior to the experiment as that is what the experiment should be testing. If the results do not support the hypothesis, that is acceptable, and often very informative. Once the experiment is complete, use the information gained to develop a new hypothesis to test.

32. D: The two types of measurement important in science are quantitative (when a numerical result is used) and qualitative (when descriptions or qualities are reported).

33. C: The chart shows two specific changes: snowfall levels from November to April and sunny days from November to April. Based on the chart alone, the only information that can be determined is that the fewest sunny days coincide with the months that have the heaviest snowfall. Anything further reaches beyond the immediate facts of the chart and moves into the territory of requiring other facts. As for answer choice D, it uses the word "relationship," which is not required in the question. The question only asks for what can be concluded.

34. D: The epiglottis covers the trachea during swallowing, thus preventing food from entering the airway. The trachea, also known as the windpipe, is a cylindrical portion of the respiratory tract that joins the larynx with the lungs. The esophagus connects the throat and the stomach. When a person swallows, the esophagus contracts to force the food down into the stomach. Like other structures in the respiratory system, the esophagus secretes mucus for lubrication.

35. B: The pads that support the vertebrae are made up of cartilage. Cartilage, a strong form of connective tissue, cushions and supports the joints. Cartilage also makes up the larynx and the outer ear. Bone is a form of connective tissue that comprises the better part of the skeleton. It includes both organic and inorganic substances. Tendons connect the muscles to other structures of the body, typically bones. Tendons can increase and decrease in length as the bones move. Fat is a combination of lipids; in humans, fat forms a layer beneath the skin and on the outside of the internal organs.

36. C: Cell layers and cell shape are the criteria for classifying epithelial tissue.

37. C: Cells come after tissues and are followed by molecules and then atoms at the very bottom of the hierarchy. Muscles are types of tissues, so muscles do not have a separate place in the hierarchy but instead fall within the types of tissues.

38. B: To determine the average number of neutrons in one atom of an element, subtract the atomic number from the average atomic mass. For Bromine (Br), subtract its atomic number (35) from its average atomic mass (79.9) to acquire the average number of neutrons, 44.9.

39. A: The number of protons is the same for every atom of a given element and is the element's atomic number: in this case, 30 for Zinc (Zn).

40. B: The conclusion was that the amount of sunlight received by the plants was affecting their growth. The independent variable was the amount of light that was given to the plants and could have been manipulated by the experimenter by moving the plants or adding equal parts of light. No control was used in this experiment.

41. B: The substance thymine cannot exist in RNA.

42. B: Each gene must match to a protein for a genetic trait to develop correctly.

43. D: Solids with a fixed shape have a crystalline order that defines and maintains that shape.

44. B: The endoplasmic reticulum is the cell's transport network that moves proteins from one part of the cell to another. The Golgi apparatus assists in the transport but is not the actual transport network. Mitochondria are organelles ("tiny organs") that help in the production of ATP, which the cells need to operate properly. The nucleolus participates in the production of ribosomes that are needed to generate proteins for the cell.

45. A: The chromosomes separate during anaphase and move to the opposite ends of the cells.

46. A: The physical expression—such as hair color—is the result of the phenotype. The genotype is the basic genetic code.

47. C: The number of 7 is the "breaking point" between basic and acidic. Above 7 solutions are considered basic; below 7 solutions are considered acidic. For instance, milk, with a pH of 6.5, is actually considered acidic. Bleach, with a pH of 12.5, is considered basic.

48. B: All of the answers use the System of International Units (SI) of measurement with the exception of gallons. A liter is the measurement of a liquid. Grams are a unit of measurement for the weight of an object, which would be measured on the triple beam balance. Meters measure length.

49. B: The transverse plane separates the body into equal upper and lower portions. The oblique plane is when a cylindrical organ is sectioned with an angular cut across the organ. The midsagittal or medial plane refers to a lengthwise cut that divides the body into equal right and left portions. The frontal or coronal plane refers to a cut that divides the body into anterior and posterior sections.

50. C: RNA has several roles, one of which is to act as the messenger and deliver information about the correct sequence of proteins in DNA. The ribosomes do the actual manufacturing of the proteins. Hydrogen, oxygen, and nitrogen work to create the bonds within DNA. And far from having a double helix shape, RNA has what would be considered a more two-dimensional shape.

51. B: Catalysts alter the activation energy during a chemical reaction and therefore control the rate of the reaction. The substrate is the actual surface that enzymes use during a chemical reaction (and there is no such term as substrate energy). Inhibitors and promoters participate in the chemical reaction, but it is the activation energy that catalysts alter to control the overall rate as the reaction occurs.

52. C: Crossing the corresponding alleles from each parent will yield a result of BB in the upper right box of this Punnett square.

53. C: Mitochondria are often called the power house of the cell because they provide energy for the cell to function. The nucleus is the control center for the cell. The cell membrane surrounds the cell and separates the cell from its environment. Cytoplasm is the thick fluid within the cell membrane that surrounds the nucleus and contains organelles.

54. B: Ribosomes are organelles that help synthesize proteins within the cell. Cilia and flagella are responsible for cell movement. The cell membrane helps the cell maintain its shape and protects it from the environment. Lysosomes have digestive enzymes.

55. B: Cells differentiate so that simple, less specialized cells can become highly specialized cells. For example, humans are multicellular organisms who undergo cell differentiation numerous times. Cells begin as simple zygotes after fertilization and then differentiate to form a myriad of complex tissues and systems before birth.

56. C: Both meiosis and mitosis occur in humans, other animals, and plants. Mitosis produces cells that are genetically identical, and meiosis produces cells that are genetically different. Only mitosis occurs asexually.

57. B: A decrease in a natural predator, such as a wolves, coyotes, bobcat, or wild dogs, would allow the population to become out of control. In a population of deer that has increased, there would be a natural decrease in a food source for the nutritional needs for the animals. Although deer have been known to share a human's developed habitat, it is often forced by reduced territory and food sources. An increase in hunting licenses would be used by local officials to try to control the population, helping to decrease the number of adults of breeding age.

58. D: A covalent bond is one in which atoms share valence electrons. Within a water molecule, one oxygen atom and two hydrogen atoms share valence electrons to yield the H2O structure.

59. A: In a closed system (when you ignore outside interactions), the total momentum is constant and conserved. The total energy would also be conserved, although not the sum of the potential and kinetic energy. Some of the energy from the collision would be turned into thermal energy (heat) for example. Nor is the total velocity conserved, even though the velocity is a component of the momentum, since the momentum also depends on the mass of the cars. The impulse is a force over time that causes the momentum of a body to change. It doesn't make sense to think of impulse as conserved, since it's not necessarily constant throughout a collision.

60. B: The speed of a wave is the product of its wavelength and frequency. V = νf. Here, ν = 12 x 3 = 36 m/s.

Image Credits

Licensed Under CC BY 4.0 (CREATIVECOMMONS.ORG/LICENSES/BY/4.0/)

Meiosis: "Meiosis Overview New" by Wikimedia user Rdbickel
(https://commons.wikimedia.org/wiki/File:Meiosis_Overview_new.svg)

Licensed Under CC BY 3.0 (CREATIVECOMMONS.ORG/LICENSES/BY/3.0/)

Biomagnification Mercury: "Mercury Food Chain" by Bretwood Higman
(https://commons.wikimedia.org/wiki/File:MercuryFoodChain.svg)

Energy Flow: "Trophic Web" by Wikimedia user Thompsma
(https://en.wikipedia.org/wiki/File:TrophicWeb.jpg)

Licensed Under CC BY-SA 3.0 (CREATIVECOMMONS.ORG/LICENSES/BY-SA/3.0/DEED.EN)

Secondary Succession: "Secondary Succession" by Wikimedia user Katelyn Murphy
(https://commons.wikimedia.org/wiki/File:Secondary_Succession.png)

How to Overcome Test Anxiety

Just the thought of taking a test is enough to make most people a little nervous. A test is an important event that can have a long-term impact on your future, so it's important to take it seriously and it's natural to feel anxious about performing well. But just because anxiety is normal, that doesn't mean that it's helpful in test taking, or that you should simply accept it as part of your life. Anxiety can have a variety of effects. These effects can be mild, like making you feel slightly nervous, or severe, like blocking your ability to focus or remember even a simple detail.

If you experience test anxiety—whether severe or mild—it's important to know how to beat it. To discover this, first you need to understand what causes test anxiety.

Causes of Test Anxiety

While we often think of anxiety as an uncontrollable emotional state, it can actually be caused by simple, practical things. One of the most common causes of test anxiety is that a person does not feel adequately prepared for their test. This feeling can be the result of many different issues such as poor study habits or lack of organization, but the most common culprit is time management. Starting to study too late, failing to organize your study time to cover all of the material, or being distracted while you study will mean that you're not well prepared for the test. This may lead to cramming the night before, which will cause you to be physically and mentally exhausted for the test. Poor time management also contributes to feelings of stress, fear, and hopelessness as you realize you are not well prepared but don't know what to do about it.

Other times, test anxiety is not related to your preparation for the test but comes from unresolved fear. This may be a past failure on a test, or poor performance on tests in general. It may come from comparing yourself to others who seem to be performing better or from the stress of living up to expectations. Anxiety may be driven by fears of the future—how failure on this test would affect your educational and career goals. These fears are often completely irrational, but they can still negatively impact your test performance.

> **Review Video: 3 Reasons You Have Test Anxiety**
> Visit mometrix.com/academy and enter code: 428468

276

Elements of Test Anxiety

As mentioned earlier, test anxiety is considered to be an emotional state, but it has physical and mental components as well. Sometimes you may not even realize that you are suffering from test anxiety until you notice the physical symptoms. These can include trembling hands, rapid heartbeat, sweating, nausea, and tense muscles. Extreme anxiety may lead to fainting or vomiting. Obviously, any of these symptoms can have a negative impact on testing. It is important to recognize them as soon as they begin to occur so that you can address the problem before it damages your performance.

> **Review Video: 3 Ways to Tell You Have Test Anxiety**
> Visit mometrix.com/academy and enter code: 927847

The mental components of test anxiety include trouble focusing and inability to remember learned information. During a test, your mind is on high alert, which can help you recall information and stay focused for an extended period of time. However, anxiety interferes with your mind's natural processes, causing you to blank out, even on the questions you know well. The strain of testing during anxiety makes it difficult to stay focused, especially on a test that may take several hours. Extreme anxiety can take a huge mental toll, making it difficult not only to recall test information but even to understand the test questions or pull your thoughts together.

> **Review Video: How Test Anxiety Affects Memory**
> Visit mometrix.com/academy and enter code: 609003

Effects of Test Anxiety

Test anxiety is like a disease—if left untreated, it will get progressively worse. Anxiety leads to poor performance, and this reinforces the feelings of fear and failure, which in turn lead to poor performances on subsequent tests. It can grow from a mild nervousness to a crippling condition. If allowed to progress, test anxiety can have a big impact on your schooling, and consequently on your future.

Test anxiety can spread to other parts of your life. Anxiety on tests can become anxiety in any stressful situation, and blanking on a test can turn into panicking in a job situation. But fortunately, you don't have to let anxiety rule your testing and determine your grades. There are a number of relatively simple steps you can take to move past anxiety and function normally on a test and in the rest of life.

> **Review Video: How Test Anxiety Impacts Your Grades**
> Visit mometrix.com/academy and enter code: 939819

Physical Steps for Beating Test Anxiety

While test anxiety is a serious problem, the good news is that it can be overcome. It doesn't have to control your ability to think and remember information. While it may take time, you can begin taking steps today to beat anxiety.

Just as your first hint that you may be struggling with anxiety comes from the physical symptoms, the first step to treating it is also physical. Rest is crucial for having a clear, strong mind. If you are tired, it is much easier to give in to anxiety. But if you establish good sleep habits, your body and mind will be ready to perform optimally, without the strain of exhaustion. Additionally, sleeping well helps you to retain information better, so you're more likely to recall the answers when you see the test questions.

Getting good sleep means more than going to bed on time. It's important to allow your brain time to relax. Take study breaks from time to time so it doesn't get overworked, and don't study right before bed. Take time to rest your mind before trying to rest your body, or you may find it difficult to fall asleep.

Review Video: The Importance of Sleep for Your Brain
Visit mometrix.com/academy and enter code: 319338

Along with sleep, other aspects of physical health are important in preparing for a test. Good nutrition is vital for good brain function. Sugary foods and drinks may give a burst of energy but this burst is followed by a crash, both physically and emotionally. Instead, fuel your body with protein and vitamin-rich foods.

Also, drink plenty of water. Dehydration can lead to headaches and exhaustion, especially if your brain is already under stress from the rigors of the test. Particularly if your test is a long one, drink water during the breaks. And if possible, take an energy-boosting snack to eat between sections.

Review Video: How Diet Can Affect your Mood
Visit mometrix.com/academy and enter code: 624317

Along with sleep and diet, a third important part of physical health is exercise. Maintaining a steady workout schedule is helpful, but even taking 5-minute study breaks to walk can help get your blood pumping faster and clear your head. Exercise also releases endorphins, which contribute to a positive feeling and can help combat test anxiety.

When you nurture your physical health, you are also contributing to your mental health. If your body is healthy, your mind is much more likely to be healthy as well. So take time to rest, nourish your body with healthy food and water, and get moving as much as possible. Taking these physical steps will make you stronger and more able to take the mental steps necessary to overcome test anxiety.

Review Video: How to Stay Healthy and Prevent Test Anxiety
Visit mometrix.com/academy and enter code: 877894

Mental Steps for Beating Test Anxiety

Working on the mental side of test anxiety can be more challenging, but as with the physical side, there are clear steps you can take to overcome it. As mentioned earlier, test anxiety often stems from lack of preparation, so the obvious solution is to prepare for the test. Effective studying may be the most important weapon you have for beating test anxiety, but you can and should employ several other mental tools to combat fear.

First, boost your confidence by reminding yourself of past success—tests or projects that you aced. If you're putting as much effort into preparing for this test as you did for those, there's no reason you should expect to fail here. Work hard to prepare; then trust your preparation.

Second, surround yourself with encouraging people. It can be helpful to find a study group, but be sure that the people you're around will encourage a positive attitude. If you spend time with others who are anxious or cynical, this will only contribute to your own anxiety. Look for others who are motivated to study hard from a desire to succeed, not from a fear of failure.

Third, reward yourself. A test is physically and mentally tiring, even without anxiety, and it can be helpful to have something to look forward to. Plan an activity following the test, regardless of the outcome, such as going to a movie or getting ice cream.

When you are taking the test, if you find yourself beginning to feel anxious, remind yourself that you know the material. Visualize successfully completing the test. Then take a few deep, relaxing breaths and return to it. Work through the questions carefully but with confidence, knowing that you are capable of succeeding.

Developing a healthy mental approach to test taking will also aid in other areas of life. Test anxiety affects more than just the actual test—it can be damaging to your mental health and even contribute to depression. It's important to beat test anxiety before it becomes a problem for more than testing.

Review Video: Test Anxiety and Depression
Visit mometrix.com/academy and enter code: 904704

Study Strategy

Being prepared for the test is necessary to combat anxiety, but what does being prepared look like? You may study for hours on end and still not feel prepared. What you need is a strategy for test prep. The next few pages outline our recommended steps to help you plan out and conquer the challenge of preparation.

STEP 1: SCOPE OUT THE TEST

Learn everything you can about the format (multiple choice, essay, etc.) and what will be on the test. Gather any study materials, course outlines, or sample exams that may be available. Not only will this help you to prepare, but knowing what to expect can help to alleviate test anxiety.

STEP 2: MAP OUT THE MATERIAL

Look through the textbook or study guide and make note of how many chapters or sections it has. Then divide these over the time you have. For example, if a book has 15 chapters and you have five days to study, you need to cover three chapters each day. Even better, if you have the time, leave an extra day at the end for overall review after you have gone through the material in depth.

If time is limited, you may need to prioritize the material. Look through it and make note of which sections you think you already have a good grasp on, and which need review. While you are studying, skim quickly through the familiar sections and take more time on the challenging parts. Write out your plan so you don't get lost as you go. Having a written plan also helps you feel more in control of the study, so anxiety is less likely to arise from feeling overwhelmed at the amount to cover.

STEP 3: GATHER YOUR TOOLS

Decide what study method works best for you. Do you prefer to highlight in the book as you study and then go back over the highlighted portions? Or do you type out notes of the important information? Or is it helpful to make flashcards that you can carry with you? Assemble the pens, index cards, highlighters, post-it notes, and any other materials you may need so you won't be distracted by getting up to find things while you study.

If you're having a hard time retaining the information or organizing your notes, experiment with different methods. For example, try color-coding by subject with colored pens, highlighters, or post-it notes. If you learn better by hearing, try recording yourself reading your notes so you can listen while in the car, working out, or simply sitting at your desk. Ask a friend to quiz you from your flashcards, or try teaching someone the material to solidify it in your mind.

STEP 4: CREATE YOUR ENVIRONMENT

It's important to avoid distractions while you study. This includes both the obvious distractions like visitors and the subtle distractions like an uncomfortable chair (or a too-comfortable couch that makes you want to fall asleep). Set up the best study environment possible: good lighting and a comfortable work area. If background music helps you focus, you may want to turn it on, but otherwise keep the room quiet. If you are using a computer to take notes, be sure you don't have any other windows open, especially applications like social media, games, or anything else that could distract you. Silence your phone and turn off notifications. Be sure to keep water close by so you stay hydrated while you study (but avoid unhealthy drinks and snacks).

Also, take into account the best time of day to study. Are you freshest first thing in the morning? Try to set aside some time then to work through the material. Is your mind clearer in the afternoon or evening? Schedule your study session then. Another method is to study at the same time of day that you will take the test, so that your brain gets used to working on the material at that time and will be ready to focus at test time.

STEP 5: STUDY!

Once you have done all the study preparation, it's time to settle into the actual studying. Sit down, take a few moments to settle your mind so you can focus, and begin to follow your study plan. Don't give in to distractions or let yourself procrastinate. This is your time to prepare so you'll be ready to fearlessly approach the test. Make the most of the time and stay focused.

Of course, you don't want to burn out. If you study too long you may find that you're not retaining the information very well. Take regular study breaks. For example, taking five minutes out of every hour to walk briskly, breathing deeply and swinging your arms, can help your mind stay fresh.

As you get to the end of each chapter or section, it's a good idea to do a quick review. Remind yourself of what you learned and work on any difficult parts. When you feel that you've mastered the material, move on to the next part. At the end of your study session, briefly skim through your notes again.

But while review is helpful, cramming last minute is NOT. If at all possible, work ahead so that you won't need to fit all your study into the last day. Cramming overloads your brain with more information than it can process and retain, and your tired mind may struggle to recall even previously learned information when it is overwhelmed with last-minute study. Also, the urgent nature of cramming and the stress placed on your brain contribute to anxiety. You'll be more likely to go to the test feeling unprepared and having trouble thinking clearly.

So don't cram, and don't stay up late before the test, even just to review your notes at a leisurely pace. Your brain needs rest more than it needs to go over the information again. In fact, plan to finish your studies by noon or early afternoon the day before the test. Give your brain the rest of the day to relax or focus on other things, and get a good night's sleep. Then you will be fresh for the test and better able to recall what you've studied.

STEP 6: TAKE A PRACTICE TEST

Many courses offer sample tests, either online or in the study materials. This is an excellent resource to check whether you have mastered the material, as well as to prepare for the test format and environment.

Check the test format ahead of time: the number of questions, the type (multiple choice, free response, etc.), and the time limit. Then create a plan for working through them. For example, if you have 30 minutes to take a 60-question test, your limit is 30 seconds per question. Spend less time on the questions you know well so that you can take more time on the difficult ones.

If you have time to take several practice tests, take the first one open book, with no time limit. Work through the questions at your own pace and make sure you fully understand them. Gradually work up to taking a test under test conditions: sit at a desk with all study materials put away and set a timer. Pace yourself to make sure you finish the test with time to spare and go back to check your answers if you have time.

After each test, check your answers. On the questions you missed, be sure you understand why you missed them. Did you misread the question (tests can use tricky wording)? Did you forget the information? Or was it something you hadn't learned? Go back and study any shaky areas that the practice tests reveal.

Taking these tests not only helps with your grade, but also aids in combating test anxiety. If you're already used to the test conditions, you're less likely to worry about it, and working through tests until you're scoring well gives you a confidence boost. Go through the practice tests until you feel comfortable, and then you can go into the test knowing that you're ready for it.

Test Tips

On test day, you should be confident, knowing that you've prepared well and are ready to answer the questions. But aside from preparation, there are several test day strategies you can employ to maximize your performance.

First, as stated before, get a good night's sleep the night before the test (and for several nights before that, if possible). Go into the test with a fresh, alert mind rather than staying up late to study.

Try not to change too much about your normal routine on the day of the test. It's important to eat a nutritious breakfast, but if you normally don't eat breakfast at all, consider eating just a protein bar. If you're a coffee drinker, go ahead and have your normal coffee. Just make sure you time it so that the caffeine doesn't wear off right in the middle of your test. Avoid sugary beverages, and drink enough water to stay hydrated but not so much that you need a restroom break 10 minutes into the test. If your test isn't first thing in the morning, consider going for a walk or doing a light workout before the test to get your blood flowing.

Allow yourself enough time to get ready, and leave for the test with plenty of time to spare so you won't have the anxiety of scrambling to arrive in time. Another reason to be early is to select a good seat. It's helpful to sit away from doors and windows, which can be distracting. Find a good seat, get out your supplies, and settle your mind before the test begins.

When the test begins, start by going over the instructions carefully, even if you already know what to expect. Make sure you avoid any careless mistakes by following the directions.

Then begin working through the questions, pacing yourself as you've practiced. If you're not sure on an answer, don't spend too much time on it, and don't let it shake your confidence. Either skip it and come back later, or eliminate as many wrong answers as possible and guess among the remaining ones. Don't dwell on these questions as you continue—put them out of your mind and focus on what lies ahead.

Be sure to read all of the answer choices, even if you're sure the first one is the right answer. Sometimes you'll find a better one if you keep reading. But don't second-guess yourself if you do immediately know the answer. Your gut instinct is usually right. Don't let test anxiety rob you of the information you know.

If you have time at the end of the test (and if the test format allows), go back and review your answers. Be cautious about changing any, since your first instinct tends to be correct, but make sure you didn't misread any of the questions or accidentally mark the wrong answer choice. Look over any you skipped and make an educated guess.

At the end, leave the test feeling confident. You've done your best, so don't waste time worrying about your performance or wishing you could change anything. Instead, celebrate the successful

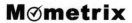

completion of this test. And finally, use this test to learn how to deal with anxiety even better next time.

Important Qualification

Not all anxiety is created equal. If your test anxiety is causing major issues in your life beyond the classroom or testing center, or if you are experiencing troubling physical symptoms related to your anxiety, it may be a sign of a serious physiological or psychological condition. If this sounds like your situation, we strongly encourage you to seek professional help.

How to Overcome Your Fear of Math

The word *math* is enough to strike fear into most hearts. How many of us have memories of sitting through confusing lectures, wrestling over mind-numbing homework, or taking tests that still seem incomprehensible even after hours of study? Years after graduation, many still shudder at these memories.

The fact is, math is not just a classroom subject. It has real-world implications that you face every day, whether you realize it or not. This may be balancing your monthly budget, deciding how many supplies to buy for a project, or simply splitting a meal check with friends. The idea of daily confrontations with math can be so paralyzing that some develop a condition known as *math anxiety*.

But you do NOT need to be paralyzed by this anxiety! In fact, while you may have thought all your life that you're not good at math, or that your brain isn't wired to understand it, the truth is that you may have been conditioned to think this way. From your earliest school days, the way you were taught affected the way you viewed different subjects. And the way math has been taught has changed.

Several decades ago, there was a shift in American math classrooms. The focus changed from traditional problem-solving to a conceptual view of topics, de-emphasizing the importance of learning the basics and building on them. The solid foundation necessary for math progression and confidence was undermined. Math became more of a vague concept than a concrete idea. Today, it is common to think of math, not as a straightforward system, but as a mysterious, complicated method that can't be fully understood unless you're a genius.

This is why you may still have nightmares about being called on to answer a difficult problem in front of the class. Math anxiety is a very real, though unnecessary, fear.

Math anxiety may begin with a single class period. Let's say you missed a day in 6th grade math and never quite understood the concept that was taught while you were gone. Since math is cumulative, with each new concept building on past ones, this could very well affect the rest of your math career. Without that one day's knowledge, it will be difficult to understand any other concepts that link to it. Rather than realizing that you're just missing one key piece, you may begin to believe that you're simply not capable of understanding math.

This belief can change the way you approach other classes, career options, and everyday life experiences, if you become anxious at the thought that math might be required. A student who loves science may choose a different path of study upon realizing that multiple math classes will be required for a degree. An aspiring medical student may hesitate at the thought of going through the necessary math classes. For some this anxiety escalates into a more extreme state known as *math phobia*.

Math anxiety is challenging to address because it is rooted deeply and may come from a variety of causes: an embarrassing moment in class, a teacher who did not explain concepts well and contributed to a shaky foundation, or a failed test that contributed to the belief of math failure.

These causes add up over time, encouraged by society's popular view that math is hard and unpleasant. Eventually a person comes to firmly believe that he or she is simply bad at math. This belief makes it difficult to grasp new concepts or even remember old ones. Homework and test grades begin to slip, which only confirms the belief. The poor performance is not due to lack of ability but is caused by math anxiety.

Math anxiety is an emotional issue, not a lack of intelligence. But when it becomes deeply rooted, it can become more than just an emotional problem. Physical symptoms appear. Blood pressure may rise and heartbeat may quicken at the sight of a math problem – or even the thought of math! This fear leads to a mental block. When someone with math anxiety is asked to perform a calculation, even a basic problem can seem overwhelming and impossible. The emotional and physical response to the thought of math prevents the brain from working through it logically.

The more this happens, the more a person's confidence drops, and the more math anxiety is generated. This vicious cycle must be broken!

The first step in breaking the cycle is to go back to very beginning and make sure you really understand the basics of how math works and why it works. It is not enough to memorize rules for multiplication and division. If you don't know WHY these rules work, your foundation will be shaky and you will be at risk of developing a phobia. Understanding mathematical concepts not only promotes confidence and security, but allows you to build on this understanding for new concepts. Additionally, you can solve unfamiliar problems using familiar concepts and processes.

Why is it that students in other countries regularly outperform American students in math? The answer likely boils down to a couple of things: the foundation of mathematical conceptual understanding and societal perception. While students in the US are not expected to *like* or *get* math, in many other nations, students are expected not only to understand math but also to excel at it.

Changing the American view of math that leads to math anxiety is a monumental task. It requires changing the training of teachers nationwide, from kindergarten through high school, so that they learn to teach the *why* behind math and to combat the wrong math views that students may develop. It also involves changing the stigma associated with math, so that it is no longer viewed as unpleasant and incomprehensible. While these are necessary changes, they are challenging and will take time. But in the meantime, math anxiety is not irreversible—it can be faced and defeated, one person at a time.

False Beliefs

One reason math anxiety has taken such hold is that several false beliefs have been created and shared until they became widely accepted. Some of these unhelpful beliefs include the following:

There is only one way to solve a math problem. In the same way that you can choose from different driving routes and still arrive at the same house, you can solve a math problem using different methods and still find the correct answer. A person who understands the reasoning behind math calculations may be able to look at an unfamiliar concept and find the right answer, just by applying logic to the knowledge they already have. This approach may be different than what is taught in the classroom, but it is still valid. Unfortunately, even many teachers view math as a subject where the best course of action is to memorize the rule or process for each problem rather than as a place for students to exercise logic and creativity in finding a solution.

Many people don't have a mind for math. A person who has struggled due to poor teaching or math anxiety may falsely believe that he or she doesn't have the mental capacity to grasp mathematical concepts. Most of the time, this is false. Many people find that when they are relieved of their math anxiety, they have more than enough brainpower to understand math.

Men are naturally better at math than women. Even though research has shown this to be false, many young women still avoid math careers and classes because of their belief that their math abilities are inferior. Many girls have come to believe that math is a male skill and have given up trying to understand or enjoy it.

Counting aids are bad. Something like counting on your fingers or drawing out a problem to visualize it may be frowned on as childish or a crutch, but these devices can help you get a tangible understanding of a problem or a concept.

Sadly, many students buy into these ideologies at an early age. A young girl who enjoys math class may be conditioned to think that she doesn't actually have the brain for it because math is for boys, and may turn her energies to other pursuits, permanently closing the door on a wide range of opportunities. A child who finds the right answer but doesn't follow the teacher's method may believe that he is doing it wrong and isn't good at math. A student who never had a problem with math before may have a poor teacher and become confused, yet believe that the problem is because she doesn't have a mathematical mind.

Students who have bought into these erroneous beliefs quickly begin to add their own anxieties, adapting them to their own personal situations:

I'll never use this in real life. A huge number of people wrongly believe that math is irrelevant outside the classroom. By adopting this mindset, they are handicapping themselves for a life in a mathematical world, as well as limiting their career choices. When they are inevitably faced with real-world math, they are conditioning themselves to respond with anxiety.

I'm not quick enough. While timed tests and quizzes, or even simply comparing yourself with other students in the class, can lead to this belief, speed is not an indicator of skill level. A person can work very slowly yet understand at a deep level.

If I can understand it, it's too easy. People with a low view of their own abilities tend to think that if they are able to grasp a concept, it must be simple. They cannot accept the idea that they are capable of understanding math. This belief will make it harder to learn, no matter how intelligent they are.

I just can't learn this. An overwhelming number of people think this, from young children to adults, and much of the time it is simply not true. But this mindset can turn into a self-fulfilling prophecy that keeps you from exercising and growing your math ability.

The good news is, each of these myths can be debunked. For most people, they are based on emotion and psychology, NOT on actual ability! It will take time, effort, and the desire to change, but change is possible. Even if you have spent years thinking that you don't have the capability to understand math, it is not too late to uncover your true ability and find relief from the anxiety that surrounds math.

Math Strategies

It is important to have a plan of attack to combat math anxiety. There are many useful strategies for pinpointing the fears or myths and eradicating them:

Go back to the basics. For most people, math anxiety stems from a poor foundation. You may think that you have a complete understanding of addition and subtraction, or even decimals and percentages, but make absolutely sure. Learning math is different from learning other subjects. For example, when you learn history, you study various time periods and places and events. It may be important to memorize dates or find out about the lives of famous people. When you move from US history to world history, there will be some overlap, but a large amount of the information will be new. Mathematical concepts, on the other hand, are very closely linked and highly dependent on each other. It's like climbing a ladder – if a rung is missing from your understanding, it may be difficult or impossible for you to climb any higher, no matter how hard you try. So go back and make sure your math foundation is strong. This may mean taking a remedial math course, going to a tutor to work through the shaky concepts, or just going through your old homework to make sure you really understand it.

Speak the language. Math has a large vocabulary of terms and phrases unique to working problems. Sometimes these are completely new terms, and sometimes they are common words, but are used differently in a math setting. If you can't speak the language, it will be very difficult to get a thorough understanding of the concepts. It's common for students to think that they don't understand math when they simply don't understand the vocabulary. The good news is that this is fairly easy to fix. Brushing up on any terms you aren't quite sure of can help bring the rest of the concepts into focus.

Check your anxiety level. When you think about math, do you feel nervous or uncomfortable? Do you struggle with feelings of inadequacy, even on concepts that you know you've already learned? It's important to understand your specific math anxieties, and what triggers them. When you catch yourself falling back on a false belief, mentally replace it with the truth. Don't let yourself believe that you can't learn, or that struggling with a concept means you'll never understand it. Instead, remind yourself of how much you've already learned and dwell on that past success. Visualize grasping the new concept, linking it to your old knowledge, and moving on to the next challenge. Also, learn how to manage anxiety when it arises. There are many techniques for coping with the irrational fears that rise to the surface when you enter the math classroom. This may include controlled breathing, replacing negative thoughts with positive ones, or visualizing success. Anxiety interferes with your ability to concentrate and absorb information, which in turn contributes to greater anxiety. If you can learn how to regain control of your thinking, you will be better able to pay attention, make progress, and succeed!

Don't go it alone. Like any deeply ingrained belief, math anxiety is not easy to eradicate. And there is no need for you to wrestle through it on your own. It will take time, and many people find that speaking with a counselor or psychiatrist helps. They can help you develop strategies for responding to anxiety and overcoming old ideas. Additionally, it can be very helpful to take a short course or seek out a math tutor to help you find and fix the missing rungs on your ladder and make sure that you're ready to progress to the next level. You can also find a number of math aids online: courses that will teach you mental devices for figuring out problems, how to get the most out of your math classes, etc.

Check your math attitude. No matter how much you want to learn and overcome your anxiety, you'll have trouble if you still have a negative attitude toward math. If you think it's too hard, or just have general feelings of dread about math, it will be hard to learn and to break through the anxiety. Work on cultivating a positive math attitude. Remind yourself that math is not just a hurdle to be cleared, but a valuable asset. When you view math with a positive attitude, you'll be much more likely to understand and even enjoy it. This is something you must do for yourself. You may find it helpful to visit with a counselor. Your tutor, friends, and family may cheer you on in your endeavors. But your greatest asset is yourself. You are inside your own mind – tell yourself what you need to hear. Relive past victories. Remind yourself that you are capable of understanding math. Root out any false beliefs that linger and replace them with positive truths. Even if it doesn't feel true at first, it will begin to affect your thinking and pave the way for a positive, anxiety-free mindset.

Aside from these general strategies, there are a number of specific practical things you can do to begin your journey toward overcoming math anxiety. Something as simple as learning a new note-taking strategy can change the way you approach math and give you more confidence and understanding. New study techniques can also make a huge difference.

Math anxiety leads to bad habits. If it causes you to be afraid of answering a question in class, you may gravitate toward the back row. You may be embarrassed to ask for help. And you may procrastinate on assignments, which leads to rushing through them at the last moment when it's too late to get a better understanding. It's important to identify your negative behaviors and replace them with positive ones:

Prepare ahead of time. Read the lesson before you go to class. Being exposed to the topics that will be covered in class ahead of time, even if you don't understand them perfectly, is extremely helpful in increasing what you retain from the lecture. Do your homework and, if you're still shaky, go over some extra problems. The key to a solid understanding of math is practice.

Sit front and center. When you can easily see and hear, you'll understand more, and you'll avoid the distractions of other students if no one is in front of you. Plus, you're more likely to be sitting with students who are positive and engaged, rather than others with math anxiety. Let their positive math attitude rub off on you.

Ask questions in class and out. If you don't understand something, just ask. If you need a more in-depth explanation, the teacher may need to work with you outside of class, but often it's a simple concept you don't quite understand, and a single question may clear it up. If you wait, you may not be able to follow the rest of the day's lesson. For extra help, most professors have office hours outside of class when you can go over concepts one-on-one to clear up any uncertainties. Additionally, there may be a *math lab* or study session you can attend for homework help. Take advantage of this.

Review. Even if you feel that you've fully mastered a concept, review it periodically to reinforce it. Going over an old lesson has several benefits: solidifying your understanding, giving you a confidence boost, and even giving some new insights into material that you're currently learning! Don't let yourself get rusty. That can lead to problems with learning later concepts.

Teaching Tips

While the math student's mindset is the most crucial to overcoming math anxiety, it is also important for others to adjust their math attitudes. Teachers and parents have an enormous influence on how students relate to math. They can either contribute to math confidence or math anxiety.

As a parent or teacher, it is very important to convey a positive math attitude. Retelling horror stories of your own bad experience with math will contribute to a new generation of math anxiety. Even if you don't share your experiences, others will be able to sense your fears and may begin to believe them.

Even a careless comment can have a big impact, so watch for phrases like *He's not good at math* or *I never liked math*. You are a crucial role model, and your children or students will unconsciously adopt your mindset. Give them a positive example to follow. Rather than teaching them to fear the math world before they even know it, teach them about all its potential and excitement.

Work to present math as an integral, beautiful, and understandable part of life. Encourage creativity in solving problems. Watch for false beliefs and dispel them. Cross the lines between subjects: integrate history, English, and music with math. Show students how math is used every day, and how the entire world is based on mathematical principles, from the pull of gravity to the shape of seashells. Instead of letting students see math as a necessary evil, direct them to view it as an imaginative, beautiful art form – an art form that they are capable of mastering and using.

Don't give too narrow a view of math. It is more than just numbers. Yes, working problems and learning formulas is a large part of classroom math. But don't let the teaching stop there. Teach students about the everyday implications of math. Show them how nature works according to the laws of mathematics, and take them outside to make discoveries of their own. Expose them to math-related careers by inviting visiting speakers, asking students to do research and presentations, and learning students' interests and aptitudes on a personal level.

Demonstrate the importance of math. Many people see math as nothing more than a required stepping stone to their degree, a nuisance with no real usefulness. Teach students that algebra is used every day in managing their bank accounts, in following recipes, and in scheduling the day's events. Show them how learning to do geometric proofs helps them to develop logical thinking, an invaluable life skill. Let them see that math surrounds them and is integrally linked to their daily lives: that weather predictions are based on math, that math was used to design cars and other machines, etc. Most of all, give them the tools to use math to enrich their lives.

Make math as tangible as possible. Use visual aids and objects that can be touched. It is much easier to grasp a concept when you can hold it in your hands and manipulate it, rather than just listening to the lecture. Encourage math outside of the classroom. The real world is full of measuring, counting, and calculating, so let students participate in this. Keep your eyes open for numbers and patterns to discuss. Talk about how scores are calculated in sports games and how far apart plants are placed in a garden row for maximum growth. Build the mindset that math is a normal and interesting part of daily life.

Finally, find math resources that help to build a positive math attitude. There are a number of books that show math as fascinating and exciting while teaching important concepts, for example: *The Math Curse; A Wrinkle in Time; The Phantom Tollbooth;* and *Fractals, Googols and Other Mathematical Tales*. You can also find a number of online resources: math puzzles and games, videos that show math in nature, and communities of math enthusiasts. On a local level, students can compete in a variety of math competitions with other schools or join a math club.

The student who experiences math as exciting and interesting is unlikely to suffer from math anxiety. Going through life without this handicap is an immense advantage and opens many doors that others have closed through their fear.

Self-Check

Whether you suffer from math anxiety or not, chances are that you have been exposed to some of the false beliefs mentioned above. Now is the time to check yourself for any errors you may have accepted. Do you think you're not wired for math? Or that you don't need to understand it since you're not planning on a math career? Do you think math is just too difficult for the average person?

Find the errors you've taken to heart and replace them with positive thinking. Are you capable of learning math? Yes! Can you control your anxiety? Yes! These errors will resurface from time to time, so be watchful. Don't let others with math anxiety influence you or sway your confidence. If you're having trouble with a concept, find help. Don't let it discourage you!

Create a plan of attack for defeating math anxiety and sharpening your skills. Do some research and decide if it would help you to take a class, get a tutor, or find some online resources to fine-tune your knowledge. Make the effort to get good nutrition, hydration, and sleep so that you are operating at full capacity. Remind yourself daily that you are skilled and that anxiety does not control you. Your mind is capable of so much more than you know. Give it the tools it needs to grow and thrive.

Thank You

We at Mometrix would like to extend our heartfelt thanks to you, our friend and patron, for allowing us to play a part in your journey. It is a privilege to serve people from all walks of life who are unified in their commitment to building the best future they can for themselves.

The preparation you devote to these important testing milestones may be the most valuable educational opportunity you have for making a real difference in your life. We encourage you to put your heart into it—that feeling of succeeding, overcoming, and yes, conquering will be well worth the hours you've invested.

We want to hear your story, your struggles and your successes, and if you see any opportunities for us to improve our materials so we can help others even more effectively in the future, please share that with us as well. **The team at Mometrix would be absolutely thrilled to hear from you!** So please, send us an email (support@mometrix.com) and let's stay in touch.

> **If you'd like some additional help, check out these other resources we offer for your exam:**
> **http://mometrixflashcards.com/nursing**

Additional Bonus Material

Due to our efforts to try to keep this book to a manageable length, we've created a link that will give you access to all of your additional bonus material.

Please visit https://www.mometrix.com/bonus948/pax to access the information.